Oxford American Handbook of

Hospice and Palliative Medicine and Supportive Care

D0813723

Published and Forthcoming Oxford American Handbooks

Oxford American Handbook of Anesthesiology
Oxford American Handbook of Cardiology
Oxford American Handbook of Clinical Dentistry
Oxford American Handbook of Clinical Exams and Practical Skills
Oxford American Handbook of Clinical Diagnosis
Oxford American Handbook of Clinical Medicine
Oxford American Handbook of Clinical Pharmacy
Oxford American Handbook of Critical Care
Oxford American Handbook of Endocrinology and Diabetes
Oxford American Handbook of Disaster Medicine
Oxford American Handbook of Emergency Medicine
Oxford American Handbook of Gastroenterology and Hepatology
Oxford American Handbook of Geriatric Medicine
Oxford American Handbook of Hospice and Palliative Medicine and
Supportive Care
Oxford American Handbook of Infectious Diseases
Oxford American Handbook of Nephrology and Hypertension
Oxford American Handbook of Neurology
Oxford American Handbook of Obstetrics and Gynecology
Oxford American Handbook of Oncology
Oxford American Handbook of Ophthalmology
Oxford American Handbook of Otolaryngology
Oxford American Handbook of Pediatrics
Oxford American Handbook of Physical Medicine and Rehabilitation
Oxford American Handbook of Psychiatry
Oxford American Handbook of Pulmonary Medicine
Oxford American Handbook of Radiology
Oxford American Handbook of Reproductive Medicine
Oxford American Handbook of Rheumatology
Oxford American Handbook of Sports Medicine
Oxford American Handbook of Surgery
Oxford American Handbook of Urology

Oxford American Handbook of
Hospice and Palliative Medicine and Supportive Care

Second Edition

Edited by

Sriram Yennurajalingam, MD
Associate Professor of Palliative Care & Rehabilitation Medicine
The University of Texas MD Anderson Cancer Center
Houston, Texas

Eduardo Bruera, MD
Professor and Chair of Palliative Care & Rehabilitation Medicine
The University of Texas MD Anderson Cancer Center
Houston, Texas

OXFORD
UNIVERSITY PRESS

OXFORD
UNIVERSITY PRESS

Oxford University Press is a department of the University of Oxford. It furthers
the University's objective of excellence in research, scholarship, and education
by publishing worldwide.Oxford is a registered trade mark of Oxford University
Press in the UK and certain other countries.

Published in the United States of America by Oxford University Press
198 Madison Avenue, New York, NY 10016, United States of America.

© Oxford University Press 2016

First Edition published in 2011
Second Edition published in 2016

Library of Congress Cataloging-in-Publication Data
Oxford American handbook of hospice and palliative medicine
Oxford American handbook of hospice and palliative medicine and supportive care /
edited by Sriram Yennurajalingam, Eduardo Bruera. — Second edition.
p. ; cm. — (Oxford American handbooks)
Handbook of hospice and palliative medicine and supportive care
Preceded by Oxford American handbook of hospice and palliative medicine /
edited by Eduardo Bruera, Sriram Yennurajalingam. 2011.
Includes bibliographical references and index.
ISBN 978-0-19-937530-1 (alk. paper)
I. Yennurajalingam, Sriram, editor. II. Bruera, Eduardo, editor. III. Title.
IV. Title: Handbook of hospice and palliative medicine and supportive care.
V. Series: Oxford American handbooks.
[DNLM: 1. Palliative Care—Handbooks. 2. Hospice Care—Handbooks.
3. Hospices—Handbooks. WB 39]
R726.8
362.17′56—dc23
2015032794

9 8 7 6 5 4 3 2
Printed by Webcom, Canada

Preface

In the United States, hospice and palliative medicine has emerged as a new subspecialty recently recognized by the American Board of Medical Specialties. During the last 10 years there has been a very significant increase in the number of inpatient and outpatient palliative care programs, as well as a major increase in the number of patients who access hospice for end-of-life care.

Unfortunately, educational efforts are lagging behind, and the vast majority of medical students, residents, and even fellows receive minimal palliative medicine education in the United States. However, these junior physicians, along with a number of busy clinical specialists, are exposed to patients with progressive incurable illnesses and their families on a daily basis.

The purpose of this handbook is to provide up-to-date, practical, and concise information to healthcare professionals delivering care to patients requiring hospice and palliative care in the United States. This includes physicians, nurse practitioners, fellows, residents, and students.

All the chapters are primarily aimed at the clinical and administrative arrangements within the American healthcare system, including the hospice Medicare benefit.

We believe this book will provide rapid access to most of the daily bedside clinical and administrative needs, and it will hopefully help our colleagues in the delivery of excellent palliative and hospice care.

We would like to acknowledge the authors of each of the chapters for having committed their time and effort to our joint project. We would also like to acknowledge the commitment to excellence by Oxford University Press and in particular Andrea Knobloch, our Senior Editor, for the excellent work in coordinating our book. Finally, we would like to acknowledge the daily effort of healthcare professionals who have contributed by their daily clinical work, education, and research to the development of the extraordinary body of knowledge that we have had the privilege to synthesize in this book.

Sriram Yennurajalingam, MD
Eduardo Bruera, MD
Houston, June 2015

Contents

Contributors

Joseph A. Arthur, MD
Department of Palliative, Rehabilitation, and Integrative Medicine
The University of Texas MD Anderson Cancer Center
Houston, Texas

Elizabeth A. Barnes, MD, FRCPC
Department of Radiation Oncology
Toronto Sunnybrook Regional Cancer Centre
Toronto, Ontario, Canada

Shirley H. Bush, MBBS, MRCGP, FAChPM
Division of Palliative Care, University of Ottawa
Bruyère Research Institute
Bruyère Continuing Care
Ottawa, Ontario, Canada

Brook A. Calton, MD, MHS
Division of Geriatrics
University of California, San Francisco
San Francisco, California

J. Randall Curtis, MD, MPH
Harborview Medical Center, University of Washington
Cambia Palliative Care Center of Excellence
Seattle, Washington

Shalini Dalal, MD
Department of Palliative, Rehabilitation, and Integrative Medicine
The University of Texas MD Anderson Cancer Center
Houston, Texas

Sara Davison, MD, MSc, FRCPC
Division of Nephrology and Immunology
University of Alberta Faculty of Medicine
Edmonton, Alberta, Canada

Egidio Del Fabbro, MD
Division of Hematology/Oncology and Palliative Care
Virginia Commonwealth University
Richmond, Virginia

Marvin Omar Delgado Guay, MD

Department of Palliative, Rehabilitation, and Integrative Medicine
The University of Texas MD Anderson Cancer Center
Houston, Texas

Rony Dev, DO

Department of Palliative, Rehabilitation, and Integrative Medicine
The University of Texas MD Anderson Cancer Center
Houston, Texas

Deborah Dudgeon, MD

Palliative Care Program
Queen's University Department of Medicine
Kingston, Ontario, Canada

James D. Duffy, MD, FAAHPM, FANPA, DABMA

Clinical Professor of Psychiatry
University of San Francisco
Kaiser Permanente Medical Group
Oakland, California

Betty R. Ferrell, PhD, RN, FAAN

Nursing Research and Education
City of Hope Comprehensive Cancer Center
Duarte, California

Joan K. Harrold, MD, MPH

Medical Services
Hospice of Lancaster County
Lancaster, Pennsylvania

David Hui, MD, MSc

Department of Palliative, Rehabilitation, and Integrative Medicine
The University of Texas MD Anderson Cancer Center
Houston, Texas

Margaret Isaac, MD

Harborview Medical Center, University of Washington
Cambia Palliative Care Center of Excellence
Seattle, Washington

Meiko Kuriya, MD

Department of Palliative, Rehabilitation, and Integrative Medicine
The University of Texas MD Anderson Cancer Center
Houston, Texas

Simeon Kwan, DO

Department of Palliative, Rehabilitation, and Integrative Medicine
The University of Texas MD Anderson Cancer Center
Houston, Texas

Kashelle Lockman, PharmD
Department of Pharmacy Practice and Science
University of Maryland School of Pharmacy
Baltimore, Maryland

Mary Lynn McPherson, PharmD, MA, BCPS, CPE
Department of Pharmacy Practice and Science
University of Maryland School of Pharmacy
Baltimore, Maryland

Valentina Medici, MD
Division of Gastroenterology and Hepatology
University of California Davis Medical Center
Sacramento, California

Frederick J. Meyers, MD, MACP
Department of Internal Medicine
University of California Davis Medical Center
Sacramento, California

Jeff Myers, MD
Division of Palliative Care
University of Toronto
Toronto, Ontario, Canada

Edward O'Donnell, MA
Clinical Management and Leadership
School of Health Sciences
The George Washington University
Washington, DC

V. S. Periyakoil, MD
Department of Medicine
Stanford School of Medicine
Stanford, California

Christina M. Puchalski, MD, FACP, FAAHPM
Department of Medicine and Health Sciences
George Washington Institute for Spirituality and Health
George Washington University School of Medicine
Washington, DC

José L. Ramos, MD
Palliative Care Specialist
University of Texas Health Sciences Center at Houston
Memorial Hermann-Texas Medical Center
Houston, Texas

Anis Rashid, MD
Department of Psychiatry
The University of Texas MD Anderson Cancer Center
Houston, Texas

Suresh K. Reddy, MD
Department of Palliative, Rehabilitation, and Integrative Medicine
The University of Texas MD Anderson Cancer Center
Houston, Texas

Christine S. Ritchie, MD, MSPH, FACP, FAAHPM
Division of Geriatrics
University of California, San Francisco
San Francisco, California

Rhonda Robert, PhD
Division of Pediatrics
Department of Pediatrics—Patient Care
The University of Texas MD Anderson Cancer Center
Houston, Texas

Mary L. S. Vachon, RN, PhD
Professor, Department of Psychiatry
Dalla Lana School of Public Health
University of Toronto
Toronto, Ontario, Canada

Marieberta Vidal, MD
Department of Palliative, Rehabilitation, and Integrative Medicine
The University of Texas MD Anderson Cancer Center
Houston, Texas

Charles F. von Gunten, MD, PhD
Vice President, Medical Affairs
Hospice and Palliative Medicine, Ohio Health
Columbus, Ohio

Tobias Walbert, MD, PhD, MPH
Hermelin Brain Tumor Center
Henry Ford Health System
Detroit, Michigan

Paul W. Walker, MD
Department of Palliative, Rehabilitation, and Integrative Medicine
The University of Texas MD Anderson Cancer Center
Houston, Texas

Kirsten Wentlandt, PhD, MD, MHSci
Palliative Care, Toronto General Hospital
University Health Network
Toronto, Ontario, Canada

Angelique Wong, MD
Department of Palliative, Rehabilitation, and Integrative Medicine
The University of Texas MD Anderson Cancer Center
Houston, Texas

Donna S. Zhukovsky, MD, FACP, FAAHPM
Department of Palliative, Rehabilitation, and Integrative Medicine
The University of Texas MD Anderson Cancer Center
Houston, Texas

Camilla Zimmermann, MD, PhD
Palliative Care, Princess Margaret Cancer Centre
University Health Network
Toronto, Ontario, Canada

Definitions and Key Elements in Palliative and Supportive Care

Sriram Yennurajalingam
and Eduardo Bruera

Introduction

The modern hospice movement started in the 1960s in the United Kingdom. Patients with progressive incurable illnesses were admitted to inpatient hospices and also received home hospice care until death. Hospices delivered care very close to the end of life (Figure 1.1). In the 1970s it became clear that many patients with severe distress were being admitted to acute care hospitals. Dr. Balfour Mount coined the term *palliative care* and adapted many of the principles of the British hospice movement to acute care hospitals, initially in Canada and then worldwide.[1] Palliative care programs[2,3] developed with three main characteristics:

- Multidimensional assessment and management of severe physical and emotional distress
- Interdisciplinary care by multiple disciplines in addition to physicians and nurses
- Emphasis on caring not only for the patients but also for their families.

Inpatient palliative care programs provided care earlier than hospice programs (Figure 1.1). However, it became clear that many of the patients with chronic progressive illnesses had severe symptom burden before they became admitted to the hospital and therefore outpatient palliative care programs were developed for early access.

In the 1990s supportive care emerged as a discipline aiming to provide predominantly cancer patients with support for the management of treatment-related adverse effects as well as disease-related symptoms. Over time, supportive care has also expanded into domains such as psychosocial and spiritual care, communication, and survivorship care.

There has been significant overlap in the described roles of supportive care, palliative care, and hospice care.[4] Figure 1.1 shows that perhaps one

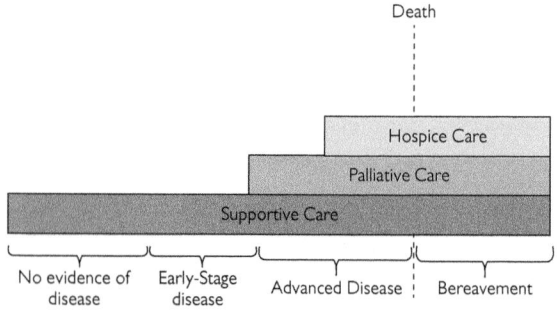

Figure 1.1. Conceptual framework toward understanding the terms *supportive care, palliative care*, and *hospice care*.

Adapted from Hui D, De La Cruz M, Mori M, Parsons H, Kwon J, Torres-Vigil I, et al. (2013). Concepts and definitions for "supportive care," "best supportive care," "palliative care," and "hospice care" in the published literature, dictionaries, and textbooks. Support Care Cancer 21(3):659–85.

of the most useful differences for clinicians relates to the proximity to death in which many of these programs are organized and delivered.

Hospice care focuses on providing care in the community setting for patients who are mainly in the last 6 months of life. Palliative care not only includes hospice care services but also acute care programs in hospitals. *Supportive care* can be seen as a more general and encompassing term that spans from survivorship to bereavement programs throughout the disease trajectory.

The sets of skills required for the delivery of hospice care, palliative care, and supportive care are essentially extremely similar, and therefore in most clinical settings they are delivered by the same group of healthcare professionals. There is evidence that using the term *supportive care* rather than the term *palliative care* for outpatient care can increase the number of referrals and can allow patients earlier access to outpatient care.

Palliative and supportive care services can be provided in a similar fashion to most other clinical problems in medicine. Primary palliative and supportive care can be delivered by the primary care physician or by specialists (oncologists, cardiologists, intensivists, etc.). Patients with more complex problems that cannot be managed by their primary physician can be seen in consultation by specialist palliative care teams. While these patients remain under the care of their primary specialists, the palliative care team can provide recommendations. This has been defined as *secondary palliative care*. Finally, a minority of patients who are unable to be well controlled at the secondary level might require treatment by specialist palliative care teams. These specialists frequently provide this care in specific centers such as palliative care units or outpatient supportive care centers. Tertiary palliative care programs, in addition to providing complex clinical care, are able to provide education and research.

References

1. O'Neill B, Fallon M (1997). ABC of palliative care: Principles of palliative care and pain control. *BMJ* 315:801–4.
2. World Health Organization (n.d.). WHO definition of palliative care. Retrieved February 12, 2015, from http://www.who.int/cancer/palliative/definition/en/.
3. National Consensus Project for Quality Palliative Care (NCP) (2013). *Clinical Practice Guidelines for Quality Palliative Care, Third Edition*. Retrieved February 12, 2015, from http://www.nationalconsensusproject.org/NCP_Clinical_Practice_Guidelines_3rd_Edition.pdf.
4. Hui D, De La Cruz M, Mori M, Parsons H, Kwon J, Torres-Vigil I, et al. (2013). Concepts and definitions for "supportive care," "best supportive care," "palliative care," and "hospice care" in the published literature, dictionaries, and textbooks. *Support Care Cancer* 21(3):659–85.

Symptom Assessment

Marvin Omar Delgado Guay

Introduction

Symptom assessment is very important because symptoms directly affect patients' distress level, quality of life (QOL), and survival.[1] Symptoms can be related to the disease itself, its treatment, and comorbid illnesses.[1] Multiple physical, psychological, and spiritually distressing factors affect QOL, a multidimensional construct with specific emotional, physical, and social aspects[2] (Figure 2.1).

The symptoms and their interference with life increase with increasing cancer stage, possibly reflecting tumor burden and treatment complications.[3] This increasing symptom burden decreases patients' QOL.[2] Symptoms affect but do not necessarily determine patients' QOL.[1]

The experience of patients living with advanced illness is complex; it includes physical symptoms, coping, financial concerns, caregiver burden, social and family changes, and spiritual concerns. In clinical practice, patients present with multiple symptoms that require simultaneous assessment and management. Clinicians must have an effective assessment strategy that respects the treatment goals and the patient's wishes.

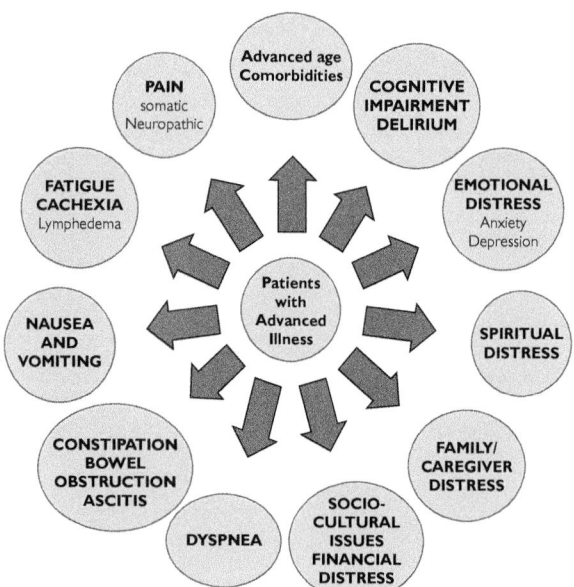

Figure 2.1. Multiple symptoms and factors associated with quality of life in patients with advanced illness.

Supportive and palliative care aim to decrease symptom burden and alleviate psychosocial distress in patients and families through multidimensional symptoms assessment and the management of distressing symptoms to improve the quality of life of patients with advanced illness as well as their caregivers.[4–7]

This chapter aims to describe the different components of multidimensional bedside clinical assessment in supportive/palliative care and its importance for symptom control, quality of life, and decision-making.

Multidimensional Assessment

It is extremely important to perform a comprehensive and multidimensional assessment in all patients with advanced illness with multiple symptoms.[8–10] The multidimensional assessment should help in the recognition of the contribution of the different dimensions to the patient's symptom expression, and thereby assist in the planning of care. Good symptom assessment precedes effective symptom treatment.

An initial step in the multidimensional assessment of the patient evaluated by the supportive and palliative care team involves a complete medical history that reviews the disease diagnosis (cancer, AIDS, end-stage chronic obstructive pulmonary disease, congestive heart failure, or renal disease, etc.), the chronology of disease-related events, previous and current therapies, and all relevant medical, surgical, and psychiatric problems. A detailed history includes current and prior use of prescription and nonprescription drugs, "alternative" medical therapies, drug allergies and previous adverse reactions, and thorough physical examination and review of the laboratory and imaging, if available. Table 2.1 describes the multidimensional assessment performed for patients with advanced illness evaluated by the supportive/palliative care teams.

Assessment tools allow for the identification of many more symptoms than do simple unstructured evaluations.[11,12] Simple assessment tools are the most appropriate for patients with advanced illnesses. These patients may be weak and experiencing symptoms that make it difficult to complete a time-consuming and complex assessment tool. Assessment tools are not only useful to diagnose and evaluate the intensity of the symptoms but also to monitor the effectiveness of therapy and to screen for side effects of medications. Assessment tools should be used regularly, especially when patients experience new symptoms, an increase in the intensity of preexisting symptoms, or when therapy changes. The results should be always documented in the patient's chart to ensure accuracy in the monitoring of the symptoms.

Efficient symptom-assessment instruments include the Edmonton Symptom Assessment Scale (ESAS), the Memorial Symptom Assessment Scale (MSAS), the Rotterdam Symptom Checklist (RSCL),[13] and the Symptom Distress Scale (SDS).

The Edmonton Symptom Assessment Scale[14–18] is used to assess 10 common symptoms (pain, fatigue, nausea, depression, anxiety, drowsiness, shortness of breath, appetite, sleep problems, and feeling of well-being) experienced by patients with cancer or chronic illness over the past 24 hours. In this scale, the patient rates the intensity of symptoms on a 0 to 10 numerical scale, with 0 representing "no symptom" and 10 representing the "worst possible symptom." It is widely used in supportive and palliative care research. Its ease of use and visual representation make it an effective and practical bedside tool[19–20] that allows the healthcare provider to track symptoms over time with regard to intensity, duration, and responsiveness to therapy. There have been independent validations of this tool in palliative care of cancer patients by a number of different authors and in a variety of different languages, for example, in English,[21–25] Italian,[26] French,[27] German,[28] Spanish,[29] Korean,[30] and Thai.[31] Two recent reviews on ESAS studies have

Table 2.1 Multidimensional Assessments of Patients with Advanced Illness Evaluated by Supportive/Palliative Care Teams

Dimension	Assessment
a. History	Stage of the cancer/illness Recent chemotherapy and/or radiotherapy or other disease-modifying therapy Self-rated symptoms scales Characteristics, intensity, location, aggravating factors of distressful symptoms
b. Performance status History of falls Use of assistant walking devices	Karnofsky Performance Scale or Eastern Co-operative Oncologic Group Scale scores
c. Activities of daily living (ADL) and instrumental activities of daily living (IADL)	Assessment of ADL (bathing, dressing and undressing, eating, transferring from bed to chair, and back, voluntarily control urinary and fecal discharge, using the toilet, and walking) Assessment of IADL (light housework, preparing meals, taking medications, shopping for groceries or clothes, using the telephone, and managing money)
d. Assessment of distressful physical symptoms (pain, fatigue, anorexia, nausea, dyspnea, insomnia, drowsiness, constipation)	Edmonton Symptom Assessment System (ESAS) Abdominal X-ray to assess constipation vs. bowel obstruction (consider abdominal CT scan)
e. Assessment of psychosocial symptoms: anxiety/depression f. Family/caregiver's distress g. Cultural and financial status	Anxiety/depression (ESAS) Identification of mood disorder during interview Assessment for family/caregiver distress during the interview Sociocultural and financial issues evaluation
h. Assessment of delirium	Memorial Delirium Assessment Scale (MDAS) Mini-Mental State Examination (MMSE) Confusion Assessment Method (CAM)
i. Assessment of spiritual distress/ spiritual pain of the patient and caregiver	Spiritual Assessment SPIRITual History; FICA Self-rated spiritual pain (pain deep in the soul/being that is not physical) Identification of spiritual distress during interview.
j. Assessment for chemical coping	CAGE questionnaire
k. Evaluation of medications and possible interactions (polypharmacy)	
l. Physical examination	

found limited psychometric evidence that supports the need for further validation studies.[32,33]

The ESAS has been validated against a widely used scale, the Hospital Anxiety and Depression Scale (HADS), for assessing the presence of depression and anxiety in advanced cancer patients.[34] The ideal cutoff point of ESAS of 2 out of 10 is sensitive for the presence of depression and anxiety in patients in the palliative care setting.

The Symptom Distress Scale (SDS) is a patient-rated instrument that assesses the intensity, frequency, and distress level associated with nine physical and two psychological symptoms.[35,36]

The Memorial Symptom Assessment Scale (MSAS), a lengthier assessment tool, is mostly used for research purposes. With the MSAS, patients rate the frequency, severity, and distress associated with 32 physical and psychological symptoms.[37] There is a short-form MSAS[38] (MSAS-SF) that captures the patient-rated distress associated with 26 physical symptoms and the frequency of 4 psychological symptoms. Another tool that can be completed in 2 to 4 minutes and contains both QOL and survival information is the condensed MSAS (CMSAS),[39] which provides equivalent information that approximates to the original 32 items. The symptoms identified by Chang et al.[38] are also included in other widely used clinical symptom assessment instruments, such as the ESAS, RSCL, and SDS. This report is also one of the first to demonstrate that scales from a shorter instrument can be predictive of survival, and that there is a core of symptoms that provide most of the information about health, QOL, and survival. It is important to recognize that the research instruments may differ from those used for clinical practice.[39]

Many larger, more complex symptom assessment tools have been developed for clinical research use. Research instruments may differ from those used in clinical practice.[39] Regardless of the type of scale used, a good symptom assessment precedes effective symptom treatment.

Instruments for the Assessment of Prognosis and Function

Functional status, an independent predictor of survival, must be considered when planning patient care at a hospice, hospital, or home.[40] The most frequently used performance status assessment scales in oncology treatment and research are the Karnofsky Performance Status (KPS) score and the Eastern Co-operative Oncology Group (ECOG) score. Both tools have reliable prognostic value.[41,42]

The Karnofsky Performance Status (KPS) score enables physicians to classify patients according to their functional impairment. This classification can be used to compare the effectiveness of different therapies and to assess prognosis in individual patients. For many patients with serious illnesses, a lower Karnofsky score indicates lower survival.[43] The Palliative Performance Scale (PPS) is a prognostic tool used in palliative care patients, which correlates with KPS (see Chapter 25, "Prognostication in Palliative Care," for details).

The ECOG score measures the intensity with which cancer affects patients' daily living abilities.[44] The ECOG scale ranges from 0 (fully active, no restrictions) to 5 (dead).

Physiotherapists and trained nurses use the Edmonton Functional Assessment Tool to determine functional performance and evaluate other factors that contribute to functional impairment in patients with advanced cancer, such as communication ability, mental status, pain level, and dyspnea intensity.[45]

The Functional Independence Measure can be used in research settings to assess the functional status of patients with advanced cancer.[46] The Functional Independence Measure includes 18 items that are used to evaluate patients' sphincter control, self-care, mobility, locomotion, communication, and social cognition.

Activities of daily living (ADL) scales are used to evaluate patients' level of physical impairment. Specifically, the Katz index of ADL assesses such activities as eating, bathing, dressing, toileting, transfer (e.g., bed to chair), and continence.[41]

The Instrumental Activities of Daily Living (IADL) questionnaire assesses how well patients perform complex life activities, such as light housework, laundry, meal preparation, transportation, grocery shopping, telephone use, medication management, and money management.[41] The IADL questionnaire helps physicians identify cognitive impairment, physical limitations, distressing symptoms, and related clinical problems in patients with advanced cancer.

Assessment of Physical Symptoms and Complications

Pain

Clinicians should comprehensively assess all patients with advanced illness who present with pain and related symptoms (such as fatigue, depression, sleep disturbance). When clinicians take the histories of patients with advanced illness who present with pain, they should ask for the location, characteristics, and intensity of the pain; about any variation in the pain with change of movement or time of the day; how the pain affects the patients' ADLs; and the possible cause(s) of the pain.[47] Using the ESAS, clinicians can identify several potential underlying symptoms and can better understand the causes of the patient's pain.

The CAGE questionnaire can be used to screen patients with advanced illnesses and pain for alcohol abuse.[48] The CAGE questionnaire consists of four questions:

1. Have you ever felt that you should Cut down on your drinking?
2. Have you been Annoyed by people criticizing your drinking?
3. Have you ever felt bad or Guilty about your drinking?
4. Have you ever had a drink to get rid of a hangover, that is, an Eye-opener?

A positive score, defined as positive answers to two or more of the four questions, has been shown to have prognostic value in opioid management in cancer patients who experience pain.

The CAGE questionnaire helps physicians identify patients who are at high risk of developing chemical coping, opioid dose escalation, and opioid-induced toxicity. Approximately 20% of cancer patients have a positive CAGE questionnaire result.[48]

Fatigue

Fatigue, a multidimensional syndrome defined as a "decrement in performance of either physical or psychological tasks,"[49] often has multiple contributing causes. Clinicians can assess patients' fatigue by characterizing its severity and temporal features (onset, course, duration, and daily pattern) and by evaluating its exacerbating, contributing, and relieving factors; its effect on patients' daily lives; and its associated distress.[49]

In palliative patients, fatigue and other symptoms such as pain and depression can be assessed with the ESAS, as detailed earlier in this chapter. Physical and/or psychological symptoms such as pain, depression, and anxiety correlate significantly with fatigue.[50]

In research settings, fatigue can be evaluated with the Functional Assessment of Chronic Illness Therapy–Fatigue (FACIT-F) subscale[51] and the Brief Fatigue Inventory, which has been validated as a measure of fatigue in cancer patients.[52]

Cachexia

Cachexia, a complex metabolic syndrome characterized by a profound loss of lean body mass, occurs in up to 80% of patients with advanced cancer.[49] Clinical assessment for cachexia should include a physical examination and a thorough history that focuses on nutritional issues.

Secondary causes of cachexia, including nausea, vomiting, constipation, ascites, swallowing problems, oral candidiasis, taste alteration, early satiety, and deconditioning, should be investigated.[49] Any loss of appetite (anorexia) expressed by the patient can be assessed with a numerical rating scale such as the ESAS or other symptom evaluation tool. Body weight should also be evaluated.

Measuring the circumference of the patient's mid-upper arm may also have prognostic value.[53] In a research setting, the 12-item Functional Assessment of Anorexia/Cachexia Therapy (FAACT) symptom-specific subscale, in addition to FACIT-F, can be used to measure patients' concerns about their anorexia and/or cachexia during the past 7 days.[52]

Nausea and Constipation

Nausea is a subjective symptom, frequently multifactorial. Nausea is commonly accompanied by pain, insomnia, anorexia, fatigue, anxiety, and/or depression. Physicians should assess patients for the presence of all these symptoms because they can contribute to or worsen nausea (thereby increasing distress in patients and their families).

To record intensity and frequency of nausea, physicians should use a validated tool such as the ESAS not only at the initial evaluation, but also at regular intervals to evaluate patients' response to nausea treatment.[41]

Constipation is difficult to assess and treat because of the wide variety of presenting symptoms.[41] Because patients with advanced disease have a greater risk for severe constipation than those with early cancer, physicians should obtain complete clinical histories of patients' bowel habits, including their bowel patterns and stool characteristics.

The Rome Criteria (romecriteria.org) can be used to help assess constipation but do not consider QOL.[41,47] An abdominal radiography can be used to help assess bowel gas patterns and rule out ileus or bowel obstruction. In addition, an abdominal X-ray film can be divided into four quadrants by drawing an "X" across the film.

Each quadrant is assigned a score of 0 to 3, with 0 indicating no stool in the lumen, 1 indicating stool occupancy of < 50%, 2 indicating > 50% occupancy, and 3 indicating complete stool occupancy of the lumen. The cumulative "constipation score" can range from 0 to 12. A score of 7 or more indicates severe constipation.[41]

Malignant Bowel Obstruction

In cases of malignant bowel obstruction, a common and distressing occurrence, particularly in patients with gastrointestinal and/or gynecologic cancer,[54] it is important to carefully assess the patient and the possible causes of the obstruction to ensure that the patient does not require emergent surgery.[54] Computed tomography (CT) can be used to help physicians decide whether a surgical or medical approach would be more effective to relieve bowel obstruction.[54]

Dyspnea

Dyspnea is defined as difficult, labored, or uncomfortable breathing as experienced by the patient.[55] The gold standard for diagnosing dyspnea is the patient's self-report, because dyspnea is a subjective symptom that has multiple potential causes, and the tachypnea and degree of oxygen saturation and other arterial blood gas results might not reflect the distress that dyspnea causes.

Dyspnea can be assessed using numeric, oral, or visual analog scales. Instruments used to assess the intensity of dyspnea include the Support Team Assessment Scale[56] and the ESAS. However, no single scale can accurately reflect the far-reaching effects of breathlessness on patients and their family or caregivers. Patients with high dyspnea scores have a poorer QOL than patients with low dyspnea scores as assessed by 0–10 severity scale (e.g., ESAS-dyspnea scale).

Delirium

The main features of delirium, a transient and potentially reversible disorder of cognition and attention, are a fluctuating course of acute-onset reduced sensorium, attention deficit, and cognitive or perceptual disturbances.[57] In patients with advanced cancer, delirium causes significant distress and frequently complicates end-of-life care.[57]

Assessment instruments with adequate psychometric properties, such as the Mini-Mental State Examination (MMSE; originally used for the diagnoses of dementia), the Confusion Assessment Method (CAM), and the Memorial Delirium Assessment Scale (MDAS), facilitate the diagnosis of delirium and impose relatively little burden on patients.[58–60]

The MDAS, a validated tool used in palliative care, measures the severity of delirium and therefore captures behavioral manifestations as well as cognitive deficits.[60] The MDAS measures relative impairment in awareness, orientation, short-term memory, digit span, attention capacity, organizational thinking, perceptual disturbance, delusions, psychomotor activity, and sleep–wake cycle. Items on the MDAS are rated from 0 (none) to 3 (severe), with a maximum possible score of 30.

A total MDAS score of 7 yields the highest sensitivity (98%) and specificity (96%) for delirium diagnosis.[60]

Assessment of Sleep Disturbance

Sleep disturbance (SD) negatively affects QOL.[61] Sleep deprivation, an underreported problem among patients with advanced cancer, heightens physical, psychological, social, and existential suffering; diminishes coping capacity; and exacerbates symptoms such as pain and discomfort by increasing the perceived level of illness severity.[61]

Several tools have been used to evaluate SD in non-cancer settings; however, there is no validated single item screening scale to identify SD in palliative population.

The Pittsburgh Sleep Quality Index (PSQI), which measures sleep quality and patterns, can be used in the research or clinical setting.[62] The PSQI differentiates "poor" from "good" sleep by measuring seven areas: subjective sleep quality, sleep latency, sleep duration, habitual sleep efficiency, sleep disturbances, use of sleeping medication, and daytime dysfunction over the previous month. Patients rate each of these seven areas on a 0 to 3 scale; the maximum combined score is 21.

A combined score of 5 or more indicates a "poor" sleeper (i.e., a patient who experiences sleep disturbance). The PSQI can be used to provide an initial assessment and/or ongoing comparative measurements in all healthcare settings. PSQI has high validity, reliability, and internal consistency.[62]

Assessment of Emotional and Spiritual Distress

Assessment of Anxiety and Depression

Although mood disorders such as depression and anxiety are among the most prevalent psychiatric illnesses experienced by patients with advanced cancer, mood disorders often remain underdiagnosed and thus under-treated.[63] However, several easy-to-administer self-reporting assessment tools have been created to improve the accuracy of screening for anxiety and depression.[64]

The Hospital Anxiety and Depression Scale (HADS) is a brief, self-administered screening tool used to measure patients' psychological distress.[65] The HADS is sensitive to change, both during the course of disease and in response to medical and psychological interventions. The HADS consists of two subscales comprising 14 items (7 for anxiety and 7 for depression). Patients use a 4-point scale to rate the degree of distress they experienced during the previous week.

The two subscales are then scored separately. Scores of 7 or less indicate non-cases of anxiety and/or depression; scores of 8–10 indicate doubt-ful cases; and scores of 11–21 indicate definite cases. Also, it has been proposed that scores of 14 or 15 or more indicate severe disorders. The HADS has good reliability and validity in assessing symptom severity, anxiety disorders, and depression in somatic, psychiatric, and primary care patients as well as the general population.[65]

Assessment of Spirituality, Religiosity, and Spiritual Distress

Spiritual and religious beliefs can affect the way patients cope with their illnesses, creating distress and worsening the burden of the illness.[66,67] Spirituality is a dimension of personhood, a part of our being, and religion is a construct of human making, which enables the conceptualization and expression of spirituality.[68,69] The spirituality and religiosity field is important to consider when we evaluate patients with advanced and terminal illness, because it can influence coping strategies and quality of life. The presence of spiritual pain can be an important component of patients with chronic and acute pain and other physical and psychological symptoms.[70]

Spiritual assessment is a conversation in which the patient is encouraged to tell and explore his or her spiritual story. As in spiritual screening, there are several options in the literature for taking a spiritual history. It is to be patient centered and guided by the extent to which the patient chooses to disclose his or her spiritual needs.

There are several tools available for taking a spiritual history, including the Systems of Belief Inventory-15R,[71] Brief Measure of Religious Coping,[72] Functional Assessment of Chronic Illness Therapy-Spiritual Well-Being,[73,74] SPIRITual History,[75] HOPE,[76] and FICA Spiritual History.[77] Some of these instruments are intended primarily for research, whereas others have been used primarily in the clinical setting for non-chaplain clinicians.

The FICA tool (Faith, Importance, Community, Address in care) developed at the George Washington Institute for Spirituality and Health has been tested and validated.[77] It is recommended that it be incorporated into the social history section of the overall history and physical. In incorporating this area into a history, providers should be conscious of not imposing their own beliefs on the patient or trying to answer any questions or concerns that the patient may have in this area. Such questions and concerns should be referred to a professional chaplain. They also should be clear that this process does not oblige them to discuss their own beliefs and practices. The main goal of this process is to understand the role of spiritual and religious beliefs and practices in the patient's life and the role they play in coping with illness. As in the screening, a basic goal of the history is to diagnose spiritual distress, which should be referred to the professional chaplain.[78] Through active listening, a relationship is established between the patient and the provider and/or the professional chaplain. The chaplain then extracts themes and issues from the story to explore further with the patient. These themes might include meaning-making, God as judge versus God as comforter, grief, despair, and forgiveness. This assessment should result in a spiritual care plan that is fully integrated into the patient's and family's total plan of care, which should be communicated to the rest of the treatment team.[78]

Conclusion

Caring for patients with advanced illnesses involves relieving distressing physical, psychosocial, and spiritual problems and empowering patients and their families to retain control while balancing the benefits and risks of treatments.

Recognizing these patients' distressing symptoms as multidimensional complexes and using appropriate and validated assessment tools help physicians manage these symptoms to improve patients' QOL and decrease caregiver burden.

Clinical Pearls

- Multiple distressing symptoms directly affect patients' level of distress, quality of life (QOL), and survival.
- Patients receiving palliative care present with multiple symptoms that require simultaneous assessment of these symptoms and management.
- A comprehensive multidisciplinary assessment provides a complete evaluation of patients with advanced and terminal illness and their caregivers.
- Patients should be assessed not only for physical symptoms that cause physical distress, but also for symptoms that cause emotional and spiritual distress.

References

1. Kirkova J, Davis M, Walsh D, et al. (2006). Cancer symptom assessment instruments: a systematic review. *J Clin Oncol* 24:1459–73.
2. Cleeland C, Reyes-Gibby C (2002). When is it "justified" to treat symptoms? Measuring symptom burden. *Oncology* 16:64–70.

3. Corner J, Hopkinson J, Fitzsimmons D, et al. (2005). Is late diagnosis of lung cancer inevitable? Interview study of patients' recollections of symptoms before diagnosis. *Thorax* 60:314–9.

4. Hui D, Elsayem A, De la Cruz M, et al. (2010). Availability and integration of palliative care at US cancer centers. *JAMA* 303(11):1054–61.

5. Yennurajalingam S, Atkinson B, Masterson J, Hui D, Urbauer D, Tu SM, Bruera E (2012). The impact of an outpatient palliative care consultation on symptom burden in advanced prostate cancer patients. *J Palliat Med* 15:20–3.

6. El-Jawahri A, Greer JA, Temel JS (2011). Does palliative care improve outcomes for patients with incurable illness? A review of the evidence. *J Support Oncol* 9(3):87–94.

7. Higginson IJ, Evans CJ (2010). What is the evidence that palliative care teams improve outcomes for cancer patients and their families? *Cancer J* 16(5):423–35.

8. Delgado-Guay MO, Bruera E (2008). Management of pain in the older person with cancer. Part 1. *Oncology* 22:56–61.

9. Basso U, Monfardinin S (2004). Multidimensional geriatric evaluation in elderly cancer patients: a practical approach. *Eur J Cancer Care* 13:424–33.

10. Hurria A, Lachs M, Cohen H, et al. (2006). Geriatric assessment for oncologists: rationale and future directions. *Crit Rev Oncol/Hematol* 59:211–7.

11. Stromgren A, Groenvold M, Pedersen L, Olsen A, Spile M, Sjogren P (2001). Does the medical record cover the symptoms experienced by cancer patients receiving palliative care? A comparison of the record and patient self-rating. *J Pain Symptom Manage* 21:89–96.

12. Stromgren A, Goldschmidt D, Groenvold M, et al. (2002). Self-assessment in cancer patients referred to palliative care: a study of feasibility and symptom epidemiology. *Cancer* 94:512–20.

13. De Haes JC, van Knippenberg FC, Neijt JP (1990). Measuring psychological and physical distress in cancer patients: structure and application of the Rotterdam Symptom Checklist. *Br J Cancer* 62: 1034–8.

14. Watanabe SM, Nekolaichuk CL, Beaumont C (2012). The Edmonton Symptom Assessment System, a proposed tool for distress screening in cancer patients: development and refinement. *Psycho-Oncology* 21:977–85

15. Stromgren AS, Groenvold M, Peterson M.A, et al. (2004). Pain characteristics and treatment outcome for advanced cancer patients during the first week of specialized palliative care. *J Pain Symptom Manage* 27:104–13.

16. Porzio G, Ricevuto E, Aielli F, et al. (2005). The Supportive Care Task Force at the University of L'Aquila: 2-years experience. *Support Care Cancer* 13:351–5.

17. Rees E, Hardy J, Ling J, Broadley K, A'Hern R (1998). The use of Edmonton Symptom Scale (ESAS) within a palliative care unit in the UK. *Palliat Med* 15:213–4.

18. Bruera E, Kuehn N, Miller MJ, Selmser P, Macmillan K (1991). The Edmonton Symptom Assessment System (ESAS): A simple method for the assessment of palliative care patients. *J Palliat Care* 7:6–9.

19. Stromgren AS, Groenvold M, Peterson MA, et al. (2004). Pain characteristics and treatment outcome for advanced cancer patients during the first week of specialized palliative care. *J Pain Symptom Manage* 27:104–13.

20. Philip J, Smith W, Craft P, Lickiss N (1998). Concurrent validity of the modified Edmonton Symptom Assessment Scale (ESAS) with the Rotterdam Symptom Checklist and the Brief Pain Inventory. *Support Care Cancer* 6:539–41.

21. Osterlind J (2003). Stablishing ESAS in daily Care. Poster communication in abstract book of the 8th Congress of the EAPC. http://www.eapcnet.eu/Corporate/Events/Abstractsarchive/Searchabstracts/tabid/217/zk/1/st/esas/Default.aspx. Access date 11.30.2015

22. Chang V, Hwang S, Feuerman M (2000). Validation of the Edmonton Symptom Assessment Scale. *Cancer* 88(9):2164–71.

23. Rees E, Jardy J, Ling J, Broadley K, A'Hern R (1998). The use of the Edmonton Symptom Assessment Scale (ESAS) within a palliative care unit in the UK. *Palliat Med* 12:75–82.

24. Watanabe S, Nekolaichuk C, Beaumont C, Mawani A (2009). The Edmonton Symptom Assessment System: What do patients think? *Support Care Cancer* 17:675–83.

25. Nekolaichuk C, Maguire P, Suarez-Almanzor M, Rogers W, Bruera E (1999). Assessing the reliability of patient, nurse, and family caregiver symptom rating in hospitalized advanced cancer patient. *J Clin Oncol* 11:3621–30.

26. Moro C, Brunelli C, Miccinesi G, et al. (2005). Edmonton symptom assessment scale: Italian validation in two palliative care settings. *Support Care Cancer* 14:30–7.

27. Pautex S, Berger A, Catelain C, Hermann F, Zulian G (2003). Symptom assessment in elderly cancer patients receiving palliative care. *Crit Rev Oncol Haematol* 47:281–6.

28. Stiel S, Matthes ME, Bertram L, et al. (2010). Validation of the new version of the minimal documentation system (MIDOS) for patients in palliative care: the German version of the Edmonton Symptom Assessment Scale (ESAS). *Schmerz* 24(6):596–604.
29. Carvajal A, Centeno C, Watson R, Bruera E (2011). A comprehensive study of psychometric properties of the Edmonton Symptom Assessment System (ESAS) in Spanish advanced cancer patients. *Eur J Cancer* 47:1863–72.
30. Kwon JH, Nam SH, Koh S, Seon Hong Y, et al. (2013). Validation of Edmonton Symptom Assessment System in Korean patients with cancer. *J Pain Symptom Manage* 46(6):947–56.
31. Jaturapatporn D (2008). Validity and cross-cultural adaptation of the Thai version of the Edmonton Symptom Assessment Scale (ESAS). *Palliat Med* 22:448.
32. Richardson L, Jones W (2009). A review of the reliability and validity of the Edmonton Symptom Assessment System. *Curr Oncol* 16:53–64.
33. Nekolaichuck C, Wataneabe S, Beaumont C (2008). The Edmonton Symptom Assessment System: a 15 year retrospective review of validation studies (1991–2006). *Palliat Med* 222:111–22.
34. Vignaroli E, Pace E, Willey J, Palmer L, Zhang T, Bruera E (2006). The Edmonton Symptom Assessment System as a screening tool for depression and anxiety. *J Palliat Med* 9:296–303.
35. McCorkle R., Young K (1978). Development of a symptom distress scale. *Cancer Nurs* 1:373–8.
36. McCorkle R., Quint-Benoliel J (1983). Symptom distress, current concerns and mood disturbance after diagnosis of life-threatening disease. *Soc Sci Med* 17:431–8.
37. Portenoy R, Thaler H, Kornblith A, et al. (1994). The Memorial Symptom Assessment Scale: an instrument for the evaluation of symptom prevalence, characteristics and distress. *Eur J Cancer* 30A:1326–36.
38. Chang V, Hwang S, Feuerman M, Kasimis B, Thaler H (2000). The Memorial Symptom Assessment Scale Short Form (MSAS-SF): validity and reliability. *Cancer* 89:1163–71.
39. Chang V, Hwang S, Kasimis B, Thaler H (2004). Shorter symptom assessment instruments: The Condensed Memorial Symptom Assessment Scale (CMSAS). *Cancer Invest* 22:526–36.
40. Viganó A, Dorgan M, Buckingham J, Bruera E, Suarez-Almazor M (2000). Survival prediction in terminal cancer patients: a systematic review of the medical literature. *Palliat Med* 14:363–74.
41. Dalal S, Del Fabbro E, Bruera E (2006). Symptom control in palliative care. Part 1: oncology as a paradigmatic example. *J Palliat Med* 9:391–408.
42. Schag C, Heinrich R, Ganz P (1984). Karnofsky Performance Status revisited: reliability validity and guidelines. *J Clin Oncol* 2:187–93.
43. Mor V, Laliberte L, Morris J.N, Wiemann M (1984). The Karnofsky Performance Status Scale: an examination of its reliability and validity in a research setting. *Cancer* 53 (9):2002–7.
44. Oken MM, Creech RH, Tormey DC, et al. (1982). Toxicity and response criteria of the Eastern Cooperative Oncology Group. *Am J Clin Oncol* 5: 649–55.
45. Kaasa T, Weesel J (2001). The Edmonton Functional Assessment Tool: further development and validation for use in palliative care. *J Palliat Care* 17:5–11.
46. Marcianiak C, Sliwa J, Spill G, Heinemann A, Semik P (2004). Functional outcome following rehabilitation of the cancer patient. *Arch Phys Med Rehab* 77:54–7.
47. Delgado-Guay MO, Bruera E (2008). Management of pain in the older person with cancer. Part 1. *Oncology* 22:56–61.
48. Bruera E, Moyano J, Seifert L, et al. (1995). The frequency of alcoholism among patients with pain due to terminal cancer. *J Pain Symptom Manage* 10:599–603.
49. Yennurajalingam S, Bruera E (2007). Palliative management of fatigue at the close of life: "It feels like my body is just worn out." *JAMA* 297:295–304.
50. Del Fabbro E, Dalal S, Bruera E (2006). Symptom control in palliative care. Part II: cachexia/anorexia and fatigue. *J Palliat Med* 9:409–21.
51. Cella D (1997). *Manual of the Functional Assessment of Chronic Illness Therapy (FACIT) measurement system.* Center on Outcomes, Research and Education (CORE). Evanston, Northwestern Healthcare and Northwestern education. Version 4, 1997.
52. Mendoza T, Wang X, Cleeland C, et al. (1999). The rapid assessment of fatigue severity in cancer patients. *Cancer* 85:1186–96.
53. Mantovani G, Maccio A, Madeddu C, Massa A (2003). Cancer-related cachexia and oxidative stress: beyond current therapeutic options. *Expert Rev Anticancer Ther* 3:381–92.
54. Ripamonti CI, Eason A, Gerdes H (2008). Management of malignant bowel obstruction. *Eur J Cancer* 44(8):1105–15.
55. Del Fabro E, Dalal S, Bruera E (2006). Symptom control in palliative care. Part III: dyspnea and delirium. *J Palliat Med* 9:422–36.

56. Bausewein C, Farquahar M, Booth S, Gysels M, Higginson I (2007). Measurement of breathlessness in advanced disease: a systematic review. *Respir Med* 101:399–410.

57. Lawlor P, Fainsinger R, Bruera E (2000). Delirium at the end of life: critical issues in clinical practice and research. *JAMA* 284:2427–9.

58. Folstein MF, Folstein SE, McHugh PR (1975). Mini-Mental State: a practical method for grading the cognitive state of patients for the clinician. *J Psychiatr Res* 12:189–98.

59. Inouye SK, van Dyck CH, Alessi CA, et al. (1990). Clarifying confusion: the Confusion Assessment Method: a new method for detection of delirium. *Ann Intern Med* 113:941–8.

60. Lawlor P, Nekolaichuk C, Gagnon B, et al. (2000). Clinical utility, factor analysis, and further validation of the Memorial Delirium Assessment Scale in patients with advanced cancer. *Cancer* 88:2859–67.

61. Fortner B, Stepanski E, Wang S, Kasprowicz S, Durence H (2002). Sleep and quality of life in breast cancer patients. *J Pain Symptom Manage* 24:471–80.

62. Buysse DJ, Reynolds CF, Monk TH, Berman SR (1989). Pittsburgh Sleep Quality Index: a new instrument for psychiatric practice and research. *Psychiatr Res* 28(2):192–213.

63. Massie MJ (2004). Prevalence of depression in patients with cancer. *J Natl Cancer Inst Monogr* 32:57–71.

64. Lloyd-Williams M, Dennis M, Taylor F (2004). A prospective study to determine the association between physical symptoms and depression in patients with advanced cancer. *Palliat Med* 18:558–63.

65. Bjelland I, Dahl AA, Haug TT, Neckelmann D (2002). The validity of the Hospital Anxiety and Depression Scale: an updated literature review. *J Psychosom Res* 52:69–77.

66. Puchalski C, Ferrel B, Virani R, et al. (2009). Improving the quality of spiritual care as a dimension of palliative care: the report of the consensus conference. *J Palliat Med* 10:885–904.

67. Pargament KI, Koenig HG, Tarakeshwar N, Hahn J (2004). Religious coping methods as predictors of psychological, physical and spiritual outcomes among medically ill elderly patients: a two year longitudinal study. *J Health Psychol* 9:713–30.

68. Puchalski C, Romer A (2000). Taking a spiritual history allows clinicians to understand patients more fully. *J Palliat Med* 3:129–37.

69. Kearney M, Mount B (2000). Spiritual care of the dying patient. In: Chochinov H., Breitbart W (eds.), *Handbook of Psychiatry in Palliative Medicine*. New York: Oxford University Press, pp. 357–73.

70. Delgado-Guay MO, Hui D, Parsons HA, Govan K, De la Cruz M, Thorney S, Bruera E (2011). Spirituality, religiosity, and spiritual pain in advanced cancer patients. *J Pain Symptom Manage* 41(6):986–94.

71. Holland JC, Kash KM, Passik S, et al (1998). A brief spiritual beliefs inventory for use in quality of life research in life-threatening illness. *Psychooncology* 7:460–9.

72. Pargament KI, Smith BW, Koenig HG, Perez L (1998). Patterns of positive and negative religious coping with major life stressors. *J Sci Study Relig* 37:710–24.

73. Brady MJ, Peterman AH, Fitchett G, Mo M, Cella D (1999). A case for including spirituality in quality of life measurement in oncology. *Psychooncology* 8:417–28.

74. Cella DF, Tulsky DS, Gray G, et al. (1993). The functional assessment of cancer therapy scale: development and validation of the general measure. *J Clin Oncol* 11:570–9.

75. Maugans TA (1996). The SPIRITual history. *Arch Fam Med* 5:11–16.

76. Anandarajah G, Hight E (2001). Spirituality and medical practice: using the HOPE questions as a practical tool for spiritual assessment. *Am Fam Physician* 63:81–9.

77. Borneman T, Ferrell B, Puchalski C (2010). Evaluation of the FICA tool for spiritual assessment. *J Pain Symptom Manag* 20(2):163–73.

78. Fitchett G, Canada AL (2010). The role of religion/spirituality in coping with cancer: evidence, assessment, and intervention. In: Holland JC (ed.), *Psycho-Oncology*, 2nd ed. New York: Oxford University Press, pp. 440–6.

Clinical Decision-Making

Eduardo Bruera

Definition

Clinical decision-making is the process used by healthcare providers to make clinical judgments and treatment decisions.[1] The way in which decisions in health care are made has been a field of study for more than 35 years, with an extensive body of knowledge.

Decision-making in health care is a process that involves different reasoning processes occurring at the same time, ranging from the most intuitive and informal to the most formal and analytical ones.[2] The art of decision-making in medicine lies in the correct balance between formal and informal decision-making strategies.

The aim of healthcare decisions in general is to determine which conduct will yield the most favorable outcome in a specific situation. The process of decision-making includes two basic phases: (1) determining the possible outcome for the possible alternative conducts, and (2) analyzing the desirability of each outcome.[3]

Palliative Care Decision-Making

In patients receiving palliative care, decisions regarding the introduction of new treatments or the withdrawal of already established therapies are almost equally frequent. As with every medical decision, palliative care decisions must reflect a balance between the ethical principles of beneficence, nonmaleficence, and patient autonomy.[4]

In particular, patient goals need to be taken into consideration, and that is why they need to be elicited very early in the relationship. For example, discussions regarding advance directives, which can significantly alter the desirability of certain outcomes, must be undertaken early in the course of life-threatening diseases. Survival estimation is unreliable at the present time, and therefore "universal preparation precautions" are important for care planning.[5]

The Five-Step Approach

Palliative care requires an extensive and structured assessment procedure, and a disciplined decision-making approach is advisable. However, every patient is unique, and the same issue might demand completely different management in different patients.

A practical approach[4] for decision-making that takes into account the patient's specificities is presented in Table 3.1 and will be further described in the sections that follow.

Step 1: Clinical Problem Identification and Exploration

Patients present to palliative care with a multitude of clinical problems that can in turn trigger new problems. For example, an infection might trigger or worsen nausea, delirium, pain, and other problems, and hypercalcemia might cause vomiting, sedation, and delirium.

The first step is tightly related with the need for structured clinical assessment in palliative care. The accurate determination of the issues that affect the patient precedes the identification of the effects of each of these issues on the patient's quality of life. Several examples are identified in Table 3.2.

Table 3.1 The 5-Step Approach

Step	Activities
1	Identify a clinical problem (i.e., bowel obstruction).
2	Establish the degree of discomfort caused by the clinical problem (i.e., emesis, lack of nutrition).
3	Identify the advantages and problems of an intervention (i.e., colostomy).
4	Balance the overall pros and cons of the intervention versus no intervention.
5	Discuss care plan with the patient, family, and care team.

Table 3.2 Some Examples of Common Palliative Care Situations

Issue	Potentially Related Problems and Side Effects
Infection	Pain, nausea, delirium, convulsions
Anemia	Fatigue, chest pain, shortness of breath, palpitations
Dehydration	Delirium, myoclonus, hallucinations, fatigue
Renal failure	Delirium, nausea, vomiting, fatigue, edema
Lymphedema	Pain, heaviness, inability to move
Constipation	Pain, nausea, vomiting, anorexia
Hypercalcemia	Sedation, confusion, delirium, nausea, vomiting
Pathological	Inability to move, pain, thrombosis/embolism, respiratory
Fracture	Infections due to being immobile
Bowel obstruction	Emesis, cachexia, dehydration

Step 2: Determination of the Patient's Discomfort

After identification of the issues that affect the patient, the patient's discomfort associated with each specific problem must be identified. This is especially important, because as the disease progresses, the impact of each symptom or problem on the patient's quality of life can change. For example, pneumonia can cause fever, fatigue, and cough with phlegm that are quite uncomfortable for a cognitively intact patient, but there may be few or no symptoms for another patient, especially if the patient has already developed hypoactive delirium due to end of life.

Step 3: Identification of Problems Associated with the Treatment

Once all clinical and psychosocial problems are identified and ranked, it is fundamental to also identify all potential advantages and problems treating a problem.

Some potential advantages of a treatment can be quite significant, such as the relief of fever, chest pain, and cough with intravenous antibiotics for pneumonia. On the other hand, the patient may need transportation to the hospital, bloodwork and X-ray, insertion of an IV, and several days of inpatient care close to the end of life. Sometimes the side effects of the correction of a problem are more bothersome to a given patient than the problem itself.

Some examples are found in Box 3.1.

Step 4: Risk–Benefit Analysis

Once the issues affecting the patient, their potential side effects, their importance and rank according to the effect on the patient's quality of life, and the side effects of treatment are identified, the palliative care provider must undertake a risk–benefit analysis, weighing all the pros and cons of specific measures (Box 3.2).

Box 3.1 Example of Situations in Which Treatment Might Be Especially Bothersome

- Hospital admission
- Intensive care unit (ICU) transfer
- Surgery risks and discomfort
- Inconvenience of multiple radiation sessions
- Side effects of chemotherapy
- Discomfort of maintaining an intravenous (IV) line
- Difficulties involved with hospital in repetitive and long visits for dialysis

Box 3.2 Important Questions to Be Answered in the Process of Decision-Making

- What is the clinical problem?
- To what extent does the problem affect the patient?
- What are the potential effects of the problem correction (desired and undesired)?
- What will be the effect of withholding the problem correction?
- Is this decision supported by the best evidence available?
- Was the decision discussed with the patient and family? Do they understand and agree with the decision?
- What are the alternatives?

Step 5: Consensus

The course of action must be discussed with the patient (whenever possible), the family, and the team in order to develop a consensus. Depending on the severity of the issues and the complexity of the relationships, family meetings or several encounters might be needed to ensure complete understanding and to reach consensus.

Flexibility on the side of the care team is needed; as conversations with the patient and family evolve, some of the previous steps may need to be re-evaluated.

Futility versus Harm

The clinician has no obligation to offer interventions that are futile and cannot ethically offer interventions that are clearly harmful. However, careful consideration should be given to these two terms with regard to some diagnostic or therapeutic interventions. Occasionally, patients or caregivers request interventions that are clinically futile but not harmful (i.e., imaging or lab work to confirm disease progression, vitamins, herbal treatments, etc.). These interventions can help the patient/caregiver emotionally. On the other hand, refusal by the clinician based solely on futility when there is no clear evidence of harm can be a source of emotional distress for the patient or caregiver and therefore harmful.

Clinical Pearls

- In palliative care, decision-making regarding the introduction of new treatments can be as frequent and important as the withdrawal of current treatments.
- Always have in mind the ethical principles: beneficence, nonmaleficence, distributive justice, and autonomy.
- The practice of evidence-based medicine involves the integration of clinical expertise with the best available evidence from clinically relevant research.
- A structured approach for decision-making in palliative care includes identification of issues, ranking of types of discomfort, determination of potential side effects, balance between intervention and nonintervention, and discussion with the patient, family, and team.

References

1. *Encyclopedia Britannica* (2009). Clinical decision making. Retrieved February 10, 2009, from http://www.britannica.com/EBchecked/topic/121745/clinicaldecsion-making.
2. Croskerry, P (2005). The theory and practice of clinical decision-making. *Can J Anesth* 52(6):8.
3. Eddy DM (1990). Clinical decision making: from theory to practice. Anatomy of a decision. *JAMA* 263(3):441–3.
4. Driver LC, Bruera E (2000). Decision-making. In: Driver LC & Bruera E (Eds.), *The MD Anderson Palliative Care Handbook*. Houston: University of Texas Health Science Printing, pp. 5–8.
5. Bruera E (2015). End-of-life diagnosis, communication, and the search for "Infectin," "Clottin," and "Heart Arrestin". *Palliat Med* 29(2):99–100.

Pain Assessment and Management

Angelique Wong and Suresh K. Reddy

Introduction

Pain is one of the main symptoms experienced by cancer patients, during both curative and palliative therapy. Pain often triggers the patient's initial medical evaluation prior to the diagnosis of malignancy. Numerous national and international surveys have found that 30%–50% of cancer patients in active therapy and as many as 60%–90% with advanced disease have pain.[1–5]

Pain, however, is undertreated. The reasons are many and include physicians' lack of knowledge, lack of availability of opioid medication, governmental regulations, physicians' fear of regulations, diversion of medication, and fear of addiction.[6,7]

Malignant diseases—both solid tumors, such as in lung or colon cancer, and liquid tumors, such as in leukemia—can lead to pain symptoms. The pain may be due to the tumor itself, either by direct involvement (e.g., of the bone, nerves, or viscera) or by indirect effects (e.g., tumor release of inflammatory mediators), or to treatments aimed at cure or palliation (see Box 4.1). Pain associated with direct tumor involvement occurs in 65%–85% of patients with advanced cancer.

Cancer therapy accounts for pain in approximately 15%–25% of patients receiving chemotherapy, surgery, or radiation therapy.[8] Pain syndromes commonly observed in the noncancer population are present in 10%–15% of cancer patients—for example, lower back pain secondary to degenerative disc disease.

Effective pain management involves an interdisciplinary approach using multimodal techniques, the goal being to relieve the patient's suffering. Precise assessment of pain and associated factors is crucial, as the objective of treatment is to treat the cause whenever possible.

In this chapter the authors discuss the most practical aspects of pain management in patients receiving palliative care. While the focus here is on pain management in patients with cancer because cancer-related pain is common and often severe, the same principles of pain management apply to patients receiving palliative care for a variety of diseases.

Box 4.1 Causes of Pain in Cancer

- Related to direct tumor involvement: 60%–65%
- Related to cancer treatment: 20%–25%
- Unrelated to cancer: 10%–15%

Definition

Cancer pain is pain as a result of cancer or its therapy. Pain is subjective and varies in expression from person to person, and these individual differences must be considered when developing a plan of symptom management (see Figure 4.1).

A useful method of treating pain is to not only respond to the patient's current symptom constellation but also anticipate the patient's symptom control needs, based on the specific cancer diagnosis and the sites of tumor involvement.

The participation of a palliative care specialist or team at a cancer center is vital to the successful management of cancer pain.

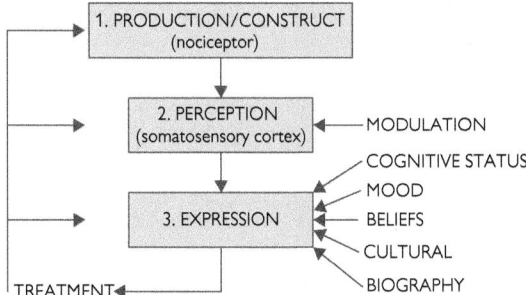

Figure 4.1. Steps involved in the expression of pain in cancer patients. Numerous factors are believed to contribute to the overall expression of pain. Many of those factors are known and summarized in this figure. The bright gray lines indicate the factors that diminish pain intensity.

Adapted from Bruera E, Kim HN (2003). Cancer pain. *JAMA* 290(18):2476–9.

Mechanisms of Pain and Pathophysiology

The pathophysiological classification of pain forms the basis for therapeutic choices. Pain states may be broadly divided into those associated with ongoing tissue damage (*nociceptive*) and those resulting from nervous system dysfunction (*neuropathic*), the latter of which may or may not be accompanied by tissue damage (see Boxes 4.2 and 4.3).

Nociceptive pain can be of the somatic or visceral type. *Somatic pain* results from the activation of nociceptors in cutaneous and deep tissues; it is described as well-localized aching, throbbing, and gnawing.

Visceral pain is caused by the activation of nociceptors resulting from distension, stretching, and inflammation of visceral organs; it is described as poorly localized deep aching, cramping, and pressure. Visceral pain may be referred—for example, pancreatic cancer pain in the abdomen with referral to the back.

Breakthrough pain is common in cancer patients and is defined as a "transitory exacerbation of pain that occurs on a background of otherwise stable persistent pain."[9] Breakthrough pain may be caused by activity or end-of-dose failure; it can also occur spontaneously. It tends to be moderate to severe and, according to one study, lasts less than 3 minutes in 43% of pain cases. The typical frequency is 1 to 4 episodes per day. Breakthrough pain tends to be prognostic of poor response to pain treatment.[10]

In many cases, the etiology of cancer pain is multifactorial. Pain may be nociceptive in origin and related to direct tumor invasion of bone and soft tissue, or related to perineural involvement, benign inflammation, or superimposed infection.

Pain may also be neuropathic in origin and secondary to peripheral or cranial nerve involvement or related to the sequelae of surgery or radiation therapy.

Clinical Pearls
- Pain can be nociceptive (visceral or somatic) or neuropathic.
- Somatic nociceptive pain is localized throbbing, gnawing; visceral pain is poorly localized cramping or pressure and is associated with autonomic symptoms.

Box 4.2 Types of Pain

Nociceptive
- Somatic: Sharp, localized, aching, throbbing, gnawing (e.g., pain in muscle, bone, soft tissues)
- Visceral: Dull, poorly localized, crampy, nauseous, squeezy, pressure (e.g., pain in the pancreas, liver, small bowel)

Neuropathic
- Burning, tingling, shooting, stabbing, itching, electric-like, numb (e.g., peripheral neuropathy, plexopathy from tumors, post-herpetic neuralgia)

Box 4.3 Cancer Pain Syndromes

Acute

- Due to cancer or related disorders
- Due to diagnostic interventions
- Due to anticancer therapy

Chronic

Nociceptive Somatic

- Bone pain
- Soft tissue
- Muscle
- Pleural pain
- Paraneoplastic syndromes

Nociceptive Visceral

- Hepatic distension syndrome
- Midline retroperitoneal syndrome
- Chronic intestinal obstruction
- Peritoneal carcinomatosis
- Malignant perineal syndrome
- Adrenal pain syndrome
- Ureteric obstruction syndrome

Neuropathic

- Leptomeningeal metastases
- Painful cranial neuralgias (e.g., glossopharyngeal neuralgia)
- Painful radiculopathy
- Painful peripheral mononeuropathies
- Paraneoplastic peripheral neuropathy
- Neuropathic pain is described as numb, shooting, or electric-like.
- More than two types of pain occur commonly in cancer.
- Breakthrough pain can occur spontaneously or can be caused by activity or end-of-dose failure.
- Cancer pain is multifactorial, requiring an interdisciplinary approach to treatment.
- A cancer pain syndrome includes acute or chronic pain, or both.
- Acute pain may be due to procedures, cancer therapy, or preexisting medical conditions.
- Chronic pain may be neuropathic, nociceptive somatic, or nociceptive visceral.
- Precise assessment of the type and cause of pain is the cornerstone of optimal pain treatment.
- Cancers have specific well-defined pain syndromes, but patients may also present with pain that is not related to the cancer. One must differentiate between the two types of pain.

Assessment of Pain

Intensity of Pain Assessment

It is crucial to assess and monitor the intensity of pain. Pain intensity can be measured by using simple visual analog, verbal, or numerical scales, or more complex pain questionnaires[11] (see Box 4.4).

Most instruments and techniques are very reliable for assessing the intensity of pain. The assessment can be made more effective by a graphic ongoing display of pain and other symptoms in the patient's chart, along with other vital sign monitoring. This establishes a baseline against which outcomes can be measured and helps the physician effectively administer appropriate care.

Current institutional pain management guidelines were established by the Joint Commission on Accreditation of Health Care Organizations (JCAHO) in 2000. On a 0 to 10 scale, mild pain can be defined as 0–3, moderate pain as 4–7, and severe pain as 8–10.

Pain assessment should always be done in the context of other cancer symptoms. In patients with a complex and evolving cancer history, visual representations of the patient's tumor sites and treatment can aid the physician in developing a tailored pain management strategy.

The Edmonton Labeled Visual Information System (ELVIS), validated in a randomized trial as a rapid and effective pictorial memorization tool, can prove useful to this end.[12]

Psychosocial Assessment

Pain as a symptom cannot be adequately evaluated in isolation from a patient's total symptom burden. The Edmonton Symptom Assessment System (ESAS) is a validated and effective tool used for identifying symptoms commonly experienced by cancer patients.[11]

Box 4.4 Pain Assessment Tools

Behavioral
- CAGE: Cut down, Annoyed, Guilty, Eye opener

Pain
- Brief Pain Inventory Short Form (SF) and Long Form (LF)
- Pain thermometer
- Wong–Baker FACES pain rating scale

Psychosocial
- Edmonton Symptom Assessment System (ESAS)
- Memorial Symptom Assessment Scale (MSAS) and MSAS–Short Form (MSAS-SF)

Cognitive
- Folstein Mini-Mental Status Exam (MMSE)
- Memorial Delirium Assessment Scale (MDAS)

Assessment of a pain complaint is not valid unless a thorough psychosocial assessment is done. The clinician should evaluate psychosocial factors such as anxiety, depression, loss of independence, family challenges, financial difficulties, social isolation, and fear of death.

Cancer patients more often meet the diagnostic criteria for adjustment disorder with anxiety and depressed mood than the criteria for major depressive disorder.[13]

The effect of pain and other symptoms on functional status must be understood to establish treatment goals. Pain, when evaluated in conjunction with other distressing psychosocial symptoms, leads to the calculation of "total pain" or "suffering."

Clinical Pearls

- Comprehensive assessment is vital for good symptom management (see Box 4.5).
- Prognostic factors and performance status need to be assessed.
- Delirium will complicate pain assessment and management. Beware of misinterpreting delirium as pain.
- Validated instruments are invaluable for measuring pain severity.
- Pain assessment must be done in the context of other symptoms contributing to the illness experience.
- Psychosocial factors affect pain reporting and expression.

Box 4.5 General Pain Management Principles

- Respect and accept the complaint of pain as real.
- Treat pain appropriately.
- Treat underlying disorder(s).
- Address psychosocial issues.
- Use a multidisciplinary approach.

Pharmacotherapy

The management of cancer pain has made significant progress in recent years, partly because of Agency for Health Care Policy and Research (AHCPR) guidelines,[14] but mostly because of an international movement to optimize symptom management in the chronically ill and dying.

Cancer pain in particular can present a challenge, necessitating accurate diagnosis and appropriate intervention. Pharmacotherapy with analgesics remains the mainstay of treating cancer pain. Most cancer pain syndromes present with moderate to severe pain and are associated with several comorbidities, requiring a multidisciplinary approach for optimal management.

The analgesics used to manage cancer-related pain can be divided into three categories:

- Non-opioid medications such as acetaminophen and nonsteroidal anti-inflammatory drugs (NSAIDs)
- Weak opioid medications such as codeine or strong opioids such as morphine
- Adjuvant medications such as tricyclic antidepressants (TCAs) and anti-epileptic drugs (AEDs).

WHO Analgesic Ladder

In 1984, the World Health Organization (WHO) proposed a simple analgesic "ladder" for the pharmacological management of cancer-related pain[15] (see Figure 4.2). Experience applying this ladder in several countries has

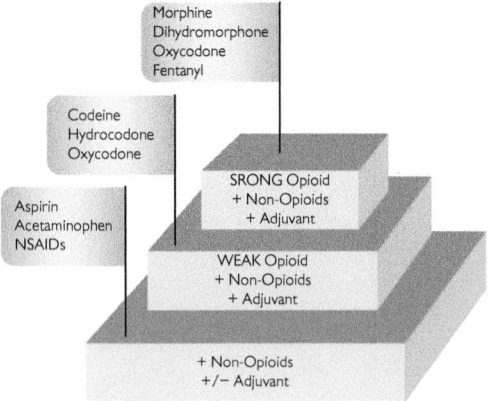

Figure 4.2. The WHO pain ladder.

Adapted by Yennurajalingam S, et al. (2005). Pain and terminal delirium research in the elderly. *Clin Geriatr Med* 21(1):93–119. Reprinted with permission from Elsevier.

shown that the simple principle of escalating from non-opioid to strong opioid analgesics is safe and effective.

Step 1

The first step of the analgesic ladder is to use a non-opioid analgesic (e.g., acetaminophen or an NSAID). Adjuvant drugs can be added to enhance analgesic efficacy, to treat concurrent symptoms that exacerbate pain, and to provide independent analgesic activity for specific types of pain. Adjuvant medications, such as TCAs, may be used at any step.

- Identify pain syndrome.
- Pain intensity: mild (0 to 3)
- Medications: acetaminophen, anti-inflammatory agents, TCAs, or AEDs
- Response: somatic and neuropathic pain syndromes respond mildly.

Step 2

If pain persists despite step 1 medications, then a mild low-potency opioid such as codeine should be added (not substituted). The pain syndrome is any or specific.

- Pain syndrome: identify
- Pain intensity: moderate (4–7)
- Medications: mild opioids, NSAIDs, TCAs, or AEDs
- Response: varies.

Step 3

If pain persists despite step 2 efforts, then a strong (high-potency) opioid such as morphine is initiated in step 3. The dose of the stronger opioid can be titrated upward according to the patient's pain, as there is no ceiling dose for morphine.

Medications for persistent or continuous pain require an around-the-clock prescription, with an extra dose available in case the patient experiences breakthrough pain.

- Identify pain syndrome.
- Pain intensity: moderate to severe, 7–10/10
- Medications: strong opioid (morphine class), plus NSAIDs, AEDs, TCAs, or other agents
- Response: good, 80%–90%.

Opioids

Opioid medications form the basis for the management of cancer-related pain, regardless of its pathophysiology. They are pharmacodynamically classified into pure agonists, mixed agonist–antagonists, and antagonists.

In clinical practice, only pure agonists are used. Mixed agonist–antagonists are not used because they exhibit a ceiling effect, at which point the benefit from agonist action on analgesia equals the side effects from antagonism, including the potential to precipitate symptoms of withdrawal.

Of the three classical opioid receptor types—mu, delta, and kappa—the mu receptor is most clinically relevant.

Low-Potency (Mild) Opioids

The list of mild or low-potency opioids includes codeine, propoxyphene, hydrocodone, and dihydrocodeine, which have a potency of between one-tenth and one-fourth that of morphine sulfate (Box 4.6).

Box 4.6 WHO Approach to Drug Therapy of Cancer Pain

Five Essential Concepts

- *By the mouth*: The oral route is preferred for simplicity in the management of nociceptive and neuropathic pain.
- *By the clock*: If the pain is persistent, then around-the-clock (atc) medication should be used, in addition to as-needed (prn) doses.
- *By the ladder*: This implies moving to the next step rather than sideways. (A next-step move would be from a non-opioid to an opioid; a sideways move would be from opioid to opioid, i.e., morphine to oxycodone.)
- *For the individual*: The dose varies from individual to individual. Hence, the right dose is the one that relieves pain without causing side effects.
- *With attention to detail*: Other factors (e.g., psychosocial distress, spiritual concerns) need to be assessed and dealt with in addition to pharmacotherapy, thereby treating total pain.

Indications for drugs from this group include mild to moderate pain not responsive to non-opioids. Examples include mild bone pain and early visceral pain.

These agents are also occasionally used for breakthrough pain in patients with constant pain who are receiving sustained-release opioids. This group of drugs is commonly formulated with acetaminophen, limiting dose escalation to the maximum allowable dose of acetaminophen. Formulations without acetaminophen can be prepared by some pharmacies.

Codeine

Codeine is commonly prescribed for both its analgesic properties and antitussive effect. It can be one of the most constipating of all drugs and is sometimes used to control diarrhea in opioid-tolerant cancer patients.

Codeine, with a plasma half-life of 2–3 hours, is metabolized by the liver to its active metabolite, morphine. Approximately 10% of the Caucasian population has mutations in the hepatic enzyme CYP2D6 and therefore cannot convert codeine to morphine, resulting in poor analgesic efficacy.

Tramadol

Codeine's synthetic analogue, tramadol, is not widely used in the treatment of cancer pain. It is a weak mu-receptor agonist, most effective for the treatment of mild to moderate pain states.

With activity via blockade of presynaptic reuptake of serotonin and norepinephrine, there is evidence that it works in neuropathic pain states.[16] It is an effective step 2 medication in the appropriate clinical scenario.

Hydrocodone

Hydrocodone is currently the most widely used opioid in the United States and is commercially available in different concentrations. Oral formulations that include either acetaminophen or ibuprofen as a co-analgesic are available.

Hydrocodone is a synthetic opioid, with a half-life of 2–3 hours, acting through conversion to hydromorphone via the CYP2D6 enzyme. Genetic mutations in CYP2D6-mediated metabolism can be associated with reduced efficacy or increased toxicity of hydrocodone, as with codeine.[17–19]

High-Potency (Strong) Opioids

This class of drugs is used for all pain types and includes oxycodone, hydromorphone, meperidine, fentanyl, and methadone.

Morphine

Morphine is the most widely used and prototype drug of its class. It is a gold-standard drug, available in all countries, and is valued for its low cost, ease of use, and analgesic potency. It is converted to morphine-3-glucuronide and mophine-6-glucuronide (M3G and M6G, respectively) by UDP-glucuronyl transferase in the liver, acting on the mu receptor in the central nervous system.

Caution should be exercised when using morphine in patients with renal impairment, as these compounds are excreted by the kidney. Only M6G has been implicated in opioid activity and side effects (e.g., sedation) in animal studies. M3G has a very low affinity for opioid receptors and is largely ineffective as an analgesic. M3G may be responsible for morphine's observed neuroexcitatory toxicities.[20]

Morphine's duration of action is 2–4 hours; however, the sustained-release form can be administered as infrequently as every 8 to 12 hours. Morphine is available for oral, rectal, intramuscular (IM), intravenous (IV), and sublingual use, as well as in epidural and intrathecal preparations.

Oxycodone

Once classified as a low-potency opioid when its dosage was limited by combination with acetaminophen or aspirin, oxycodone is now available as a stand-alone preparation. With a sustained-release as well as an immediate-release form, it has gained widespread popularity in the treatment of cancer pain.

Oxycodone is considered equipotent to, if not more potent than, morphine. It is available only in the oral form in the United States and has a higher oral bioavailability than that of morphine.

Oxymorphone

Oxymorphone (oxymorphone hydrochloride, or 14-hydroxydihydromorphinone) is a semi-synthetic mu-opioid receptor agonist available in immediate- and extended-release formulations.[21] It is considered a more potent opioid than its parent compound, morphine.

Taking oxymorphone with food can increase serum levels by up to 50%; thus, it is recommended to be taken at least 1 hour before or 2 hours after a meal.[22,23] Co-ingestion of alcohol with extended-release oxymorphone can raise serum levels (from 70% up to 270% in some patients) in an unknown manner and, thus, should be avoided.[22]

Hydromorphone

Hydromorphone is a useful, short-acting opioid, 6–7 times more potent than morphine. It is available for administration via all routes, including neuraxial.

Hydromorphone is available in immediate-release and sustained-release oral formulations. The long-acting formulation of hydromorphone is coated in a casing to minimize abuse and diversion but can be associated with medication bezoars.[24]

Meperidine

Meperidine is commonly used throughout the world as an opioid analgesic, although it is not used as often as morphine. It is predominantly a mu-opioid receptor agonist, available in oral and IV formulations. It undergoes hepatic metabolism to normeperidine and is excreted by kidney.

In the oral form, its potency is one-tenth that of morphine, which makes it less efficacious in most patients. Increased doses required to achieve morphine-equianalgesic levels are associated with the risk of normeperidine accumulation.

With the potential for increased central nervous system excitability and convulsions, it should be used with extreme caution in renally impaired and elderly patients.

Fentanyl

Fentanyl is a semi-synthetic opioid available in parenteral, transdermal, and oral preparations. The prototype of a semi-synthetic opioid, it is the only drug of this class available in parenteral form. Its rapid onset and relatively short duration of action make it a good choice for the control of acute pain and for use in patient-controlled analgesia (PCA) pumps.

Unlike other opioids, a sustained-release form (transdermal) was developed long before its breakthrough non-parenteral counterpart, oral transmucosal fentanyl.[24–26] The sustained-release, transdermal form has been used successfully for stable pain.

Once applied, it forms a depot under the skin and is slowly released into the circulation. This limits its use in emergency situations, though, since it takes up to 18 hours to reach peak.[27] Patch is changed every 72 hours, which is convenient in patients whose pain is stable. Its use is difficult, however, in patients requiring frequent dose titration.

Oral transmucosal fentanyl has been approved for use in cancer patients with breakthrough pain, based on its rapid absorption via the oral mucosa.[28] A new oral preparation uses a novel effervescent drug delivery shown to enhance absorption across the buccal mucosa.[29] Intranasal fentanyl spray and fentanyl pectin nasal spray have been approved for use in breakthrough cancer pain.[30,31]

Sufentanil

This synthetic derivative of fentanyl is 5–10 times more potent than fentanyl itself. Its use has been mostly limited to anesthetic purposes.

As clinical familiarity increases and more routes of administration become available (only an injectable form is available now), it is expected that the use of sufentanil will increase in patients with cancer pain, especially those who are highly tolerant to opioids. It has shown good results when used intravenously in PCAs and in subcutaneous (SC) infusions in the context of palliative care.[32]

According to one report, it can be used successfully for breakthrough pain when applied sublingually.[33] Neuraxial application of sufentanil is an option in select patients.

Methadone

Because of its low cost and well-understood pharmacological properties, methadone is now accepted as a second-line opioid for the treatment of cancer-related pain.

Methadone is tightly bound to α-1-acid-glycoprotein, shows high lipid solubility, and given its significant tissue distribution, sustains a steady level in plasma during chronic treatment. No active metabolites are currently known.

It is generally available as a racemic mixture containing both D and L isomers. Levo-methadone, with twice the potency of the racemic form, is available in some countries.

The frequently observed interindividual variation in methadone pharmacokinetics has been attributed to differences in metabolism by the cytochrome P450 hepatic enzyme family. At least four heterologous expressed P450 proteins have been shown to catalyze the N-demethylation of methadone, for which the P450 3A4 type appears to be the main enzyme.

Caution should be observed with the co-administration of other drugs that interact with the cytochrome P450 system. Cytochrome P450 inhibitors include certain antibiotics, antifungals, antivirals, and antidepressants. Induction of the P450 system may be caused by anticonvulsants, rifampin, and corticosteroids.

Despite a wide range in interindividual pharmacokinetic variations of methadone, there are two phases identified: a rapid and extensive distribution phase (half-life of 2–3 hours), followed by a slow elimination phase (half-life of 15–60 hours). This extended elimination phase is of particular clinical importance since it can result in accumulation and toxicity. Adverse effects include sedation, nausea, and respiratory depression.

One limitation with the use of methadone is how it is viewed by society. Methadone is stigmatized because of its traditional use in the management of opioid addiction. It was termed a "killer drug" by the *New York Times* because of an increase in its use by recreational drug users and the associated rise in overdoses and subsequent deaths.[34]

Despite its questionable reputation, methadone has many advantages in palliative care. It can be administered orally, rectally, and intravenously, and is an effective alternative to morphine, hydromorphone, and fentanyl for treating cancer-related pain.

Finally, methadone is inexpensive and thus may be of particular interest for developing countries. It is also considered to be an NMDA receptor antagonist and may have a role in the management of opioid-resistant and neuropathic pain.

Methadone currently has two main indications in palliative care: (1) treatment of patients with opioid resistance and neuropathic pain, and (2) as a second-line agent in opioid rotation.

An optimal conversion method, rotating commonly used opioids to methadone and vice versa, has not yet been established.

Patients usually benefit from rotations from a previous opioid to methadone over 3 days, progressively reducing the dose of the previous opioid and increasing the dose of methadone (PO doses). The usual ratio from methadone to morphine is 4:1 in patients requiring < 90 mg/day of morphine; 8:1 the ratio is 90–300 mg/day, and 12:1 when the dose is > 300 mg/day (see Table 4.1).

This method was used in a prospective, multicenter study of 108 patients.[35] Although the multicenter study dealt mainly with the rotation from morphine to methadone, identical approaches have been used for the rotation of other opioids to methadone.

Studies examining the frequency of administration, including every 8, 12, and 24 hours, have had different results. One prospective study rotated 52 patients receiving oral morphine to oral methadone every 8 hours using different dose ratios. Patients were switched because of poor analgesia or adverse effects related to morphine. Switching to methadone was considered effective in 42 (80%) of the patients. The average period after which results were achieved was 3.65 days.

Future prospective studies are needed to explore equianalgesic conversion ratios for rotation from opioids to methadone and vice versa, including the influence of methadone on neuropathic pain and fast-developing tolerance induced by other opioids.

Bruera et al. proposed the following considerations for the future development of equianalgesic tables:[36] first, methadone appears to be more potent than previously accepted; second, conversion ratios relative to methadone depend on the dose of the previously used opioid. Also, conversion ratios falter at extremes of doses.

In addition to an equianalgesic conversion factor, strong emphasis should be placed on the physician's clinical experience, the patient's clinical condition, the use of other interacting drugs, and the use of other simultaneous interventions for pain relief, which may include radiation, surgery,

Table 4.1 Method of Rotation to Methadone

	Morphine	Methadone Dose*
Day 1–Day 3	Reduce the dose of morphine over the period of 3 days†	Increase the dose of methadone over the period of 3 days† 4:1 morphine < 90 mg/day 8:1 morphine 90–300 mg/day 12:1 morphine > 300 mg/day Rescue [breakthrough] dose: one-sixth of daily dose up to 3 allowed per day

* Methadone dose divided and administered every 8 hours. Ratio given is for morphine: methadone ratio.

Reprinted from Bruera E, Sweeney C (2002). Methadone use in cancer patients with pain: a review. *J Palliat Med* 5(1):127–38.

† Consider 50% on Day 1, 30% on Day 2 and 20% on Day 3

chemotherapy, or a combination thereof, as well as the use of other analgesics.

After the administration of methadone, its side effects, in particular sedation and impaired cognition, should be monitored carefully. Monitoring should be continued for several days after successful rotation to another opioid because of potential accumulation of the drug and late toxicity.

For further details on pharmacological properties and the use of methadone in cancer patients, we refer the reader to some of the recent extensive reviews of methadone and international guidelines.[37–39]

Methadone's tendency to prolong the QTc interval, increasing the risk for conversion to torsade de pointes, has led to a black-box warning.[40] Studies have shown a QTc increase between 9.5 ms and 20 ms on initiation of methadone therapy. This is of particular concern in patients with a history of cardiac conduction abnormalities, patients with a prolonged QTc (> 450 ms) at baseline, or patients receiving other commonly used medications that are cytochrome p450 inhibitors or are known to prolong the QTc.

A recent study did not show QTc prolongation in patients given methadone in a palliative care setting.[41] Routine EKG screening of all patients in a palliative care setting may not be necessary; however, if circumstances permit, a routine EKG screening prior to the initiation of methadone therapy is recommended.

Levorphanol

Levorphanol, a morphinian derivative, is available in oral, IV, and SC forms. It exerts its effects via mu, delta, and kappa opioid receptors; by inhibition of norepinephrine and serotonin uptake; and by NMDA receptor antagonism.[42]

Levorphanol is glucuronidated in the liver with its glucuronidated products renally excreted. Levorphanol's half-life of approximately 12–16 hours must be considered in patients with hepatic or renal dysfunction.

Clinical Pearls

- Most pain can be satisfactorily controlled using relatively simple medication regimens.
- Personalized treatment goals should be discussed with patients and their families.
- The WHO ladder concept of escalating from non-opioid to strong opioid analgesics is safe and effective.
- Analgesics include non-opioids and opioids.
- Pure opioid formulations are preferred to combinations with low-potency analgesics (i.e., acetaminophen with oxycodone).
- Opioid medications form the basis of the management of cancer pain, regardless of the pathophysiology of the pain.
- Mu-opioid receptors are the most clinically relevant of the three classical opioid receptor types (mu, delta, and kappa).
- The pain regimen should be tailored to the type and intensity of pain.
- The clinician should schedule around-the-clock (atc) and adequate breakthrough dosing.
- Appropriate adjuvant analgesics should be considered.
- Anti-emetics and laxatives should be prescribed proactively.

- Familiarization with opioid conversion principles is critical.
- Clinicians must recognize the signs and symptoms of opioid-induced delirium and overdose.
- Clinicians must use caution in prescribing benzodiazepines for anxiety-induced pain.
- Clinicians must identify and anticipate the potential for drug interactions and polypharmacy.
- Nonpharmacological approaches (i.e., anesthetic and neurosurgical procedures) should be considered where appropriate.
- Balanced analgesia is the key to good cancer pain management.
- Clinicians must be able to differentiate between tolerance and physical and psychological dependence.
- Clinicians should always consider the "total pain" concept and treat accordingly.

Steps to Treating Cancer Pain

Pain severity, previous opioid use, dosing, and side effects, as well as any preexisting conditions, guide the principles of pain treatment.

Step 1

Assess Pain Severity

Pain severity serves as a guide in the decision-making process with regard to choosing a low-potency opioid versus a high-potency drug like morphine. Most low-potency opioids are less suitable for severe pain because of their dose limitations and the presence of the ceiling effect.

Most cancer pain situations call for high-potency opioids. If a patient has an optimal trial with oral opioids, including rotation to a different opioid, or has experienced dose-limiting side effects, an alternative route such as IV or neuraxial may be tried.

Pain severity reported on a verbal numeric scale should be interpreted in the context of other psychosocial symptoms.

Step 2

Assess Opioid History and Side Effects

Patient-to-patient variability in response to a specific opioid has been widely appreciated and documented.[43] Some patients may respond well to one opioid after other opioids fail or are intolerable.

This phenomenon is likely explained by the drugs' action on different receptors or genetic factors in opiate receptor constitution and will influence the selection of drugs within the same class.[43,44]

Step 3

Previous Opioid Dosing and Pharmacokinetics

"Opioid-naïve" patients will require lower doses at least initially, reflecting the degree of tolerance. Opiate-tolerant patients are more likely to require longer-acting agents, while an as-needed-only regimen is recommended for patients with incident pain syndromes.

Opioid-tolerant patients may require stronger and higher than conventional doses of opioids from the beginning.

Opioid medications exhibit a wide interindividual variation, possibly because of differences in intrinsic activity and action at different receptors and receptor subtypes.[43,44] Hence, opioid rotation is a worthwhile exercise when dose-limiting side effects are encountered.

The generally accepted method is to treat side effects before opioid switching. There is no general consensus on the number of opioid rotations, but in the authors' experience at least two or three opioid rotations, which should include methadone at some stage, need to be attempted.

Administration Strategies

Around the Clock (atc)

Around-the-clock (atc) administration is required in patients with continuous or frequent episodic pain. It is given to maintain a steady-state level and depends on the half-life of the drug chosen. Sustained-release oral preparations (morphine, oxycodone, oxymorphone) and transdermal patches (fentanyl) have gained popularity for their convenience.

Opioid-tolerant patients may require more frequent dosing regardless of the preparation used, to avoid end-of-dose failure.

Breakthrough (prn, or as needed)

Since fluctuations in the pain level occur in most patients on long-acting preparations, the need for shorter-acting agents is present in almost every case to provide coverage during surges. Rescue doses can be prescribed for as often as once every hour orally, or even once every 15–20 minutes when the IV route is used.

Traditionally, 10%–20% of the total opioid dose in a 24-hour period is given as a breakthrough dose. For patients experiencing less frequent episodic pain or pain related only to activity, only short-acting opioid medications are used, preferably on a preemptive basis.

Most of the short-acting opioids are not suitable for pain episodes lasting only a few minutes; however, transmucosal fentanyl preparations can be used for breakthrough cancer pain in these settings, with rapid onset and short clinical half-life.[45] High cost limits its use and accessibility.

Patient-Controlled Analgesia

Delivery of opioids by patient-controlled analgesia (PCA) is occasionally indicated in refractory pain syndromes with acute exacerbations of pain. It is also used in patients unable to tolerate oral preparations. It can be delivered either intravenously or subcutaneously.

Although opioids are traditionally delivered intravenously in hospitalized patients, PCAs are available for use on an outpatient basis with appropriate supervision. In the outpatient or home setting, the SC route may be considered because of its convenience and ease of use.

The pharmacodynamics for both SC and IV delivery tends to be similar once steady state is achieved.

Presence of Other Symptoms

Sometimes symptoms of delirium, anxiety, and depression may be interpreted as physical pain, and opioid escalation is done with worsening of delirium. Hence, assessment of these symptoms is mandatory to avoid overdosing of opioids.

Step 4

Assess Opioid Side Effects

A thorough knowledge of opioid side effects is necessary. While some side effects are common to all opioids, some patients may exhibit side effects unique to a specific drug and its metabolic end products.

Diminution or elimination of side effects is an important part of opioid therapy. Every effort should be made to treat side effects prophylactically (e.g., treat constipation with laxatives, and nausea with anti-emetics). The opioid-switching phenomenon likely emerged in an effort to treat the side effects of opioids.

Whenever possible, dose readjustment should be the first measure in managing adverse reactions. Some common opioid side effects are described as follows (for a more detailed review of each symptom, please refer to relevant chapters in this Handbook).

Sedation

Sedation is a commonly encountered side effect that often signifies excessive dosing. Downward titration of the dose to the level of analgesia is usually desirable. Drug combinations with opioids and other adjuvant medications may allow for an opioid-sparing effect, thereby minimizing sedation.

If sedation tends to be refractory to these maneuvers, the addition of a central nervous system stimulant (e.g., methylphenidate or dextroamphetamine) with upward titration could be helpful.[46] Methylphenidate is started with an initial dose of 5 mg on wakening and 5 mg at noon, with upward titration to response.

The development of sedation following a period of adequate pain control may indicate improvement in or resolution of the original painful stimulus (e.g., decreased tumor burden after antineoplastic therapy). Downward titration of the opioid to the level of analgesia would again be recommended.

Tolerance

Tolerance is the second most common side effect and usually occurs within the first few days of opioid administration. It is defined as a reduction in the effectiveness of central or peripheral opioid activity, including analgesia, despite further attempts at dose escalation.

The dominant mechanism (central versus peripheral) should be determined in order to guide therapeutic choices (i.e., neuroleptics vs. motility agents, respectively).

Nausea and Vomiting

Opioids can trigger nausea and vomiting directly by decreasing gastrointestinal (GI) motility and indirectly by inducing constipation. Patients with advanced malignancy can have decreased GI peristalsis secondary to circulating inflammatory mediators, with opioids compounding this effect.

Metoclopramide is frequently used to treat nausea and vomiting because it has multiple mechanisms of action that antagonize opioids, at both the central chemoreceptor trigger zone and the GI tract. Other agents include prochlorperazine, diphenhydramine, butyrophenones, benzodiazepines, steroids, and serotonin antagonists, such as ondansetron.

In patients who are receiving chemotherapy, a more aggressive approach should be used that is based on anticipated emetogenicity. This includes the use of aprepitant, a neurokinin-1 (NK-1) receptor antagonist.

Constipation

Constipation is one of the most common and easy-to-anticipate side effects. It often masquerades as other symptoms, presenting as intractable nausea and vomiting, increased abdominal pain, delirium, anorexia, or overflow diarrhea.

Since tolerance develops very slowly, if at all, patients will likely require regular laxative treatment from the inception and throughout the duration of opioid therapy. Dehydration, impaired mobility, autonomic dysfunction, and chemotherapy (e.g., vinca alkaloids) may compound the effects of opioid-induced constipation.

A bowel stimulant (e.g., senna) with a softening agent (e.g., docusate) is the most commonly used combination.[47] Multi-agent prophylaxis with gradual incremental dose increases may be necessary to reach the desired effect, based on patient subjective reports and clinical examination.

A kidney, ureters, and bladder (KUB) or flat-plate X-ray of the abdomen provides useful objective information regarding the degree of constipation when the clinical history or exam is inconclusive.[48]

Preparations such as polyethylene glycol (PEG) are tasteless, well tolerated, and useful as an adjunct to daily regular laxative therapy with senna and docusate. Resorting to an osmotic laxative such as lactulose or bowel preparations (magnesium citrate) is usually reserved for severe cases and could produce diarrhea.

As a backup measure, bowel lavage can be used in refractory cases until regular bowel movements are restored. A simple Fleet Enema, milk and molasses enema, or a manual maneuver may be the first remedies tried in these situations.

Caution should be used in patients whose constipation could be due to ileus, intestinal obstruction, or spinal cord compression, which is not uncommon in abdominopelvic malignancies and metastatic disease.

Neostigmine has been administered successfully in refractory cases, but caution should be exercised in cases of bowel obstruction and in patients with cardiac abnormalities. Oral naloxone has been used to manage severe cases of constipation.[49]

Recently, IV methylnaltrexone was approved for the management of refractory constipation in patients receiving opioid therapy. This drug has been shown to exert peripheral effects on the GI tract without reversing central analgesia.[50]

Important and commonly encountered considerations in patients undergoing active chemotherapy are neutropenia and thrombocytopenia. In patients with neutropenia (absolute neutrophil count < 1000/µL blood), therapy is limited to the oral route, since rectal manipulation of any kind can lead to bacterial translocation and sepsis.

Thrombocytopenia (defined as < 50,000 platelets/µL blood) also limits the physician to an oral route secondary to bleeding risks.

Cognitive Impairment

Other causes of cognitive impairment should be aggressively sought before opioid medications are implicated. Impaired cognition, presenting as delirium, hallucinations, agitation, or somnolence, has been observed with sepsis, leptomeningeal disease, brain metastases, metabolic derangements (i.e., hypercalcemia), chemotherapy (e.g., ifosfamide-induced encephalopathy[51]), antifungal therapy (i.e., voriconazole), radiation (e.g., radiation-induced encephalopathy[52]), and hepatic encephalopathy.

Cancer patients often receive a variety of psychotropic medications for depression and other conditions, which alone or in conjunction with opioids may produce mental status changes. Benzodiazepines in combination with opioids and other psychotropic drugs can complicate matters.

When opioid-induced cognitive impairment is suspected, the initial step should be to lower the dose, which can also be diagnostic. It is highly recommended not to add another medication to treat agitation or other symptoms without this step.

If manipulation of the analgesic regimen, including opioid rotation, is ineffective, then haloperidol or a drug from the same class may be considered.

Urinary Retention

Urinary retention is a relatively rare adverse reaction. It is usually observed in patients at extremes of age and is more likely to occur when medications with anticholinergic properties are administered concurrently with opioids.

It is commonly observed in patients receiving neuraxial opioids. Tolerance usually develops, but occasional patients may need temporary catheterization.

Myoclonus

Myoclonus is a dose-dependent phenomenon presumably related to opioid metabolites, more often those of morphine and meperidine. This phenomenon can occur with all opioids. It results from central motor excitability and could be a sign that a patient's level of tolerance has been overwhelmed.

A simple dose adjustment may abate the symptoms; however, rotating the opioid or temporarily adding a benzodiazepine may be necessary.

Respiratory Depression

Respiratory depression is a rare occurrence in patients on chronic opioid therapy, as tolerance to this opioid action usually develops in a short time. However, accidental overdose or the addition of another sedative agent can trigger respiratory depression.

As long as respiratory function is not significantly impaired, temporary discontinuation and recommencement at a lower dose are recommended.

Opioids in combination with benzodiazepines are a common cause of respiratory depression. In cases where respiration is compromised, leading to derangements in arterial blood gas values, the opioid antagonist naloxone can be titrated to response. It is given in 40 mcg increments rather than as a bolus to avoid acute opioid withdrawal.

Cases of tachyarrhythmias leading to myocardial compromise as well as pulmonary edema have been observed with bolus doses of 400 µg of naloxone.

Given the short half-life of naloxone, a continuous infusion of naloxone diluted in a liter of saline or dextrose solution may be required to prevent recurrence of respiratory depression.

Pruritis

The type of opioid medication and route of administration determine the likelihood of developing pruritis.[53] For example, local administration of an opioid medication (i.e., SC or transdermal) can lead to a localized allergic wheal-and-flare reaction, whereas systemic administration (i.e., oral or IV) can lead to more generalized pruritus.

The mechanism behind opioid-induced pruritis is not completely understood. Peripheral and central pathways have been implicated, peripherally via histamine release and centrally via action of mu-opioid receptors.

Whereas histamine release can be treated with H2 antagonists such as diphenhydramine and ranitidine, centrally mediated pathways are more difficult to treat, requiring use of mu-opioid receptor antagonists such as naloxone for intractable pruritis. In less severe cases, opioid rotation in conjunction with antihistamines or ranitidine should be attempted prior to naloxone reversal.

Clinical Pearls

- If the patient had an optimal trial with oral opioids, including rotation to a different opioid, or has experienced dose-limiting side effects, an alternative such as the IV or neuraxial route may be considered.
- Opioid escalation without identification of symptoms potentially augmenting pain expression can lead to worsening delirium.
- Common opioid side effects should be treated prophylactically (e.g., laxatives for constipation).
- Opioids trigger nausea and vomiting directly by decreasing gastrointestinal motility and indirectly through the induction of constipation.
- Myoclonus is a dose-dependent phenomenon presumably related to opioid metabolites.
- Naloxone is used for opioid overdose and respiratory depression.
- Naloxone is given at 40-mcg increments rather than as a bolus to avoid acute opioid withdrawal.

Opioid Rotation

Opioid rotation is the switch from one opioid to another when treatment-limiting toxicity results in poor responsiveness.[36,43,54] Opioid rotation is based on the concept of incomplete cross-tolerance between opioids: changing to an alternative drug may yield a far better balance between analgesia and side effects.

Guidelines for opioid rotation are intended to reduce the risk of relative overdosing or underdoing as one opioid is discontinued while the second one is started (see Box 4.7). These guidelines require a working knowledge of an equianalgesic dose table (see Table 4.2).

The most common reasons for opioid rotation include cognitive failure, hallucinations, myoclonus, uncontrolled pain, and nausea.

Clinical Scenarios and Examples of Opioid Rotation

Case 1

A 56-year-old woman has mid-back pain from thoracic soft-tissue metastases from breast cancer. She is taking morphine sulfate immediate release (IR) 15 mg every 4 hours on an as-needed basis. She used 90 mg in the last 24 hours. She is being discharged home. If one needs to start sustained-release (SR) morphine, what will be the starting dose and what would be the breakthrough dose and frequency?

- *Step 1*: Take the total dose of short-acting morphine in 24 hours and divide it into two equal parts. Since the patient used 90 mg in the last 24 hours, the SR morphine dose would be 45 mg every 12 hours.
- *Step 2*: The breakthrough dose is 15%–20% of the 24-hour morphine dose, or about 15 mg every hour as needed.

Box 4.7 Practical Steps for Opioid Rotation

Five Essential Concepts

- Use the equianalgesic table to calculate the dose of the new opioid that is roughly equivalent to the dose of the current opioid.
- Determine the clinically relevant starting point. If switching to an opioid other than methadone or fentanyl, decrease the equianalgesic dose by 25%–50%.
- Consider further dose adjustments based on medical condition and pain. If the patient is elderly or has significant organ failure, consider further dose reduction. If the patient has severe pain, consider a lesser dose reduction.
- If a rescue dose is to be used, calculate it as 15%–20% of the total daily dose and administer at an appropriate interval. The exception is oral transmucosal fentanyl citrate, which should be started at a dose of 200 mcg or 400 mcg. Take into account simultaneous treatments that can potentially reduce pain (i.e., steroids, radiation, and surgery).
- Reassess and titrate the new opioids according to therapeutic response and side effects.

Table 4.2 Equianalgesic Dose Ratio Table*

Opioid	From Parenteral Opioid to Parenteral Morphine	From Same Parenteral Opioid to Oral Morphine	From Oral Opioid to Oral Morphine	From Oral Morphine to Oral Opioid
Morphine [†]	1	2.5	1	1
Hydromorphone	5	2	5	0.2
Meperidine	0.13	4	0.1	10
Levorphanol	5	2	5	0.2
Codeine	–	–	0.15	7
Oxycodone	–	–	1.5	0.7
Hydrocodone	–	–	1	1

* As per clinical guidelines in a comprehensive cancer center.

[†] Approximate: (a) Fentanyl patch in mcg/hour x 2 = daily morphine in mg orally. (b) Fentanyl parenteral 10 mcg = morphine 1 mg parenteral

Reprinted from *MD Anderson Palliative Care Handbook*.

Case 2

A 66-year-old man with a history of squamous cell carcinoma of the lung has been receiving an IV morphine infusion of 2 mg/hour and also 5 mg IV/hour for breakthrough pain. He received 4 breakthrough doses in the last 24 hours. He is being discharged home and is able to take pills by mouth. What doses does he need for SR and for IR morphine?

- Step 1: Total morphine in 24 hours = (2 mg x 24 hours) + (5 mg x 4 doses) = 68 mg IV morphine, which is also 68 x 2.5 = 170 mg of oral morphine or approximately 90 mg of SR morphine every 12 hours.
- Step 2: Breakthrough dose is 15%–20% of 170 mg or approximately 30 mg orally every hour as needed.

Case 2.1

If the above patient is unable to swallow pills, how do you convert to a transdermal fentanyl patch?

- Step 1: From the equianalgesic table, fentanyl patch x 2 = oral morphine PO. If the oral morphine equivalent daily dose (MEDD) is 170 mg, divide by 2. The fentanyl patch would therefore be 75 mcg/hour. This formula takes into account incomplete tolerance; thus, no further reduction is needed.
- Step 2: For breakthrough dosing, try concentrated liquid morphine (20 mg:1 mL) at the same dose as above, 30 mg every hour as needed.

Case 3

A 46-year-old woman with a history of gastric carcinoma is admitted with severe abdominal pain, myoclonus, sedation, and delirium. Her pain is currently treated with a fentanyl patch delivering 200 mcg/hour and with hydromorphone 8 mg oral every 2 hours as needed. She required 6 doses in the last 24 hours. The patient is being switched to PCA hydromorphone. What are the starting settings on PCA?

- Step 1: Convert fentanyl to hydromorphone. According to the conversion table, 200 mcg/hour patch of fentanyl is 400 mg oral morphine or 160 mg of IV morphine (400 mg divided by 2.5). This is equal to 30 mg of IV hydromorphone (160 mg IV morphine divided by 5). Reducing by 50% for incomplete tolerance, it will be 15 mg IV hydromorphone over 24 hours, or 0.6 mg/hour of hydromorphone (15 mg divided by 24 hours).
- Step 2: Breakthrough dose: Calculate 15%–20% of 15 mg, yielding a starting dose of 2 mg every hour as needed for breakthrough pain.

Case 4

A 52-year-old woman diagnosed with recurrent cervical carcinoma has been on SR morphine 120 mg orally every 12 hours and IR morphine 45 mg orally every 2 hours as needed for breakthrough pain. She received 8 doses of 45 mg within the last 24 hours. She had bilateral hydronephrosis with percutaneous nephrostomy tubes.

Her blood urea nitrogen (BUN) is 48 mg/dL and creatinine is 2.2 mg/dL. She presents with mental status changes and severe pain in the left lower extremity, radiating down the buttock into the little toe laterally. She is also on gabapentin 900 mg four times a day.

The spectrum of symptoms indicates a need for opioid rotation in the setting of opioid toxicity; methadone is chosen because the patient has renal insufficiency. How would you rotate from morphine to methadone?

- Step 1: Total morphine in 24 hours is 600 mg.
- Step 2: Because of incomplete tolerance, reduce the MEDD by 50%, yielding a new dose of 300 mg MEDD.
- Step 3: Conversion to methadone will be 15 mg orally every 12 hours. Calculation: (300 mg MEDD divided by 10) divided by 2 to obtain the dose given every 12 hours. Usually this is done over 3 days.
- Step 4: Breakthrough dose of morphine, if continued, would be 45–60 mg every hour as needed (or 15%–20% of 300 mg MEDD).
- Step 5: Reduce the dose of gabapentin to account for altered renal function.

Case 5

A 44-year-old man with progressive metastatic sarcoma is transitioning to hospice care. He has been receiving IV PCA hydromorphone at a basal rate of 0.5 mg/hour, prn PCA demand dose of 0.5 mg every hour, and a prn nursing bolus dose of 2 mg every hour for severe breakthrough pain. IV hydromorphone intake for the last 24 hours totaled 35 mg.

The referring doctor asks you to transition the patient to an appropriate regimen. The patient is able to tolerate liquids but cannot swallow tablets. What would you recommend?

- Step 1: Calculate the MEDD from 35 mg IV hydromorphone I 35 x 10, or MEDD of 350 mg.

- *Step 2*: Choose a regimen the patient will tolerate, taking into consideration his inability to swallow tablets. Consider a fentanyl patch for basal pain control and high-concentration morphine (20 mg/mL) for prn dosing.
- *Step 3*: Using prior 24-hour requirements (no dose reduction needed when converting to fentanyl patch[*]), fentanyl-patch dosing would be 350 MEDD divided by 2, or 175 mcg/hour. The prn dose would be 15%–20% of MEDD, or 15% of 350, or 50 mg of morphine elixir (if 20 mg/mL, it would be 2.5 mL every 1 hour prn).

Opioid Conversion Exercises

a. PO morphine 300 mg. Convert to PO hydromorphone =
b. IV hydromorphone 50 mg. Convert to morphine PO =
c. PO morphine 100 mg over 24 hours (MEDD). Convert to transdermal fentanyl =
d. Fentanyl transdermal 100 mcg/hour. Convert to IV morphine =

ANSWERS: (a) 60 mg; (b) 500 mg; (c) 50 mcg/hour; (d) 80 mg.

Clinical Pearls

- Opioid rotation should be considered when dose-limiting side effects are encountered.
- As a general rule, treat side effects before opioid switching.
- Common side effects triggering rotation include cognitive impairment, hallucinations, and myoclonus.
- The rationale for opioid rotation is based on incomplete cross-tolerance between opioids.
- Working knowledge of an equianalgesic dose table is critical to successful opioid rotation.

---

[*] As both clinical experience and survey data suggest, no reduction is needed for conversion to a transdermal fentanyl system (TFS). In addition, in the development of this formulation, conversion guidelines were developed that incorporated a safety factor, obviating the need for additional dose reductions in most patients.[54a]

Approximate: (a) fentanyl patch in mcg/hour × 2 = daily morphine in mg orally. (b) Fentanyl parenteral 10 mcg = morphine 1 mg parenteral. (c) Cases of withdrawal reported with use of package insert for conversion.

Analgesic Adjuvants

Adjuvant analgesics are non-opioid medications with analgesic properties, used for specific pain syndromes in conjunction with other medications, sometimes used as first-line agents in cancer pain management. They are recommended at every step of the WHO ladder. The main categories are TCAs and AEDs, but may include steroids and bisphosphonates.

Acetaminophen

Acetaminophen, or paracetamol, is an antipyretic analgesic with an unclear mechanism of action. It may inhibit cyclooxygenase (COX) in the central nervous system, with inhibitory effects on the serotonergic system.[55] It has little or no anti-inflammatory action and is usually combined with low-potency opioids.

Guidelines for the use of acetaminophen in cancer pain are empiric and are based mostly on clinical experience.[56] The dose of acetaminophen varies widely between countries, with a dose of 0.5–1 g every 4 or 6 hours most commonly used. In the United States, given the concerns of liver toxicity, doses are limited to < 4 g in a 24-hour period.

In a study by Stockler et al.[57] on the treatment of cancer pain, adding up to 6 g of acetaminophen to morphine for cancer pain can be safe.

In another study, volunteers taking acetaminophen alone or in combination with opioids had an increase in alanine aminotransferase up to three times the upper limit after 4 g of acetaminophen per day.[58] This study raises questions regarding the safety of acetaminophen use at higher doses.

The benefits of adding acetaminophen possibly outweigh the risks in countries where morphine availability continues to be a problem. Acetaminophen is freely available and affordable.

However, the use of acetaminophen should be individualized. It should be used with caution in chronic pain states, and liver function tests should be performed at regular intervals.

NSAIDs

NSAIDs is limited to the inhibitors of the enzyme cyclooxygenase (COX), inhibiting the synthesis of prostaglandins, which are mediators of pain and inflammation. This group is subdivided into nonspecific COX inhibitors and selective COX-2 inhibitors.

Nonselective inhibitors are medications like ibuprofen and naproxen. However, these drugs continue to cause concern about the integrity of gastric mucosa and alteration in renal function.

These medications are only useful as step 1 drugs or as adjuncts to opioid therapy in more advanced cases. They are very useful agents for treating bone pain and as adjuvants to opioid medications in a wide variety of pain syndromes.

In general, their use in cancer pain is limited because of the ceiling effect and the long-term side-effect profile. Their use is controversial in patients with thrombocytopenia, who constitute a large proportion of those receiving antineoplastic therapy.

Gastric and duodenal ulceration is another potential problem that could result from long-term use of aspirin and other nonselective NSAIDS. Other problems include salt and water retention and renal failure.

Ketorolac is formulated for parenteral administration and thus is considered unique, but there is concern over its effect on the integrity of the gastric mucosa.

COX-2 Inhibitors

A more selective group of drugs, COX-2 inhibitors,[59] block the COX-2 enzyme with very little action on COX-1, thereby having minimal effect on the integrity of the gastric mucosa and platelet aggregation.

In clinical trials, these agents exhibited a safety profile comparable to that of placebo when compared to nonselective COX inhibitors. However, the efficacy remains the same as that of conventional NSAIDs. The COX-2 inhibitor drugs offer significant advantages in cancer patients undergoing chemotherapy.[60]

Controversy over increased cardiac events and strokes in patients taking the COX-2 inhibitor rofecoxib resulted in the US Food and Drug Administration (FDA) withdrawing the drug from the market.[61] Controversy remains over both NSAIDs and selective COX-2 inhibitors regarding risk of cardiac events.[62–64]

TCAs (Amitriptyline and Nortriptyline)

TCAs are the main group of antidepressants used for the management of neuropathic pain syndromes. They have postulated action via serotonin and norepinephrine reuptake inhibition at nerve endings in the spinal cord and brain.

It is now widely accepted that the mechanism of action is independent of their mood-altering effects, resulting from an inherent influence over the nervous system or via the modulation of opioid pathways.[65,66]

TCAs are not universally tolerated, especially at the initiation of therapy, and often have to be discontinued or their dosage decreased because of dose-limiting side effects, most commonly anticholinergic and sedative effects.

Amitriptyline and nortriptyline (with a lower cardiovascular side effect profile) are felt to be the most efficacious agents and are more often used.

The nonanalgesic properties of these agents are particularly useful in patients with depression and/or insomnia, symptoms frequently experienced by cancer patients. The tricyclic dose should be escalated gradually, with full benefit experienced in 3 to 4 weeks.

Anticonvulsants (Anti-Epileptic Drugs)

Anticonvulsants are traditionally used with good results in the treatment of diabetic neuropathy, post-herpetic neuralgia, trigeminal neuralgia, phantom pain, and similar syndromes,[66] all of which can coexist in cancer patients. Space-occupying lesions, due to new tumor growth or extension, may cause significant pain secondary to brachial and lumbosacral plexopathies.

Anticonvulsant agents are commonly used in the management of peripheral neuropathies resulting from chemotherapy (i.e., platinum agents, vinca alkaloids, and taxanes).

Traditional anti-epileptic drugs (AEDs; e.g., phenytoin, valproate, and carbamazepine) have been used as anticonvulsants. Given the side effects and safety concerns, their use in pain control has been limited to neuropathic pain states.

Gabapentin has become the gold-standard, prototypical drug in this category to treat neuropathic pain.[67,68] With its wide therapeutic window, lack of need for blood monitoring, and comparable efficacy to that of other anticonvulsants, gabapentin is easier to manage than other drugs in its class. Sedation is a noted side effect that can be reduced by starting therapy at a low dose and titrating upward to the desired effect.

Newer AEDs are more widely used for noncancer pain syndromes but have started to gain popularity in cancer pain situations. Such newer agents include pregabalin, oxcarbamazepine, and Lamictal (lamotrigine). Pregabalin has been studied in Indian patients with peripheral neuropathy and has shown favorable results.[69]

Miscellaneous

In refractory pain situations, drugs from other classes have the potential to achieve clinically meaningful responses. These alternative agents include psychotropic drugs,[70,71] benzodiazepines,[72] bisphosphonates, steroids, lidocaine, ketamine, capsaicin, radiopharmaceuticals (strontium-89, samarium-153), and antibiotics for infection.

Pamidronate or zoledronic acid, both bisphosphonates, can be used routinely for pain control and hypercalcemia associated with metastatic bone disease, especially in patients with breast cancer or multiple myeloma.[73]

Lidocaine

Analgesia can be achieved with systemic administration of lidocaine, presumably through its inhibitory action on sodium channels. Compared with other types of pain, more benefit has been observed in the treatment of neuropathic pain and phantom pain syndromes with a predominance of central features.[74,75]

Low infusion rates have been used as third- or fourth-line treatment in opioid-tolerant patients at doses of 2.5–4 mg/kg. Incremental rate infusions over 20–30 minutes can be used as a therapeutic test before starting the oral form, mexiletine, especially in patients for whom anticonvulsants are not effective.

Cardiac monitoring is mandatory during IV therapy. Transdermal lidocaine patches are indicated for allodynia related to post-herpetic neuralgia.[76,77]

Ketamine

This anesthetic agent, an NMDA receptor antagonist, has well-documented analgesic properties; it is available in IV, oral, and rectal forms. Several reports have been published regarding its use in sub-anesthetic doses as an analgesic in cancer patients.[78,79]

Ketamine could be considered in cases of extreme opioid tolerance and may be used long term in palliative care situations. The recommended starting dose is 150 mg daily by SC infusion.

Capsaicin

Because of its high-toxicity profile, capsaicin is used only as a topical cream for the management of neuropathic pain.[80] It acts by inhibiting substance P formation at the skin and is effective in only 50%–60% of patients.

Clinical Pearls

- Consider adjuvant medications where appropriate (e.g., AEDs for neuropathic pain).
- Avoid opioid combinations with acetaminophen as an analgesic adjuvant, as hepatotoxicity is a concern.
- Develop awareness of potential drug interactions and side-effect profiles of these groups of drugs.
- Avoid multiple adjuvant medications at the same time.
- Consider dose reductions in the setting of renal failure.

Spinal Opioid Therapy

Neurointerventional procedures such as neuraxial therapy have been increasingly used in the treatment of cancer pain,[81] especially for patients who develop pain refractory to opioid treatment. Spinal opioids work by binding to the mu receptor in the substantia gelatinosa and can be administered epidurally or intrathecally.

Options for delivering epidural or intrathecal opioids include percutaneous catheters, tunneled catheters, or implantable programmable pumps. Catheter obstruction and epidural fibrosis are more common with the epidural route.[82] Intrathecal administration has the advantage of being less affected by the presence of extensive epidural metastasis.[83]

A simple checklist can be followed prior to proceeding with neurointerventional procedures for cancer pain in patients with advanced cancer:[84]

- Is pain expression exclusively due to nociception? Initial pain assessment needs to rule out the presence of non-nociceptive factors capable of influencing pain expression, such as somatization related to depression or anxiety,[85] delirium with disinhibition of symptom expression,[86,87] and chemical coping.[88,89] If one of these factors is identified as a major contributor to the expression of pain, it needs to be treated prior to using an interventional approach to pain control.
- Does the patient have refractory pain? If patients have not had (1) adequate opioid titration, (2) trial of opioid rotation, or (3) consideration of adjuvant drugs, pain should not be considered refractory.
- Is the pain syndrome likely to respond to spinal opioids? To make this determination, physicians should rule out central deafferentation and the involvement of pain origination at higher anatomical locations that are less likely to benefit from spinal opioid treatment. Before permanent placement of an intrathecal opioid delivery system, an adequate response should be obtained with a trial administration of intrathecal spinal opioids.[90]
- Are there logistical problems? This consideration requires ensuring that patients are able to continue their treatment via a community hospice program. If such care is not available, the patient and family need to be informed that the patient may not be able to be discharged home, and this should be discussed prior to initiating the intervention.

Nonpharmacological Treatment

Nerve Blocks

The loss of normal sensory input, as occurs when a peripheral nerve is severed, may lead to a deafferentation pain. Some patients obtain relief from electrical stimulation, which augments non-nociceptive input.

Neurostimulation may be applied transcutaneously or via implanted devices to peripheral nerves, the spinal cord, or the brain. Carefully selected patients may benefit from the surgical implantation of stimulation devices.[91,92]

Neuroablation, or destruction of nerve tissue, may be accomplished by chemical or surgical means. The goal of this technique is to isolate the site of somatic pain from the central nervous system. The efficacy of each procedure must be weighed against the risks.

A significant percentage of patients who fail to respond to oral therapy may be helped with appropriate nerve blocks. It is not known which patients might benefit from earlier procedures.[93,94]

Somatic nerve blocks may be diagnostic (i.e., to determine the indication for permanent neurolysis or somatic nerves), facilitative, prophylactic, or therapeutic. Visceral blocks (such as celiac plexus block) have been demonstrated to be effective for specific pain syndromes.[95]

Sympathetically maintained pain is suggested when signs of marked sympathetic dysfunction accompany typical diffuse burning or deep aching pain. Sympathetic blockade may then be diagnostic and therapeutic. In some cases of refractory generalized pain, pituitary adenolysis has been effective.

Some of the useful nerve blocks for head and neck pain include stellate ganglion block, trigeminal nerve block, mandibular nerve block, maxillary nerve block, gasserian ganglion block, and glossopharyngeal nerve block. These blocks should be attempted using local anesthetic first, and then, based on a favorable risk–benefit ratio, a neurolytic agent like alcohol, phenol, or glycerine may be used.

Side effects to watch for following neurolytic blocks include brainstem anesthesia, convulsions (with volumes as low as 0.5 mL), hematoma, respiratory distress, recurrent laryngeal block, phrenic nerve block, pneumothorax, systemic toxicity, and unintended subarachnoid or epidural injection.

Evidence for the efficacy of nerve blocks in head and neck cancer is lacking. Most reports are based on anecdotal case reports or on clinical experience.

Somatic Nerve Blocks (Root, Brachial Plexus, Psoas Compartment)

Somatic nerve blocks are effective for nociceptive somatic pain in the territory of root, plexus, or peripheral nerve. Blocks can be short lasting when a local anesthetic is employed.

These temporary blocks have a limited role in cancer pain management, but may act as a precursor to permanent neurolysis. Examples include root block, brachial plexus block, and psoas compartment block.

Neurolytic Blocks

When taking into account their risk–benefit ratio, neurolytic blocks are generally favored in advanced cancer patients with limited life expectancy.

Sympathetic blocks such as celiac plexus block have been demonstrated to be effective for pancreatic cancer pain and other abdominal visceral pain syndromes.[96]

Contrary to an earlier study demonstrating improved survival,[97] Wong et al. showed that although pain was better controlled in the celiac plexus block group, there was no significant difference in survival or quality of life.[98]

Occasionally, a subarachnoid neurolytic block[99] or a neurolytic intercostal block may be employed. The risks of neurological deficits that may result from these blocks must be weighed against the possible benefits.

In a recent study by Smith et al.[100] randomizing patients to intrathecal opioid therapy versus conservative management, the intrathecal group had improved survival; however, concerns were raised regarding the comprehensive medical management group.[101,102] Perhaps more studies with a better inception cohort are needed to confirm the findings.

Neurosurgical Procedures

Surgical Ablation

Surgical ablation[103] may be accomplished by rhizotomy (section of nerve root) or dorsal root entry zone lesions (DREZ). Spinal anterolateral tractotomy or cordotomy, mesencephalotomy, medullary tractotomy, and cingulotomy should be reserved for carefully selected cases. Vertebroplasty, which involves injecting cement into metastatic compression fractures, is gaining wide popularity.[104,105]

Percutaneous cordotomy employed for intractable pain of the lower extremity has been useful in select patients.[106] Radiofrequency lesioning of bone metastases has recently been shown to be another modality to treat bone pain.[107]

The loss of normal sensory input, as occurs when a peripheral nerve is severed, may lead to deafferentation pain. Some patients obtain relief from electrical stimulation, which augments non-nociceptive input. Neurostimulation may be applied transcutaneously or via implanted devices to peripheral nerves, the spinal cord, or the brain. Carefully selected patients may benefit from surgical implantation of stimulation devices.[108]

Neuroablation, or destruction of nerve tissue, may be accomplished by chemical or surgical means. The goal of this technique is to isolate the site of somatic pain from the central nervous system. The efficacy of each procedure must be weighed against the risks.

Ablative and neurointerventional procedures provide options for the management of refractory cancer pain. However, prior to invasive procedures or placement of permanent pain pumps, a rigorous interdisciplinary team assessment and treatment of total pain (physical, psychological, spiritual, social, and practical) are recommended.

Psychological Techniques for Pain Control

The following are brief descriptions of techniques that can enable patients to accept the responsibility of managing their pain so that they can begin to cope and function more effectively. These techniques include, but are not limited to, biofeedback, relaxation training, hypnosis, and cognitive and operant approaches.

Biofeedback

The aim of biofeedback techniques is to enable patients to bring involuntary physiological events into voluntary control using electronic equipment. Biofeedback can modify certain physiological processes that underlie pain disorders, for example, electromyographic (EMG) feedback to treat muscle contraction headaches.

Affected physiological processes include the relaxation response (decreases in autonomic arousal will lead to reductions in pain) and self-regulation (patients become aware of their contribution to the pain experience and their ability to reduce it).

Biofeedback methods include EMG biofeedback, skin temperature or thermal biofeedback, alpha EEG, and cephalic blood volume pulse feedback.

Relaxation Training

Relaxation training is used to control pain and increase body awareness. All techniques elicit the relaxation response, with the goal of achieving pain reduction and decreases in sympathetic activity, oxygen consumption, heart rate, and blood lactate concentration. Relaxation methods include progressive muscle relaxation, breathing therapy, and guided imagery.

Focused concentration reduces persistent intrusive thoughts, relaxes muscles, and reduces pain. In progressive muscle relaxation, the most common approach, patients are taught to tense and relax muscles that contribute to pain, techniques that are used in such activities as yoga.

Relaxation training is particularly useful in controlling migraines, muscle contraction headaches, temporomandibular joint pain, chronic back pain, and myofascial pain.

Hypnosis

Hypnosis is a heightened state of responsiveness to suggestions and ideas. Pain relief may be dramatic in some cases and is not related to endorphin action. Hypnosis involves cognitive processes such as narrowing of attention, mental relaxation, and increased suggestibility.

Even though pain relief through hypnosis is of short duration and shows a variable response among individuals, it can provide a sense of peacefulness and comfort, helping relieve organic pain more than psychogenic pain.

Hypnosis can be modified by operant training, biofeedback, and sensory deprivation.

Cognitive Behavioral Therapy

Cognitive behavioral therapy (CBT) is based on the premise that cognition influences both emotion and behavior. Several cognitive styles, or thinking patterns, have been identified as particularly maladaptive and related to poor outcomes, distress, and likelihood of injury.

CBT is a multimodal treatment aimed at replacing maladaptive thinking patterns with more adaptive patterns and replacing maladaptive behavior patterns with functional alternatives. The therapy has been shown to affect emotions, pain behavior, and healthcare use outcomes.

Cognitive approaches affect expectations, attitudes, and beliefs about pain, helping patients gain better control over their pain. Since behavior and actions are affected by how individuals see the world, correction of faulty thought processes decreases suffering and disability; maladaptive beliefs are replaced with new, more adaptive ones.

Cognitive approaches can be action oriented, limited, or structured, and they can be administered in group or individual settings.

Operant Approaches

Operant approaches are based on the principle that a person's behavior is governed by both the positive and negative consequences of it. Positive reinforcement increases the likelihood of a behavior recurring, and negative reinforcement decreases that likelihood. The goal is to replace learned behaviors with "healthy" behaviors, ones that are incompatible with and in contrast to the "sick role."

Family members and healthcare providers are instructed to reinforce healthy behavior and to discourage pain behaviors, narcotic use, and inactivity. Other forms of therapy can be incorporated, including marital counseling, family therapy, and vocational training. The desired end state is decreased medication use and increased activity.

Physical Modalities for Pain Control

Therapeutic Heat and Cold

Heat reduces muscle spasms, and an increase in muscle temperature reduces spindle afferent sensitivity and firing. The addition of cold to sensory terminals also tends to decrease the muscle spindle response.

While heat increases local blood flow, cold decreases it. In cases of acute injury, cold is preferred to reduce swelling. Heat reduces joint stiffness by increasing the extensibility of collagen tissue.

Superficial heating modalities (with no effect beyond a depth of 1 cm) include hot packs, paraffin baths, hydrotherapy, and radiant heat. Although heat may be applied locally, it may still cause a reflex effect on other parts of the body (e.g., reduction in smooth muscle activity of the visceral organs when heat is applied to the abdomen). Available modalities use the principles of conduction, convection, and radiation.

Deep heating modalities (heating structures to a depth of 3–5 cm) include ultrasound techniques and short- and microwave diathermy. Ultrasound converts high-frequency acoustic vibrations into heat, selectively heating bone and tissue without risk of superficial thermal burn. Absorption is determined by the protein content of the tissues.

Since ultrasound does not travel through air, topical application of gel or water is required to transmit the heat. Ultrasound may also produce nonthermal effects, increasing the extensibility of collagen and muscle. Nonthermal effects of concern include pseudocavitation, which is the production of gas bubbles that carry a risk of subsequent tissue destruction.

In short-wave diathermy, high-frequency current is used to heat subcutaneous and deep tissues. It should not be used in the presence of a metal implant, as this may lead to burns in the surrounding tissues.

Microwave diathermy uses electromagnetic radiation, with heat production depending on interface reflection and absorption characteristics of underlying tissues. Its use is limited mostly to hepatic lesions and is contraindicated in fluid-filled areas such as eyes or joints.

The use of therapeutic heat is contraindicated over anesthetic or ischemic areas, in delirious patients, near gonads or developing fetuses (except ultrasound), and in the presence of cardiac pacemakers or metal implants (especially shortwave and microwave diathermy).

Therapeutic cold reduces metabolism, the inflammatory response, nerve conduction velocity, and muscle spindle activity. It is used to reduce pain, inflammation, and edema in cases of acute injury. Commonly used techniques include cold packs (10–20 minutes); ice massage (through the stages of coolness, burning, and numbness); cold baths (13°–18°C); vapocoolant spray (ethyl chloride and fluorimethane); and the spray and stretch technique on trigger points.

Therapeutic cold is contraindicated in patients with Raynaud's phenomenon or hypersensitivity to cold.

Transcutaneous Electrical Nerve Stimulation

In transcutaneous electrical nerve stimulation (TENS), electrical energy is transmitted across the skin surface to the nervous system, stimulating large, myelinated A fibers and closing the gate for pain coming from C fibers.

Traditional TENS methodology is of low intensity and high frequency (pulse width of 50–80 microseconds and frequency of 80–100 Hz) with an immediate effect, mediated by serotonin but not reversible with naloxone. High-intensity and low-frequency ("acupuncture-like," pulse width > 200 microseconds, frequency < 10 Hz) methodologies may be reversed by naloxone, with a delayed effect (20–30 minutes).

Clinical indications include acute pain (such as that from sprains, lacerations, and fractures), postoperative pain, labor pain, and chronic pain (such as lower back pain, arthritis, phantom limb pain, neuropathies, and cancer pain).

Acupuncture

Acupuncture is the practice of inserting one or more needles into specific sites on the body surface for therapeutic purposes. In addition to needle insertion, acupuncture points can also be "stimulated" with heat, electrical currents, pressure, laser light, or shock waves.

Acupuncture works by stimulating A-delta fibers in the skin and muscles, conducting impulses to the spinal gray matter, and inhibiting painful stimuli from the periphery, thereby reducing pain perception. The activation of encephalin-containing interneurons in the substantia gelatinosa of the spinal gray matter inhibits conduction of pain signals to the brain.

Subsequent neuromodulatory effects include the release of beta-endorphin and met-encephalin in the brain, the activation of two descending pain control systems in the midbrain, and modulatory effects on the central pain network in the hypothalamus and the limbic system.

Acupuncture also induces relaxation by affecting a person's emotional state, evoking a pleasant sensation through theorized action on the reward system of dopamine and serotonin.

It may reduce gastric acid secretion and correct gastric arrhythmia, thereby reducing nausea and vomiting, and may also reduce bladder urgency and incontinence caused by an overactive or unstable bladder.

Evidenced-based studies of acupuncture benefits are limited. In a 2006 review article by Derry et al.[109] analyzing 35 systematic reviews of acupuncture that were published between 1996 and 2005, 17 of the reviews found no evidence of benefit, 12 found some benefit, and none could demonstrate evidence of benefit when strict criteria of quality, validity, and size were applied.

Nonserious adverse effects occur in 7%–11% of all acupuncture patients, including severe tiredness and exhaustion, pain at the site of needling, and headache. Serious adverse effects include rare instances of pneumothorax or cardiac tamponade and infections such as hepatitis C or HIV.

Clinical Pearls

- Physical modalities to reduce pain and muscle spasm should be considered in every patient.
- Explore cognitive behavioral therapies in all patients.
- Explore expressive supportive counseling in patients with psychosocial problems.
- Consider anesthetic and neurosurgical procedures where appropriate (e.g., celiac plexus block for pancreatic cancer pain).
- Counsel patients and explore spiritual issues complicating pain.
- A multidisciplinary approach is the key to successful pain management.

Risk Evaluation and Mitigation Strategies for Opioid Medications

With a concerning trend toward increasing opioid-related deaths and opioid misuse and addiction in the United States, the FDA has proposed extending Risk Evaluation and Mitigation Strategies (REMS) to opioid medications. The Food and Drug Administration Amendments Act of 2007 gave the FDA the authority to require REMs from manufacturers of certain prescription medications to "ensure that the benefits of a drug or biological product outweigh its risks."[110]

Initially targeting both long- and short-acting preparations, the application of REMS to opioids is now limited to long-acting preparations. The FDA hopes that stricter controls on opioid prescribing will increase safety and minimize risks. From the prescriber's and the patient's standpoint, decreased access to opioids as a result of stricter controls could potentially create a new barrier to effective pain control.

REMS for a particular opioid will require special certification and enrollment of pharmacists and healthcare practitioners who dispense and prescribe a drug. The practitioner would only dispense the drug to patients with evidence of safe-use conditions (i.e., documentation of consent and understanding, as well as pregnancy and blood chemistry testing). Each patient using the drug will be enrolled in a registry and will be subject to regular monitoring by a physician.

Ongoing discussions between the Industry Working Group (IWG), a committee composed of opioid manufacturers, and the FDA are geared toward the collaborative development of new safety standards for opioid medications.[111] IWG recommendations to the FDA during a December 4, 2009, open hearing included developing a medication guide for patients and a detailed communication plan for prescribers to follow.

Recommendations also included the development of special certification or training for prescribers, unless already possessing specialty or subspecialty certification in such areas as hospice and palliative medicine.

A prescriber–patient agreement would provide information regarding opioid prescribing, storage, and use; a patient medication information sheet would make such information available to patients.

Recognizing the challenge of developing REMS for opioids, the FDA has been receptive to public contributions.

References

1. Foley KM (1979). *Pain syndromes in patients with cancer.* In: Bonica JJ, Ventafridda V (eds.), *Advances in Pain Research and Therapy.* New York: Raven Press, pp. 59–75.

2. Bonica JJ (1990). *Cancer pain.* In: Bonica JJ (ed.), *The Management of Pain.* Philadelphia: Lea & Febiger, p. 400.

3. Twycross RG, Fairfield S (1982). Pain in far-advanced cancer. *Pain* 14:303–10.

4. World Health Organization (1986). *Cancer Pain Relief.* Geneva: World Health Organization.

5. Levin D, Cleeland CS, Dar R (1985). Public attitudes toward cancer pain. *Cancer* 56:2337–9.

6. Koshy RC, Rhodes D, Devi S, Grossman SA (1998). Cancer pain management in developing countries: a mosaic of complex issues resulting in inadequate analgesia. *Support Care Cancer* 6(5):430–7.

7. Rajagopal MR, Joranson DE, Gilson AM (2001). Medical use, misuse, and diversion of opioids in India. *Lancet* 358(9276):139–43.

8. Higginson IJ (1997). Innovations in assessment: epidemiology and assessment of pain in advanced cancer. In: Jenson TS, Turner JA, Wiesenfeld-Hallin Z (eds.), *Proceedings of the 8th World Congress on Pain, Progress in Pain Research and Management.* Vol. 8. Seattle, WA: IASP Press, pp. 707–16.

9. Portenoy RK, Hagen NA (1990). Breakthrough pain: definition, prevalence, and characteristics. *Pain* 41:273–81.

10. Bruera E, MacMillan K, Hanson J, et al. (1989). The Edmonton staging system for cancer pain: preliminary report. *Pain* 37:203–9.

11. Bruera E, Kuehn N, Miller MJ, Selmser P, MacMillan K (1991). The Edmonton Symptom Assessment System: a simple method for the assessment of palliative care patients. *J Palliat Care* 7:6–9.

12. Walker P. (2001). Impact of the Edmonton Labeled Visual Information System on the physician recall of metastatic cancer patient histories: a randomized controlled trial. *J Pain Symptom Manage* 21(1):4–11.

13. Derogatis LR, Marrow GR, Fetting J, et al. (1983). The prevalence of psychiatric disorders among cancer patients. *JAMA* 249:754.

14. Jacox A, Carr DB, Payne R, et al. (1994). *Management of Cancer Pain.* Clinical Practice Guidelines No. 9. AHCPR Publication 94–0592. Rockville, MD: US Department of Health and Human Services, Agency for Health Care Policy and Research.

15. World Health Organization (1990). Cancer pain relief and palliative care: report of a WHO Expert Committee. *World Health Organ Tech Rep Ser* 804:11–2.

16. Sindrup SH, Andersen G, Madsen C, Smith T, Brosen K, Jensen TS (1999). Tramadol relieves pain and allodynia in polyneuropathy: a randomized, double-blind, controlled trial. *Pain* 83(1):85–90.

17. Madadi P, Hildebrandt D, Gong IY, et al. (2010). Fatal hydrocodone overdose in a child: pharmacogenetics and drug interactions. *Pediatrics* 126(4):e986–90.

18. Foster A, Mobley E, Wang Z (2007). Complicated pain management in a CYP450 2D6 poor metabolizer. *Pain Pract* 7(4):352–6.

19. Susce MT, Murray-Carmichael E, de Leon J (XXXX). Response to hydrocodone, codeine and oxycodone in a CYP2D6 poor metabolizer. *Prog Neuropsychopharmacol Biol Psychiatry* 30(7):1356–8.

20. Andersen G, Christrup L, Sjogren P (2003). Relationships among morphine metabolism, pain and side effects during long-term treatment: an update. *J Pain Symptom Manage* 25(1):74–91.

21. Prommer, E (2006). Oxymorphone: a review. *Support Care Cancer* 14(2):109–15.

22. Endo Pharmaceuticals. *Oxymorphone ER (Opana ER) Prescribing Information.* http://www.endo.com/PDF/OPANA_3R_PI.pdf.

23. Endo Pharmaceuticals. *Oxymorphone IR (Opana) Prescribing Information.* http://www.endo.com/PDF/OPANA_IR_PI.pdf.

23. Mallinckrodt Brand Pharmaceuticals (2010). Exalgo: Hydromorphone HCL extended-release tablets [package insert]. Hazelwood, MO, Mallinckrodt Brand Pharmaceutical.

24. Portenoy RK, Taylor D, Messina J, Tremmel L (2006). A randomized, placebo-controlled study of fentanyl buccal tablet for breakthrough pain in opioid-treated patients with cancer. *Clin J Pain* 22(9):805–11.

25. Portenoy RK, Payne R, Coluzzi P, Raschko JW, Lyss A, Busch MA, Frigerio V, Ingham J, Loseth DB, Nordbrock E, Rhiner M (1999). Oral transmucosal fentanyl citrate (OTFC) for the treatment of breakthrough pain in cancer patients: a controlled dose titration study. *Pain* 79(2-3):303–12.

26. Tennant F, Hermann L (2002). Self-treatment with oral transmucosal fentanyl citrate to prevent emergency room visits for pain crises: patient self-reports of efficacy and utility. *J Pain Palliat Care Pharmacother* 16(3):37–44.

27. Skaer TL. (2006). Transdermal opioids for cancer pain. *Health Qual Life Outcomes* 4:24.

28. Gordon DB (2006). Oral transmucosal fentanyl citrate for cancer breakthrough pain: a review. *Oncol Nurs Forum* 33(2):257–64.

29. Portenoy RK, Messina J, Xie F, Peppin J (2007). Fentanyl buccal tablet (FBT) for relief of breakthrough pain in opioid-treated patients with chronic low back pain: a randomized, placebo-controlled study. *Curr Med Res Opin* 23(1):223–33.

30. Dietrich E, Gums JG. (2012). Intranasal fentanyl spray: a novel dosage form for the treatment of breakthrough cancer pain. *Ann Pharmacother* 46(10):1382–91.

31. Taylor D, Galan V, Weinstein SM, et al. (2010). Fentanyl pectin nasal spray in breakthrough cancer pain. *J Support Oncol* 8(4):184–90.

32. Paix A, Coleman A, Lees J, et al. (1995). Subcutaneous fentanyl and sufentanil infusion substitution for morphine intolerance in cancer pain management. *Pain* 63:263–9.

33. Kunz K, Thiesen J, Schroder M (1993). Severe episodic pain management with sublingual sufentanil [letter]. *J Pain Symptom Manage* 8:189–90.

34. Belluck P (2003). Methadone, once the way out, suddenly grows as a killer drug. *New York Times*, February 9.

35. Mercadente S, Casuccio A, Fulfaro F, et al. (2001). Switching from morphine to methadone to improve analgesia and tolerability in cancer patients: a prospective study. *J Clin Oncol* 19(11):2898–904.

36. Bruera EB, Pereira J, Watanabe S, et al. (1996). Systemic opioid therapy for chronic cancer pain: practical guidelines for converting drugs and routes. *Cancer* 78:852–7.

37. Shaiova L, Berger A, Blinderman CD, et al., (2008). Consensus guideline on parenteral methadone use in pain and palliative care. *Palliat Support Care* 6(2):165–76.

38. Weschules DJ, Bain KT (2008). A systematic review of opioid conversion rations used with methadone for the treatment of pain. *Pain Med* 9(5):595–612.

39. Nicholson AB (2007). Methadone for cancer pain. *Cochrane Database Syst Rev* 17(4): CD003971.

40. Krants M, Martin J, Stimmel B, Haigney MC (2009). QTc interval screening in methadone treatment. *Ann Intern Med* 150(6):387–95.

41. Reddy S, Hui D, El Osta B, et al. (2010). The effect of oral methadone on the QTc interval in advanced cancer patients: a prospective pilot study. *J Palliat Med* 13:33–8.

42. Prommer, E (2007). Levorphanol: the forgotten opioid. *Support Care Cancer* 15(3):259–64.

43. Galer BS, Coyle N, Pasternak GW, Portenoy RK (1992). Individual variation in the response to different opioids: report of five cases. *Pain* 49:87–91.

44. Hanks G, Forbes K (1997). Opioid responsiveness. *Acta Anesthesiol Scand* 41:154–8.

45. Mystakidou K, Katsouda E, Parpa E, Vlahos L, Tsiatas ML (2006). Oral transmucosal fentanyl citrate: overview of pharmacological and clinical characteristics: *Drug Deliv* 13(4):269–76.

46. Bruera E, Chadwick S, Brenneis C, Hanson J, MacDonald RN (1987). Methylphenidate associated with narcotics for the treatment of cancer pain. *Cancer Treat Rep* 71(1):67–70.

47. Starreveld JS, Pols MA, Van Wijk J, Bogaard JW, Poen H, Smout AJ (1990). The plain abdominal radiograph in the assessment of constipation. *Z Gastroenterol* 28:335–8.

48. Bruera E, Suarez-Almazor M, Velasco A, Bertolino M, MacDonald SM, Hanson J (1994). The assessment of constipation in terminal cancer patients admitted to a palliative care unit: a retrospective review. *J Pain Symptom Manage* 9(8):515–9.

49. Sykes NP (1996). An investigation of the ability of oral naloxone to correct opioid-related constipation in patients with advanced cancer. *Palliat Med* 10:135–44.

50. Thomas J, Karver S, Cooney GA, Chamberlain BH, Watt CK, Slatkin NE, Stambler N, Kremer AB, Israel RJ (2008). Methylnaltrexone for opioid-induced constipation in advanced illness. *N Engl J Med* 358(22):2332–43.

51. Merimsky O, Reider-Grosswaser I, Wiggle N, Chaitchik S (1992). Encephalopathy in ifosfamide-treated patients. *Acta Neurol Scand* 86(5):521–5.

52. Crossen JR, Garrod D, Glatstein E, Neuwelt EA (1994). Neurobehavioral sequelae of cranial irradiation in adults; a review of radiation-induced encephalopathy. *J Clin Oncol* 12(3):627–42.

53. Reich A, Szepietowski JC (2009). Opioid-induced pruritus: an update. *Clin Exp Dermatol* 35(1):2–6.

54. Cherny NJ, Chang V, Frager G, et al. (1995). Opioid pharmacotherapy in the management of cancer pain: a survey of strategies used by pain physicians for the selection of analgesic drugs and routes of administration. *Cancer* 76:1288–93.

54 a. Indelicato RA, Portenoy RK (2002). Opioid rotation in the management of refractory cancer pain. *J Clin Oncol* 20(1):348–52.

55. Pickering G, Loriot MA, Libert F, Eschalier A, Beaune P, Dubray C (2006). Analgesic effect of acetaminophen in humans: first evidence of a central serotonergic mechanism. *Clin Phamacol Ther* 79:371–8.

56. Saito O, Aoe T, Yamamoto T (2005). Analgesic effects of nonsteroidal anti-inflammatory drugs, acetaminophen, and morphine in a mouse model of bone cancer pain. *J Anesth* 19(3):218–24.

57. Stockler M, Vardy J, Pillai A, Warr D (2004). Acetaminophen (paracetamol) improves pain and well-being in people with advanced cancer already receiving a strong opioid regimen: a random-ized, double-blind, placebo-controlled cross-over trial. *J Clin Oncol* 22(16):3389–94.

58. Watkins PB, Kaplowitz N, Slattery JT, Colonese CR, Colucci SV, Stewart PW, Harris SC (2006). Aminotransferase elevations in healthy adults receiving 4 grams of acetaminophen daily: a ran-domized controlled trial. *JAMA* 296(1):87–93.

59. Lane NE (1997). Pain management in osteoarthritis: the role of COX-2 inhibitors. *J Rheumatol* 24:20–4.

60. Fine PG, et al. (2002). The role of rofecoxib, a cyclooxygenase-2-specific inhibitor, for the treat-ment of non-cancer pain: a review. *J Pain* 3(4):272–83.

61. Bresalier RS, Sandler RS, Quan H, Bolognese JA, Oxenius B, Horgan K, Lines C, Riddell R, Morton D, Lanas A, Konstam MA, Baron JA (2005). Adenomatous Polyp Prevention on Vioxx (APPROVE) Trial Investigators. Cardiovascular events associated with rofecoxib in a colorectal adenoma chemoprevention trial. *N Engl J Med* 352(11):1092–102.

62. Zhang J, Ding EL, Song Y. (2006). Adverse effects of cyclooxygenase 2 inhibitors on renal and arrhythmia events: meta-analysis of randomized trials. *JAMA* 296(13):1619–32.

63. McGettigan P, Henry D. (2011). Cardiovascular risk with non-steroidal anti-inflammatory drugs: systematic review of population-based controlled observational studies. *PLoS Med* 8(9):e1001098.

64. Trelle S, Reichenbach S, Wandel S, et al. (2011). Cardiovascular safety of non-steroidal anti-inflammatory drugs: network meta-analysis. *BMJ* 342:c7086.

65. Magni G (1991). The use of antidepressants in the treatment of chronic pain: a review of current evidence. *Drugs* 42:730–48.

66. Kolke M, Hoffken K, Olbrich H, Schmidt CG (1999). Antidepressants and anticonvulsants for the treatment of neuropathic pain syndromes in cancer patients. *Onkologie* 14:40–3.

67. Rowbotham M, Harden N, Stacey B, Bernstein P, Magnus-Miller L (1998). Gabapentin for the treatment of postherpetic neuralgia: a randomized controlled trial. *JAMA* 280:1837–42.

68. Backonja M, Beydoun A, Edwards KR, et al. (1998). Gabapentin for the symptomatic treatment of painful neuropathy in patients with diabetes mellitus: a randomized controlled trial. *JAMA* 280:1831–6.

69. Lyrica Study Group (2006). Pregabalin for peripheral neuropathic pain: results of a multicenter, non-comparative, open-label study in Indian patients. *Int J Clin Pract* 60(9):1060–7.

70. Brietbart W (1998). Psychotropic adjuvant analgesics for pain in cancer and AIDS. *Psychooncology* 7:333–45.

71. Patt R, Propper G, Reddy S (1994). The neuroleptics as adjuvants analgesics. *J Pain Symptom Manage* 9:446–53.

72. Reddy S, Patt RB (1994). The benzodiazepines as adjuvant analgesics. *J Pain Symptom Manage*. 9:510–14.

73. Thiebaud D, Leyvarz S, von Fliedner V, et al. (1991). Treatment of bone metastases from breast cancer and myeloma with pamidronate. *Eur J Cancer* 27:37–41.

74. Nagaro T, Shimizu C, Inoue H, et al. (1995). The efficacy of intravenous lidocaine on various types of neuropathic cancer pain. *Masui* 44(6):862–7.

75. Brose W, Cousins M (1991). Subcutaneous lidocaine for the treatment of neuropathic cancer pain. *Pain* 45(2):145–8.

76. Rowbotham MC, Davies PS, Verkempinck C, Galer BS. (1996). Lidocaine patch: double-blind controlled study of a new treatment method for post-herpetic neuralgia. *Pain* 65(1):39–44.

77. Rowbotham MC, Fields HL. (1996). The relationship of pain, allodynia and thermal sensation in post-herpetic neuralgia. *Brain* 119(2):347–54.

78. Clark JL, Kalan GE (1995). Effective treatment of severe cancer pain of the head using low-dose ketamine. *J Pain Symptom Manage* 10(4):310–14.

79. Mercadante S, Lodi F, Sapio M, et al. (1995). Long-term ketamine subcutaneous infusion in neuropathic cancer pain. *J Pain Symptom Manage* 10(7):564–8.

80. Ellison N, Loprinzi CL, Kugler J, et al. (1997). Phase 3 placebo-controlled trial of capsaicin cream in the management of surgical neuropathic pain in cancer patients. *J Clin Oncol* 15(8):2974–80.

81. Kedlaya D, Reynolds L, Waldman S (2002). Epidural and intrathecal analgesia for cancer pain. *Best Pract Res Clin Anaesthesiol* 16:651–5.

82. Aldrete JA (1995). Epidural fibrosis after permanent catheter insertion and infusion. *J Pain Symptom Manage* 10:624–31.

83. Applegren L, Nordberg C, Sjoberg M, et al. (1997). Spinal epidural metastasis: implications for spinal analgesia to treat refractory cancer pain. *J Pain Symptom Manage* 13:25–42.

84. Yennurajalingam S, Dev R, Walker PW, Reddy SK, Bruera E (2010). Challenges associated with spinal opioid therapy for pain in patients with advanced cancer: a report of three cases. *J Pain Symptom Manage* 39(5):930–5.

85. Hopwood P, Stephens RJ (2000). Depression in patients with lung cancer: prevalence and risk factors derived from quality-of-life data. *J Clin Oncol* 18:893–903.

86. Klepstad P, Hilton P, Moen J, et al. (2002). Self-reports are not related to objective assessments of cognitive function and sedation in patients with cancer pain admitted to a palliative care unit. *Palliat Med* 16:513–19.

87. Bruera E, Fainsinger RL, Miller MJ, Kuehn N (1992). The assessment of pain intensity in patients with cognitive failure: a preliminary report. *J Pain Symptom Manage* 7:267–70.

88. Parsons HA, Delgado-Guay MO, El Osta B, et al. (2008). Alcoholism screening in patients with advanced cancer: impact on symptom burden and opioid use. *J Palliat Med* 11:964–68.

89. Fainsinger RL, Nekolaichuk CL, Lawlor PG, et al. (2005). A multicenter study of the revised Edmonton Staging System for classifying cancer pain in advanced cancer patients. *J Pain Symptom Manage* 29:224–37.

90. Krames ES (2002). Implantable devices for pain control: spinal stimulation and intrathecal therapies. *Best Pract Res Clin Anaesthesiol* 16:619–49.

91. Mayerson BA (1983). Electrostimulation procedures: effects, presumed rationale, and possible mechanisms. In: Bounce JJ, et al. (eds.), *Advances in Pain Research and Therapy*. New York: Raven Press, pp. 495–534.

92. Duncan GH, Bushnell MC, Marchand S (1991). Deep brain stimulation: a review of basic research and clinical studies. *Pain* 45:49–60.

93. Arner S (1982). The role of nerve blocks in the treatment of cancer pain. *Acta Anaesthesio Scand* 74:104–8.

94. Cousins MJ, Bridenbaug PO (eds.) (1988). *Neural Blockade*, 2nd ed. Philadelphia: J. B. Lippincott.

95. Brown DL, Bulley CK, Quiel EL (1987). Neurolytic celiac plexus block for pancreatic cancer pain. *Anesth Analg* 66:869–73.

96. (2004). Neurolytic celiac plexus block for pancreatic cancer pain? *J Watch Gastroenterology* 2004(414):6.

97. Lillemoe KD, Cameron JL, Kaufman HS, Yeo CJ, Pitt HA, Sauter PK (1993). Chemical splanchnicectomy in patients with unresectable pancreatic cancer: a prospective randomized trial. *Ann Surg* 217(5):447–55; discussion 456–7.

98. Gilbert Y. Wong MD, Darrell R, et al. (2004). Effect of neurolytic celiac plexus block on pain relief, quality of life, and survival in patients with unresectable pancreatic cancer: a randomized controlled trial. *JAMA* 291:1092–99.

99. Patt RB, Payne R, Farhat GA, Reddy SK (1995). Subarachnoid neurolytic block under general anesthesia in a 3-year-old with neuroblastoma. *Clin J Pain* 11(2):143–6.

100. Smith TJ, Staats PS, Deer T, et al. (2002). Randomized clinical trial of an implantable drug delivery system compared with comprehensive medical management for refractory cancer pain: impact on pain, drug-related toxicity, and survival. *J Clin Oncol* 20(19):4040–9.

101. Davis MP, Walsh D, Lagman R, LeGrand SB (2003). Randomized clinical trial of an implantable drug delivery system. *J Clin Oncol* 21(14):2800–1.

102. Ripamonti C, Brunelli C (2003). Randomized clinical trial of an implantable drug delivery system compared with comprehensive medical management for refractory cancer pain: impact on pain, drug-related toxicity, and survival. *J Clin Oncol* 21(14):2801–2.

103. Meyerson BA (1982). The role of neurosurgery in the treatment of cancer pain. *Acta Anaesthesiol Scand* 74:109–13.
104. Weill A, Chiras J, Simon JM, Rose M, Soal-Martinez T, Enkaoua E (1996). Spinal metastases: indications for and results of percutaneous injection of acrylic surgical cement. *Radiology* 199:241–7.
105. Cotton A, Boutry N, Cortet B, et al. (1998). Percutaneous vertebroplasty: state of the art. *Radiographic* 18:311–22.
106. Macalusco C, Foley KM, Arbit E (1988). Cordotomy for lumbosacral, pelvic and lower extremity pain of malignant origin: safety and efficacy. *Neurology* 38:110.
107. Goetz MP, Callstrom MR, Charboneau JW, et al. (2004). Percutaneous image-guided radiofrequency ablation of painful metastases involving bone: a multicenter study. *J Clin Oncol* 15;22(2):300–6.
108. Mayerson BA (1983). Electrostimulation procedures: effects, presumed rationale, and possible mechanisms. In: Bounce JJ, et al. (eds), *Advances in Pain Research and Therapy*. New York: Raven Press, pp. 495–534.
109. Derry CJ, Derry S, McQuay HJ, Moore RA (2006). Systematic review of systematic reviews of acupuncture published 1996–2005. *Clin Med* 6(4):381–6.
110. US Food and Drug Administration (2010). *Approved Risk Evaluation and Mitigation Strategies (REMS)*. http://www.fda.gov/Drugs/DrugSafety/PostmarketDrugSafetyInformation forPatientsandProviders/ucm111350.htm.
111. Muir JC (2010). Opioid REMS—tension between two competing public health crises: undertreatment of pain versus increased opioid-related deaths in the United States. *AAHPM Bull* Spring, pp. 6–7.

Fatigue

Sriram Yennurajalingam

Definition and Prevalence

The National Comprehensive Cancer Network defines cancer-related fatigue as "a distressing, persistent, subjective sense of *physical, emotional*, and/or *cognitive* tiredness or exhaustion related to cancer or cancer treatment that is not proportional to recent activity and interferes with usual functioning." From 48% to 85% of cancer patients report or experience fatigue, and fatigue is most severe near the end of patients' lives.[1,2]

Fatigue is a more common and severe symptom in patients receiving palliative care[3] than in early cancer and cancer survivors.[3] However, it is still underdiagnosed and undertreated.[4] Fatigue has substantial adverse physical, psychosocial, and economic consequences for patients and caregivers and is an important predictor of patients' quality of life.[3,4]

Due to its subjective nature and multifactorial causes, assessing and treating fatigue in the palliative setting can be complex. In this chapter we review the definition and prevalence of fatigue, its causes, clinical evaluation, and treatment in palliative care settings.

Most of the evidence presented in this chapter relates to studies in cancer patients. However, similar principles can be applied to fatigue in patients with other diseases.

Causes

Fatigue is a multidimensional syndrome, often with multiple contributing causes (Figure 5.1). Studies have shown that fatigue is correlated with the severity of psychological symptoms (e.g., anxiety and depression), pain, sleep disturbances, dyspnea, anorexia, anemia, and opioid dose (if used).[2]

Pro-Inflammatory Cytokines

Pro-inflammatory cytokines can induce fatigue by affecting mood, muscle mass, cognition, and metabolic status.[5,6] These cytokines can be induced by disease process or its treatment and can trigger alterations of immune homeostasis and neuroendocrine axis. Inflammatory cytokines (specifically interleukin-6, interleukin-1β, and tumor necrosis factor-α) also induce

Figure 5.1. Possible contributors to fatigue.

disturbances in the hypothalamic-pituitary axis that affect corticotrophin-stimulating and adrenocorticotropic hormone levels, which in turn influence adrenocorticoid secretion.[6] However, the exact mediating role of inflammatory cytokines in the causation of fatigue in advanced cancer is still unclear.[6]

Anemia

Anemia causes fatigue in patients receiving cancer therapy, and treating anemia in these patients has been shown to reduce their fatigue and improve their quality of life.

However, as the severity of other contributing factors—anxiety and depression, pain, cachexia, drug side effects, inactivity, infections, and hypogonadism—tends to increase progressively at the end of a patient's life, anemia's relative contribution to fatigue diminishes.[7]

Symptoms Caused by Cancer and Its Treatment

Various correlative studies have established fatigue's association with pain, dyspnea, anorexia, sleep disturbances, and psychological symptoms such as anxiety and depression. (Figure 5.1). However, the intensity of an individual symptom in a given patient may determine its ultimate contribution to the cause of the patient's fatigue.[2]

Drug Interactions

The combination of opioids and other medications (such as anticholinergics, antihistamines, anticonvulsants, neuroleptics, central α-adrenergic antagonists, β-blockers, diuretics, selective serotonin reuptake inhibitors [SSRIs], tricyclic antidepressants [TCAs], muscle relaxants, and benzodiazepines) or the interaction between these medications may contribute to drowsiness and fatigue.

Clinical Assessment

The clinical assessment of fatigue relies on complete evaluation in three areas: patient history, physical examination, and lab evaluation.[2,8]

Patient History

Characterizing the Fatigue

A variety of clinical assessment tools, including 0–10 on visual analog scales, can be used to assess the intensity of a patient's fatigue, its onset and duration, and its effect on a patient's function and overall quality of life (Table 5.1).

However, one patient who presents with a fatigue score of 9 on a 0–10 scale may have fatigue caused mainly by anemia and cachexia, while another patient who presents with the same intensity may have fatigue caused primarily by depression. Hence, using a simple Edmonton Symptom Assessment Scale or other multidimensional tool may help provide a more comprehensive assessment of a patient's fatigue.

Identifying Possible Causes and Contributing Factors

Patients should be evaluated for the following major reversible factors in fatigue: mood disorders (specifically depression and anxiety), cognitive disorders (dementia and delirium), pain, anemia, malnutrition, and deconditioning. Other contributing factors may include sleep patterns, weight changes, infections, trauma, self-medication with over-the-counter drugs, prescription drugs, tobacco, alcohol or illicit drugs, diet, and social changes (such as retirement).

Environmental assessment should be considered if necessary.

Physical Examination

Physical examination should include an evaluation for orthostatic changes, an inspection of mucous membranes for pallor or icterus, and examination for lymphadenopathy, hepatosplenomegaly, murmurs, or bruits. A detailed neurological examination, including an assessment of cognition, should be performed.

Laboratory Investigations

Laboratory investigations should include any blood tests and diagnostic imaging as suggested by the physical examination or history.[2]

Table 5.1 Fatigue Assessment Tools for Patients with Cancer or Other Conditions*

Measure/Scale	Reliability (Cronbach Coefficient)	Validity	Population Base	Number of Items	Comments
Multidimensional Fatigue Inventory	0.80	Validity ($r \leq 0.78$)	Cancer patients receiving radiotherapy, patients with chronic fatigue syndrome, medical students, army recruits, and junior physicians	20-item self-report instrument	Multidimensional scale, including general fatigue, physical fatigue, mental fatigue, reduced motivation, and reduced activity
Multidimensional Assessment of Fatigue	0.93		Adults with rheumatoid arthritis, HIV, multiple sclerosis, coronary heart disease, or cancer	16 items, self-administered, 5 minutes	Subjective aspects of fatigue, including quantity, degree, distress, impact, and timing, are assessed.
Multidimensional Fatigue Symptom Inventory (short form)	0.87–0.96		Patients with different types of cancer	30-item instrument	Global, somatic, affective, cognitive, and behavioral symptoms of fatigue
Revised Piper Fatigue Scale	0.85–0.97		Patients with cancer-related fatigue; or chronic hepatitis C infections	22-item measure	Multidimensional; assesses global fatigue severity to evaluate the efficacy of intervention strategies
Brief Fatigue Inventory	0.82–0.97		Cancer and cancer treatment	9 items, self-administered, 5 minutes	Severity and impact of fatigue on daily functioning in the past 24 hours

(continued)

Table 5.1 (Continued)

Measure/Scale	Reliability (Cronbach Coefficient)	Population Base	Number of Items	Comments
Fatigue Symptom Inventory	0.90	Cancer and cancer treatment	13 items, self-administered	Fatigue intensity and duration and interference with QOL in the past week
Functional Assessment of Chronic Illness Therapy—Fatigue (FACIT-F)	0.93–0.95 Test-retest reliability r = 0.87 over 3–7 days	Cancer and cancer treatment	41 items, self-administered or interview, 10 minutes	Multidimensional fatigue subscales of Functional Assessment of Cancer Therapy (FACT); assesses global fatigue severity and QOL
Edmonton Symptom Assessment Scale (ESAS) (Figure 5.1)	0.79 Test-retest reliability 0.65	Elderly palliative care patients	Patients rate the severity of 9 symptoms, including fatigue (visual analogue scales); self-administered or interview, 5 minutes	Global fatigue severity
Profile of Mood States (vigor and fatigue)	0.89 Test-retest reliability r = 0.65	Cancer patients; patients with many other chronic conditions	8 items (vigor), 7 items (fatigue)	Global fatigue severity
Short Form–36–Version 1 Vitality (Energy/Fatigue) Subscale	0.87	Adults with cancer and other populations	1–2 minutes for 4-item subscale	Vitality (energy level and fatigue)

Management

Optimal fatigue management involves comprehensive symptom assessment and aggressive treatment of reversible causes, if possible (Figure 5.2).[2] If the cause is not reversible or apparent, the fatigue should be treated symptomatically (Figure 5.2).

Ideally, fatigue treatment should involve an interdisciplinary team with active participation by the physician, nurse, psychiatric counselor, social worker, chaplain, physical therapist, and occupational therapist, as appropriate.

Treatment of Causes

Anemia

Anemia in palliative care patients is best managed by treating its underlying cause or (if the cause is not known) by treating it symptomatically with

Figure 5.2. Treatments for fatigue and its underlying causes.

transfusions of packed red blood cells. Patients who receive repeated transfusions risk blood-borne infection, acute transfusion reaction, transfusion-associated graft-versus-host disease, subtle immune modulation that occurs with transfusion, and iron overload.

If repeated blood transfusions are not an option, recombinant human erythropoietin (rhEPO) therapy can help relieve fatigue and thus improve the quality of life in chronically anemic patients who have AIDS or end-stage renal disease or who are undergoing chemotherapy. However, rhEPO therapy is expensive, and although treating anemia with rhEPO has been shown to decrease fatigue in patients receiving chemotherapy, concerns about the safety of rhEPO arose after several phase III studies showed increased mortality and thromboembolic complications in rhEPO-treated patients compared to controls.

Pain and Opioid-Induced Neurotoxicity

Treating pain and opioid-induced neurotoxicity may benefit patients with chronic disorders and patients at the end of life. Successful management requires either reducing the opioid dose or administering a different opioid, as well as addressing other reversible precipitants such as dehydration. If opioid-induced sedation is persistent, a trial of methylphenidate may be helpful.

Because the combination of opioids and medications from different drug classes and the interaction of these medications may contribute to drowsiness and fatigue, it is appropriate to cease these medications or adjust their doses to reduce fatigue.

Depression

Antidepressants, counseling, and exercise can reduce the vegetative symptoms caused by depression. Clinical observations suggest that antidepressant therapy can increase energy levels without altering a patient's mood to the same degree.

Methylphenidate has been shown to reduce fatigue in cancer patients with depression. Counseling and exercise are the other modalities of treatment that are found to be effective in the treatment of fatigue and depression in patients with cancer.[2]

Delirium and Cognitive Dysfunction

To successfully manage delirium and cognitive dysfunction, the physician must identify and correct the underlying reversible causes and the symptoms. Thus, the practitioner should evaluate the patient for opioid toxicity, dehydration, infection, medication interactions or adverse effects, metabolic disturbances, thyroid dysfunction, and anemia.

In an end-of-life setting, the intensity of the diagnostic workup and the treatment strategies for cognitive dysfunction and delirium must be individualized.

Weight Loss

Fatigue and cachexia coexist in the great majority of patients with advanced cancer, and it is likely that malnutrition is a major contributor to fatigue. The inflammation in response to progressive cancer and loss of muscle mass resulting from progressive cachexia provide a reason for profound weakness and fatigue.

Treatment of Fatigue as a Symptom

Because of the complex nature of fatigue and the limited number of randomized controlled studies that have been performed in the palliative care setting, there are few pharmacological options for effective fatigue treatment (Table 5.2). In this section, we review established drug therapies, investigational agents, and nonpharmacological treatment options.

Established Pharmacological Agents

Corticosteroids

Preliminary studies have shown that corticosteroids can reduce symptoms such as fatigue, pain, poor appetite, and nausea and can improve the overall quality of life in patients with advanced cancer. It is unclear if there are any differences between types of corticosteroids, because dexamethasone appears to be the most intensively investigated.[2] The overall adverse reaction profile of dexamethasone is well understood. It appears that the severity of most of its toxic effects is dose dependent. Side effects may include infection, oral thrush, insomnia, mood swings, myalgia, and elevation of blood glucose.

Prolonged use of dexamethasone (for more than 1 month) in some patients will cause gastritis (particularly if the patient is concurrently using nonsteroidal anti-inflammatory drugs [NSAIDs]), hiccups, edema, hyperglycemia, increased risk for infections, muscle weakness, easy bruising, dizziness, unusual hair growth, and slow wound healing. In a randomized double blind placebo-controlled trial of 84 evaluable patients with advanced cancer, dexamethasone 4 mg twice a day orally for 14 days was associated with significant improvement of fatigue.[10] There was no significant increase in the side effects in the dexamethasone as compared to the placebo group. In another recent randomized placebo controlled double blind study in patients with advanced cancer, oral methylprednisolone (32mg/day) for a period of 7 days significantly improved fatigue.[11] However, further studies are needed to test the exact dose, type, and duration to treat fatigue for prolonged periods with minimal side effects.[11]

Megestrol Acetate

In randomized controlled trials, megestrol acetate (160–480 mg/day) increased appetite, activity levels, and overall well-being compared to placebo in anorexia patients with advanced cancer. However, further larger studies are needed. Megestrol is dosed orally, once daily. The response increases as the dose rises from 160 to 800 mg/day.

Investigational Drugs

Psychostimulants

In patients receiving palliative care, sedation due to opioids and depression can be treated with psychostimulants such as methylphenidate or modafinil. Advanced cancer patients with fatigue with additional symptoms such as anxiety, depression, or sedation may benefit from a trial of psychostimulants.[11]

Psychostimulants act rapidly, are well tolerated, and are generally safe. However, they should be used with caution in patients with heart disease or cognitive disturbances (e.g., delirium). The role of psychostimulants in the

Table 5.2 Medications for Symptomatic Treatment of Fatigue at the End of Life

Drug and Indication	Initial Dose	Side Effects
Corticosteroids: Disease-related fatigue (off-label use)	Dexamethasone: 8 mg/day for 2 weeks	Severity of most toxic effects is dose dependent. Adverse effects include infection, oral thrush, insomnia, mood swings, myalgia, and elevation of blood glucose. Prolonged use (> 1 month): gastritis (especially with concurrent use of NSAIDs), hiccups, edema, muscle weakness, easy bruising, dizziness, hirsutism, and slow wound healing.
Methylphenidate: Cancer-related fatigue (off-label use)	5 mg/day	Common adverse effects include loss of appetite, slurred speech, abnormal behavior, and restlessness. Serious adverse effects include hypertension, tachyarrhythmia, thrombocytopenia, and hallucinations.
Megestrol acetate: FDA-approved treatment for cachexia in patients with AIDS and as a treatment for breast and endometrial cancer; also used for treating cancer-associated cachexia and anorexia (off-label use)	480–800 mg/day	Common adverse effects include hypertension, sweating, hot flashes, weight gain, dyspepsia, nausea, vomiting, insomnia, mood swings, and impotence. Serious adverse effects include thrombophlebitis, adrenal insufficiency, and pulmonary embolism.
Modafinil: Fatigue related to cancer and multiple sclerosis (off-label use)	200 mg/day	Common adverse effects include diarrhea, nausea, dizziness, headache, insomnia, agitation, anxiety, nervousness, and rhinitis. Serious adverse effects include cardiac dysrhythmia, hypertension, and infectious disease.

management of fatigue in terminally ill patients needs to be defined further due to the mixed results from recent randomized controlled trials.[11]

Methylphenidate

In patients with cancer, methylphenidate has been effective against opioid-induced sedation, cognitive failure associated with brain tumors, and depression. It stimulates the CNS by blocking presynaptic norepinephrine and dopamine reuptake.

Methylphenidate is usually administered orally twice a day, at breakfast and lunch, to minimize insomnia. Because of its rapid onset of action and short half-life, methylphenidate is effective at relieving fatigue. In an open-label study of 31 patients with advanced cancer who experienced fatigue, methylphenidate every 2 hours as needed significantly reduced fatigue.

In contrast, a recent randomized controlled trial of 141 patients with advanced cancer showed that although patients using methylphenidate plus nursing telephone intervention and patients using placebo and the intervention both experienced a significant reduction in fatigue after treatment for 14 days, there was no significant difference in improvements between the groups.[11]

Modafinil

Modafinil, a psychostimulant, is an effective and well-tolerated agent used to treat excessive daytime sleepiness in patients with narcolepsy and other conditions such as Parkinson's disease and obstructive sleep apnea. The exact mechanism of action is unclear; however, a recent preclinical house study implicated non-noradrenergic, dopamine-dependent adrenergic signaling in promoting wakefulness.

In a recent randomized controlled study of advanced non-small cell lung cancer patients, fatigue improved in both modafinil and matched placebo groups. However, there was no significant improvement of fatigue in the modafinil group compared to the placebo group.[12]

Testosterone Replacement in Hypogonadic Males

Hypogonadism occurs in two-thirds of men with advanced cancer; low testosterone levels in men with cancer are associated with fatigue, anorexia, depression, and insomnia. Testosterone replacement has shown beneficial effects on fatigue and quality of life in patients with non-cancer conditions. A preliminary study examined 29 advanced cancer patients who were treated with either intramuscular testosterone or placebo for 14 days for the primary outcome at day 29.[13] Although no statistically significant difference was found for fatigue (FACIT-F) scores between arms at 4 weeks, Sexual Desire Inventory Score and performance status improved in the testosterone group, and fatigue subscale scores from the Edmonton Symptom Assessment Scale were significantly better in those treated with testosterone by day 72. Further studies are needed.

Nonpharmacological Approaches

Physical Activity or Exercise

Well-powered randomized controlled trials have demonstrated that exercise is an effective nonpharmacological treatment for fatigue. Physical activity helps patients maintain their sense of well-being and enhances their quality of life.[5]

Most palliative care patients experience multiple symptoms (e.g., fatigue, pain, dyspnea, and nausea) that may lead to diminished physical activity and thereby lead to deconditioning. Exercise rehabilitation during or after curative or palliative treatment is now considered an effective means of restoring patients' physical and psychological functioning. Most recent evidence points to significant benefits of other nonpharmacological measures such as yoga, acupuncture, and other complementary therapies. However, there are limited studies in patients with advanced cancer.

Psychosocial Interventions

Psychosocial interventions have been found to be effective treatments for cancer-related fatigue. Randomized clinical trials have shown that both group and individual supportive interventions, such as cognitive behavioral therapies, education and stress management groups, coping strategies training, and behavioral interventions, can help cancer patients manage their fatigue.[9]

Combined Therapies

In view of the recent evidence and guidelines,[14] personalized strategies should be considered for patients in whom fatigue is refractory to available treatments (i.e., treatment of the reversible causes or a trial of steroids or psychostimulants in addition to non pharmacological management such as physical activity). These personalized strategies may target the predominant symptoms in addition to fatigue. Possible examples include clinical trials of psychostimulants and physical activity in subgroups of patients with fatigue with high levels of sedation or depression, or clinical trials of steroids and counseling in patients with high levels of C-reactive protein, pro-inflammatory cytokines, and/or other measures of inflammation, and clinical trials of testosterone in patients with fatigue and hypogonadic states. Further studies are needed.

Clinical Pearls

- Fatigue is a subjective, complex, multidimensional symptom.
- Routine screening and assessment of the predominant dimensions of fatigue may help in diagnosis and treatment.
- Management should include an interdisciplinary approach.
- Identification and treatment of reversible causes should be considered.
- Nonpharmacological treatments such as physical activity should be offered to all patients.
- Multimodal approaches personalized to a given patient should be considered in refractory cases.

References

1. Lawrence DP, Kupelnick B, Miller K, et al. (2004). Evidence report on the occurrence, assessment, and treatment of fatigue in cancer patients. *J Natl Cancer Inst Monogr* 32:40–50.
2. Yennurajalingam S, Bruera E (2007). Palliative management of fatigue at the close of life: "It feels like my body is just worn out." *JAMA* 297:295–304.
3. Cella D, Davis K, Breitbart W, Curt G, for the Fatigue Coalition (2001). Cancer-related fatigue: prevalence of proposed diagnostic criteria in a United States sample of cancer survivors. *J Clin Oncol* 19:3385–91.

4. Curt GA, Breitbart W, Cella D (2000). Impact of cancer-related fatigue on the lives of patients: new findings from the Fatigue Coalition. *Oncologist* 5:353–60.
5. Bower JE (2014). Cancer-related fatigue: mechanisms, risk factors, and treatments. *Nat Rev Clin Oncol* 11(10):597–609.
6. Saligan LN, Olson K, Filler K, et al. (2015). The biology of cancer-related fatigue: a review of the literature. *Support Care Cancer* (8):2461–78.
7. Munch TN, Zhang T, Willey J, Palmer JL, Bruera E (2005). The association between anemia and fatigue in patients with advanced cancer receiving palliative care. *J Palliat Med* 8:1144–9.
8. Dittner AJ, Wessely SC, Brown RG (2004). The assessment of fatigue: a practical guide for clinicians and researchers. *J Psychosom Res* 56:157–70.
9. Wagner LI, Cella D (2004). Fatigue and cancer: causes, prevalence and treatment approaches. *Br J Cancer* 91:822–8.
10. Yennurajalingam S, Frisbee-Hume S, Palmer JL, et al. (2013). Reduction of cancer-related fatigue with dexamethasone: a double-blind, randomized, placebo-controlled trial in patients with advanced cancer. *J Clin Oncol* 31(25):3076–82.
11. Yennurajalingam S, Bruera E (2014). Review of clinical trials of pharmacologic interventions for cancer-related fatigue: focus on psychostimulants and steroids. *Cancer J* 20(5):319–24.
12. Spathis A, Fife K, Blackhall F, et al. (2013). Modafinil for the treatment of fatigue in lung cancer: results of a placebo-controlled, double-blind, randomized trial. *J Clin Oncol* 32(18):1882–8.
13. Del Fabbro E, Garcia JM, Dev R, et al. (2013). Testosterone replacement for fatigue in hypogonadal ambulatory males with advanced cancer: a preliminary double-blind placebo-controlled trial. *Support Care Cancer* 21:2599.
14. Bower JE, Bak K, Berger A, et al. (2014). Screening, assessment, and management of fatigue in adult survivors of cancer: an American Society of Clinical Oncology Clinical Practice Guideline Adaptation. *J Clin Oncol* 32:1840–50.

Cachexia

Egidio Del Fabbro

Definition

Cachexia is a multifactorial syndrome characterized by involuntary weight loss, regardless of caloric intake or appetite. Patients often experience a combination of muscle wasting, progressive functional impairment, loss of body fat, and poor appetite, resulting in the cachexia–anorexia syndrome (CAS).

Cachexia should be distinguished from starvation and sarcopenia (see Table 6.1). However, all three conditions could be present to some degree in an individual.

Cachexia may be found in many seemingly disparate conditions, including cancer,[1] HIV, tuberculosis and malaria, rheumatoid arthritis, chronic obstructive pulmonary disease (COPD)[1,2] congestive heart failure,[2,3] chronic kidney disease, and liver failure.

Table 6.1 Distinguishing Between Cachexia, Sarcopenia, and Starvation[*]

	Starvation	Cachexia	Sarcopenia
Weight loss/BMI	↓↓	↓↓	↓/↔
Inflammatory markers (CRP and cytokines)	↔	↑↑	↑/↔/↓
Resting energy expenditure (REE)	↓↓	↑↑/↔/↓[†]	↑/↔/↓
Protein synthesis	↓↓	↓/↑[‡]	↓↓
Muscle/fat loss insulin	↓/↓↓	↓↓/↓	↓/↔
Insulin	↓↓	↑↑	↔
Cortisol	↔	↑	↔
Effect of caloric intake on muscle mass	↑↑	↔	↔

[*] An individual patient may have components of all three conditions. Most patients with cancer cachexia are also sarcopenic, but most sarcopenic individuals are not considered cachetic.
[†] Cachexia patients may be hyper-, hypo-, or eumetabolic.
[‡] Increased acute-phase response proteins, decreased myosin (muscle)
↓ = decreased; ↔ = no change; ↑ = increased; / = and/or.

Mechanisms of Cachexia–Anorexia Syndrome

An aberrant inflammatory response generated by the disease–host interaction is probably the dominant mechanism[3]. Cytokine-induced catabolism causes impaired synthesis and increased degradation of muscle and fat. Other disease-specific factors (e.g., lipid mobilizing factor in cancer) may also be involved (see Figure 6.1).

There is also neurohormonal dysfunction. A loss of endocrine homeostasis impairs anabolism and appetite. Abnormalities associated with the CAS include elevated cortisol levels, ghrelin and insulin resistance, low serum testosterone, and sympathetic activation.

Pro-inflammatory cytokines play a role in propagating these irregularities and alter hypothalamic sensitivity to orexigenic and anorexigenic peptides.

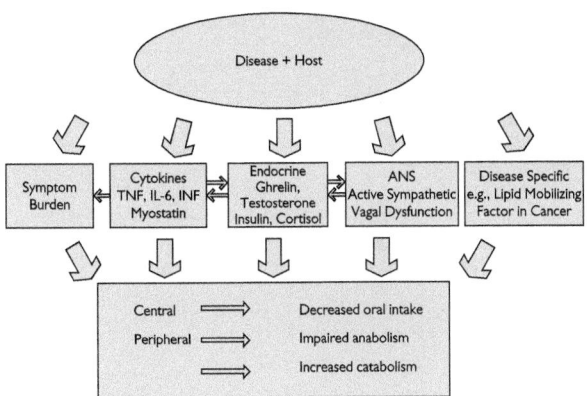

Figure 6.1. Mechanisms of cachexia–anorexia syndrome.
ANS = autonomic nervous system.

Exacerbating Factors

Appetite loss experienced by many patients can be aggravated by symptoms such as severe pain, nausea, early satiety, constipation, and depression. Elderly or sedentary patients may have underlying sarcopenia and poor muscle reserves.

Deficiencies of particular substrates, such as amino acids and, L-carnitine, may also play a role (Figure 6.2).

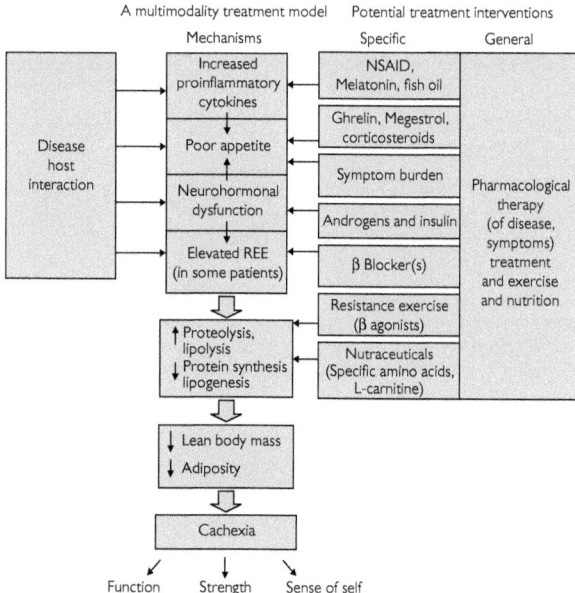

Figure 6.2. Model of multimodality therapy directed at the mechanisms of cachexia.

Clinical Assessment

Patient History

Patient history can be used to identify patients with involuntary weight loss of > 5% within the past 6 months (if no prior weights are available). Ideally, these patients should be identified even earlier in the disease trajectory in order for interventions to produce the greatest impact.

Prior comorbid conditions such as endocrine abnormalities (hyper- or hypothyroidism, adrenal insufficiency, diabetes) and vitamin deficiencies (vitamin B_{12}, vitamin D) need to be determined.

Symptoms contributing to decreased oral intake are also important factors. A symptom assessment tool such as the Edmonton Symptom Assessment Scale (ESAS) can be used to identify symptoms such as pain, depression, and nausea. Additional factors may include early satiety, oral ulcers, dental problems, dry mouth, and dysphagia.

Patient goals are crucial in determining the choice of therapy. For most patients, an improvement in strength and function is the goal. Others may want an improved appetite above all, to enjoy meals with family and friends. For some, body image may be more important, since cachexia is a very visible manifestation of illness.

Examination

Muscle wasting is often readily apparent but may be disguised in patients who were obese prior to their illness. Body mass index (BMI = body weight divided by height in kg/m^2) is not useful in evaluating body composition or lean body mass.

Monitor the impact of therapy with relatively low-burden tests, such as arm muscle area:

(mid-arm circumference [MAC] in centimeters) − π
× tricipital skin fold thickness [in millimeters])^2/(4 × π)

minus a correction factor of 10 for men and 6.5 for women.

Electrical bioimpedance analysis (BIA) can conveniently measure fat-free mass (FFM). The fat-free mass index (FFMI = FFM divided by height in kg/m^2) is especially useful in patients with COPD. Edema affects the accuracy of BIA. BIA may be useful for prognostication.

Dual energy X-ray absorptiometry (DEXA) and computerized tomographic (CT) scanning for measuring muscle mass are possible in the research setting.

Physical Strength and Function

- These should be assessed for longitudinal follow-up.
- Choose tests that are least burdensome to the patient.
- Use a 6-minute walk or 50-meter walk for assessing an intervention's impact on endurance.
- Use a hand-grip dynamometer and gait speed.

Investigations

These depend on the history and exam, but could include all of the following.

Laboratory

- Complete blood count (CBC) to monitor polycythemia/anemia (androgen replacement, anti-inflammatory use)
- Electrolytes, creatinine, BUN, and glucose
- Calcium—hypercalcemia produces poor appetite and fatigue
- Liver function tests
- C-reactive protein (CRP) for prognostication in cancer
- Vitamin B_{12}, folate, vitamin D
- Thyroid-stimulating hormone (TSH) for hypothyroidism (especially in the elderly and after radiation for head and neck cancer), monitor replacement therapy
- Testosterone—early morning, preferably bioavailable (free and weakly bound). Decreased levels common in COPD, HIV, and cancer cachexia (75%)
- Cortisol—early morning (< 3 mcg/dL is diagnostic, > 18 mcg/dL is normal, mid-range requires additional tests of dynamic adrenal function)
- Albumin has prognostic value, particularly in renal-failure cachexia.

Radiology

- Abdominal X-ray to evaluate for mechanical obstruction (cancer) or severe constipation.

Metabolism

- Indirect calorimetry, if possible
  - Resting energy expenditure (REE) and caloric needs are more accurately measured than by equations such as the Harris–Benedict Equation.

Treatment

Nutrition

The ideal goal of 34 kcal/kg/day or 1.5 x REE may not be realistic,[7] depending on the patients' condition. Usually, frequent small meals that are calorie dense are advised. Counseling by a dietician can increase caloric intake.

Specific amino acids given in patients with HIV and cancer cachexia (arginine-, glutamine-, and leucine-related products such as Beta hydroxyl Beta methylbutyrate) may increase lean body mass.

Antioxidants and polyphenols in open-label combination therapy improved outcomes for cancer cachexia.

A systematic review[5] found that omega-3 oils had no benefit for cachexia in advanced cancer. There may be benefit to the earlier use of fish oil when patients are newly diagnosed and receiving chemotherapy.[6]

Symptoms and Conditions Contributing to Poor Appetite

- Oral: poor dentition, infection, mucositis, xerostomia
- Dygeusia: trial of zinc for 2 weeks
- Nausea: 5HT3 antagonists during chemotherapy, metoclopramide for non-chemotherapy-related nausea
- Early satiety: metoclopramide
- Pain: opioid, nonsteroidal anti-inflammatory drugs (NSAIDs)
- Depression: tricyclic antidepressants, mirtazapine
- Constipation: laxatives
- Dysphagia: endoscopic intervention, enteral and parenteral nutrition if starvation is a large component of the weight loss
- Treat conditions contributing to CAS (see lab investigations).

Drugs for Cachexia

No single pharmacological intervention is consistently effective for treating CAS. Multiple medications have demonstrated benefit in small trials.

Some disease-specific drugs, for example, β-blockers for congestive heart failure (CHF), could modulate the mechanisms of cachexia in other conditions, such as hypermetabolic cancer cachexia.

Conventional Drugs

Corticosteroids are effective for multiple symptoms (poor appetite, fatigue, nausea) in the short term. Prolonged use increases the risk of infections and myopathy. They may be best for the last 2 months of life.

With megestrol acetate treatment, a systematic review[2] found appetite improved and weight increased slightly (predominantly fat/fluid). Benefit was shown in patients with cancer, HIV, or COPD. The risk of thromboembolism is dose dependent and increases with chemotherapy. Hypogonadism and hypoadrenalism may require replacement therapy.

Investigational Drugs

- Cannabinoids are no better than placebo for cancer cachexia[8] but improve taste in cancer patients and appetite in HIV patients. They may be more effective at higher doses but are limited by side effects.
- NSAIDs are given alone or combined[5] with appetite stimulants for cancer cachexia. Ibuprofen in combination with megestrol increased lean

mass in patients with solid tumors. Celecoxib[9] as part of multimodality therapy was also effective in small open-label trials, but NSAID use should be reserved for investigational studies.

- Melatonin was effective in preventing and treating cancer cachexia in open-label trials but not in a randomized controlled trial[10] in advanced cancer.
- β-blockers, angiotensin-converting enzyme (ACE) inhibitors, and angiotensin II receptor blockers (ARBs) are the standard of care for CHF and may prove to be useful in other conditions, for example, cancer cachexia.
- Androgens and selective androgen receptor modulators (SARMs) have shown benefit in small trials of HIV, COPD, and cancer cachexia.
- Muscle anabolism: beta agonists, myostatin inhibitors in the future.
- Thalidomide is useful in HIV, tuberculosis, and preliminary cancer cachexia trials.[11]
- Ghrelin and ghrelin mimetics/agonists[12] show benefit in treating cachexia in cancer, and COPD in preliminary trials. Their safety needs to be established in larger studies.
- Growth hormone is used for HIV cachexia. Patient tolerance may be a problem.
- Parenteral nutrition is used when starvation is a major component, the tumor is slow growing, and there is > 6 weeks survival.

Exercise

There is preliminary evidence of greater muscle strength with resistance training in patients with sarcopenia, chronic renal insufficiency, rheumatoid arthritis, HIV, or COPD.

Outcomes

Effective therapies should (ideally) achieve all of the following:
- Increased lean body mass
- Improved function (activities of daily living [ADL], see functional tests)
- Increased appetite
- Weight gain

Prognosis

- Weight loss > 5% (CHF, HIV)
- BMI < 20
- CRP > 10 mg/L[13]
- Hypoalbuminemia (renal cachexia)
- Combination in cancer cachexia may be more accurate: weight loss ≥ 10%, CRP ≥ 10 mg/L, food intake ≤ 1500 kcal/day.

What Families and Patients Need to Know

Many patients and families believe poor appetite and weight loss are the most burdensome issues they face. Unfortunately, their concerns are seldom addressed by healthcare providers.

Opening a dialogue with patients and their families may resolve family conflict, increase confidence in healthcare providers, and avoid unnecessary interventions. Explaining the mechanisms of cachexia without medical jargon may help families appreciate that increased caloric intake will not necessarily result in muscle gains or functional improvement.

An understanding of this counterintuitive concept could help avoid unnecessary enteral or parenteral supplementation and relieve pressure on patients perceived as not trying "hard enough" to eat.

Clinical Pearls

- A pro-inflammatory state is likely the dominant mechanism causing muscle wasting.
- Frequently used medications such as corticosteroids and megestrol are associated with dose-dependent side effects.
- C-reactive protein levels are useful for prognosis.
- Multimodality therapy (including pharmacological, nutritional, and exercise interventions) should always be considered.
- Nutritional issues are important to patients and their families and need to be addressed (even when therapeutic options are not available or indicated).

References

1. Fearon K, Strasser F, Anker SD, Bosaeus I, Bruera E, Fainsinger RL, et al. (2011). Definition and classification of cancer cachexia: an international consensus. *Lancet Oncology* 12(5):489–95.
2. Ceelen JJ, Langen RC, Schols AM. (2014). Systemic inflammation in chronic obstructive pulmonary disease and lung cancer: common driver of pulmonary cachexia? *Curr Opin Support Palliat Care* 8(4):339–45.
3. von Haehling S, Steinbeck L, Doehner W, Springer J, Anker SD (2013). Muscle wasting in heart failure: an overview. *Int J Biochem Cell Biol* 45(10):2257–65.
4. Molfino A, Gioia G, Rossi Fanelli F, Muscaritoli M (2013). Beta-hydroxy-beta-methylbutyrate supplementation in health and disease: a systematic review of randomized trials. *Amino Acids* 45(6):1273–92.
5. Ries A, Trottenberg P, Elsner F, Stiel S, Haugen D, Kaasa S, Radbruch L (2012). A systematic review on the role of fish oil for the treatment of cachexia in advanced cancer: an EPCRC cachexia guidelines project. *Palliat Med* 26(4):294–304.
6. Murphy RA, Mourtzakis M, Chu QS, Baracos VE, Reiman T, Mazurak VC (2011). Nutritional intervention with fish oil provides a benefit over standard of care for weight and skeletal muscle mass in patients with nonsmall cell lung cancer receiving chemotherapy. *Cancer* 117(8):1775–82.
7. Ruiz Garcia V, López-Briz E, Carbonell Sanchis R, Gonzalvez Perales JL, Bort-Marti S (2013). Megestrol acetate for treatment of anorexia-cachexia syndrome. *Cochrane Database Syst Rev* 3:CD004310.
8. Cannabis-In-Cachexia-Study-Group, Strasser F, Luftner D, Possinger K, Ernst G, Ruhstaller T, et al. (2006). Comparison of orally administered cannabis extract and delta-9-tetrahydrocannabinol in treating patients with cancer-related anorexia-cachexia syndrome: a multicenter, phase III, randomized, double-blind, placebo-controlled clinical trial from the Cannabis-In-Cachexia-Study-Group. *J Clin Oncol* 24(21):3394–400.
9. Macciò A, Madeddu C, Gramignano G, Mulas C, Floris C, Sanna E, et al. (2012). A randomized phase III clinical trial of a combined treatment for cachexia in patients with gynecological cancers: evaluating the impact on metabolic and inflammatory profiles and quality of life. *Gynecol Oncol* 124(3):417–25.
10. Del Fabbro E, Dev R, Hui D, Palmer L, Bruera E (2013). Effects of melatonin on appetite and other symptoms in patients with advanced cancer and cachexia: a double-blind placebo-controlled trial. *J Clin Oncol* 31(10):1271–6. PMC3607670.
11. Reid J, Mills M, Cantwell M, Cardwell CR, Murray LJ, Donnelly M (2012). Thalidomide for managing cancer cachexia. *Cochrane Database Syst Rev* 4:CD008664.
12. Ali S, Chen JA, Garcia JM (2013). Clinical development of ghrelin axis-derived molecules for cancer cachexia treatment. *Curr Opin Support Palliat Care* 7(4):368–75. PMC4121852.
13. Douglas E, McMillan DC (2014). Towards a simple objective framework for the investigation and treatment of cancer cachexia: the Glasgow Prognostic Score. *Cancer Treat Rev* 40(6):685–91.

Dehydration

Shalini Dalal

Introduction

The vast majority of patients in the terminal phase of their illness experience severely reduced oral intake before death, which may arise due to a variety of causes related to their diagnosis or its treatment.

Commonly experienced symptoms such as decreased appetite, nausea and vomiting, bowel obstruction, dysphagia, cognitive impairment, and depression predispose to deficits in fluid status, which in turn can lead to distressful symptoms (such as confusion, fatigue) and/or death (see Figure 7.1). In this chapter, we offer recommendations for an individualized approach in the management of fluid deficits in terminally ill patients that is based on symptom burden, patient and family preferences, and goals of care.

Figure 7.1. Theoretical model of the effects of fluid deficits in terminally ill patients and the role of parenteral hydration on symptom distress and delirium.

Reprinted with permission from Dalal S, Del Fabbro E, Bruera E (2009). Is there a role for hydration at the end of life? *Curr Opin Support Palliat Care* 3:72–8.

Fluid Homeostasis

Fluid homeostasis is dependent on the maintenance of a relatively constant and stable composition of body fluids. It is achieved in normal individuals by matching daily water intake to fluid losses from the body.

In normal, healthy adults, water constitutes approximately 60% of total body weight (TBW) in men and 55% in women. This amount declines with aging, with shifts in body composition resulting in a 10%–15% reduction of total body water.

Water in the body is in a constant state of motion, shifting between the various fluid compartments of the body. Two-thirds of the total body water is present in tissue cells. The remaining third is present as extracellular fluid and is divided between the plasma (intravascular compartment) and interstitial compartment. The amount of these fluids is highly variable, and these compartments are generally ignored when considering body fluids.

Dehydration

Classically, the medical literature has distinguished two forms of total body water fluid loss: (1) dehydration, which refers to a loss of body water mainly from the intracellular compartments, and (2) volume depletion, referring to a loss of extracellular fluid clinically affecting the vascular tree and interstitial compartment.

Dehydration can be defined as a complex condition resulting in a reduction in total body water. This can be due primarily to a water deficit (water loss dehydration) or both a salt and water deficit (salt loss dehydration). In most cases, dehydration is due to disease and/or the effects of medication and not primarily due to lack of access to water. Clinically, it cannot be defined by a single symptom, sign, or laboratory value.[1]

The fluid requirement in terminal patients may be less; however, they are at an increased risk of fluid deficit, often precipitated by minor variations in fluid intake, infections, and other conditions.

Many patients are elderly, with renal and neurohormonal functions deteriorated by age and thereby not as effective as in younger individuals. The thirst mechanism diminishes with age, significantly impairing the ability of the elderly to maintain homeostasis and increasing the risk for dehydration. An age-related decrease in maximal urinary concentrating ability further increases the risk for dehydration.

Symptoms

Fluid deficits may cause cognitive impairment, altered behavior, decreased energy level, confusion, delirium, fainting, or syncope.[2] Confused patients may be a danger to themselves or at risk for falls, or have aberrant behavior with paranoid delusions or hallucinations. They can also appear significantly distressed to their caregivers.

Studies noting a high prevalence of thirst and dry mouth in patients with advanced cancer have failed to show an association between these symptoms and biochemical markers of fluid deficit or dehydration.

Dry mouth can be alleviated by simple measures such as oral care, small sips of water, and lubrication.

Persistent subclinical dehydration is associated with anxiety, panic attacks, and agitation. Fluctuation in tissue hydration results in inattention, hallucinations, and delusions. Severe dehydration leads to somnolence, psychosis, and unconsciousness.[1]

Mechanisms include increased local cytokine production, glutamate toxicity, mitochondrial dysfunction, altered pharmacokinetics of drugs, and increased anticholinergic burden.[3]

Assessment of Hydration Status

Initial Assessment
Determine the presence of fluid deficits.

History
- Urine output, third spacing, hemorrhage
- Cognitive impairment
- Altered behavior
- Constipation

Physical Examination
- Dry mucous membranes
- Reduced skin turgor
- Sunken eyes
- Dry axillae
- Postural hypotension, tachycardia, increased capillary refill time
- Cyanosis, mottling, reticulation

Laboratory
Clarification of the goals of treatment is important prior to ordering laboratory tests, as some may not be useful in determining treatment.
- Increased plasma protein
- Increased hematocrit
- Increased sodium
- Increased blood urea nitrogen and serum creatinine

Symptom Effects
Determine the symptom burden (using multidimensional assessment tools).
Determine the impact of symptoms on quality of life, patient and family distress, and function.
- Thirst and dry mouth are distressing symptoms for both the patient and family.
- Symptoms are not exclusive to dehydration.
- May be a consequence of medication, radiation, mouth breathing, or thrush.

Determine benefits versus burden of artificial hydration.
- Hydration may be beneficial if there are cognitive changes or delirium in select patients, such as those on opioids.
- Hydration was not shown to benefit hospice patients who were in their last 3 weeks of life.
- Hydration may not be beneficial for symptoms of thirst or dry mouth.
- Determine disadvantages (hospitalization, mobility, discomfort).

Determine Patient and Family Preferences and Goals
- Discuss both the benefits and burdens of hydration.
- Disclose uncertainties.
- Discuss a trial of hydration to assess benefit.
- Provide alternatives if hydration is not considered.

- Provide emotional support.
- Inform the patient and family that hydration can be ethically withheld and withdrawn.

If Hydration Is Considered

- Consider hypodermoclysis.
- Administer appropriate volumes (< 1000 mL/day).
- Consider discontinuation if there are no perceived benefits.

Intravenous

The traditional route for hydration has been intravenous (IV) and usually via a peripheral line. In some patients with terminal illness, central venous access devices (CVADs) are placed. These CVADs are associated with an increased risk of complications during placement as well as ongoing use.

Patients have an increased frequency of local infections and catheter-associated bacteremia.[4] Management of these catheters can be a difficult option in the home care setting.

The IV route should be limited to situations where subcutaneous (SC) administration of fluids is contraindicated, such as in patients with generalized edema or major coagulation disorders or who already have an IV line or CVAD in place for other purposes.

Enteral

This route is indicated for any malnourished patient with a functional GI tract who is unable to orally ingest sufficient nutrients as long as access can be achieved safely. This route is simpler, safer, more physiologic, and less costly than parenteral.

Common indications include dysphagia due to head and neck cancer, esophageal obstruction, gastric outlet obstruction, or critical illness requiring prolonged mechanical ventilation.

The choice of access device is dependent on anticipated duration of use, the underlying pathophysiology and anatomy, patient preference, and local expertise. Nasogastric (NG) tubes are best for patients who require enteral support for less than 30 days.

Placement of a percutaneous feeding tube is indicated in patients who will require long-term support.

Hypodermoclysis

Hypodermoclysis is the infusion of fluids into the SC space and can be used in reference to medication infusion. Several recent studies in patients with terminal illness and for infusion of analgesics have demonstrated its safety, efficacy, and practical advantages over IV routes.[5]

Hypodermoclysis involves the insertion of a butterfly needle subcutaneously and attaching a line for fluids to be administered via an infusion pump or gravity in the home setting. In ambulatory patients, the abdomen, upper chest, and area above the breast may be used as the SC infusion site. In bedridden patients, preferred sites are the thighs, abdomen, and outer aspects of the upper arm. These sites can be used for 5–7 days.[6]

Approximately 1 L of fluid is sufficient for a 24-hour period and allows for normal urine output and adequate hydration in most patients. In home settings, these fluids can be administered via gravity at a rate of 1–2 mL per minute at one site, allowing up to 1.5 L in a 24-hour period. Patients can receive overnight infusions or several 1-hour boluses, which will allow for mobility and freedom from tubing for most of the day.

Commonly administered electrolyte fluid solutions, such as normal (0.9%) and half-normal (0.45%) saline, saline-dextrose combinations such as one-third saline with two-thirds glucose (5%), have been used in studies involving hypodermoclysis and can be safely administered.[7]

The use of non-electrolyte solutions is not recommended for hypodermoclysis as they can cause sloughing of tissue, mostly in pediatric patients.

Rapid or large-volume SC infusion of electrolyte-free solutions can cause circulatory collapse. Side effects can include local skin irritation and occasional itching, site bleeding, and infection. Colloidal and hyperosmolar solutions should not be given.

Hypodermoclysis is contraindicated in patients with generalized edema or clotting disorders. Patients at increased risk of pulmonary edema should be treated with caution and monitored to prevent respiratory distress due to fluid overload.

The risks of hypodermoclysis are minimal when it is administered within accepted indications and guidelines.

Proctolysis

Proctolysis is the rectal administration of fluids. This is an alternative for patients who require hydration but are unable to receive it by another route. The procedure is invasive, requiring insertion of a catheter about 40 cm into the rectum.

Disadvantages include enema effect with maximal rates of infusion, leakage of fluids, and pain during insertion of catheter and infusion of fluids.

Clinical Pearls

- Hydration may benefit symptoms of delirium, fatigue, and opioid neurotoxicity in patients who are not in the last 2–3 weeks of life.
- Hydration may not be beneficial for symptoms of thirst or dry mouth.
- Hypodermoclysis is an excellent alternative to intravenous hydration because of its simplicity, low cost, and feasibility.

References

1. Thomas DR, Cote TR, Lawhorne L, et al. (2008). Understanding clinical dehydration and its treatment. *J Am Med Dir Assoc* 9:287–8.
2. Dalal S, Del Fabbro E, Bruera E (2009). Is there a role for hydration at the end of life? *Curr Opin Support Palliat Care* 3:72–8.
3. Wilson MM, Morley JE (2003). Impaired cognitive function and mental performance in mild dehydration. *Eur J Clin Nutr* 57:S24–9.
4. Dalal S, Bruera E (2004). Dehydration in cancer patients: to treat or not to treat. *J Support Oncol* 2:467–79.
5. Bruera E, Legris MA, Kuehn N, et al. (1990). Hypodermoclysis for the administration of fluids and narcotic analgesics in patients with advanced cancer. *J Pain Symptom Manage* 5:218–20.
6. Bruera E, Hu S, Dalal S et al. (2013). Parenteral hydration in patients with advanced cancer: a multicenter, double-blind, placebo-controlled randomized trial. *J Clin Oncol* 31:111–8.
7. Slesak G, Schnurle JW, Kinzel E, et al. (2003). Comparison of subcutaneous and intravenous rehydration in geriatric patients: a randomized trial. *J Am Geriatr Soc* 51:155–60.

Anxiety and Depression

Paul W. Walker and Anis Rashid

Introduction

Changes in mood and coping are expected when a person is diagnosed with a devastating illness such as cancer. The treatment of cancer is complex, and managing all aspects of treatment may be overwhelming. From diagnosis of cancer to survivorship is a long battle with emotional ups and downs. How to best manage these emotions, and when to medicate the patient for anxiety and depression, are important consideration for clinicians.[1,2]

Understanding the differences between typical adjustment reactions and major depressive disorder is important. *Adjustment reactions* occur with an acute stressor such as a diagnosis of a serious illness or with other setbacks such as recurrences or relapses.

The patient often reacts with increased anxiety or depression that fluctuates and is usually limited to a period of weeks. This is generally an acute emotional reaction to the stressor and improves with time and psychotherapeutic support.

Depression is a serious disorder that requires careful attention to diagnosis and management. It is important to note that depression is underdiagnosed and undertreated. A survey of patients receiving palliative care for cancer revealed that 60% of patients with major depressive disorder were not being treated with antidepressants. In cancer patients, depression may mistakenly be considered as a normal response to a cancer diagnosis as well as to the side effects of chemotherapy and may not be considered for treatment.

Depression

Prevalence

Variable rates of depression are reported for patients in the palliative setting, ranging from 1.5% to 50%. In the past, studies focused on cancer patients, but other diseases are now coming under the purview of hospice and palliative care.

Of these non-cancer diseases, patients with myocardial infarction show a prevalence of depression of 16%–23%. Patients with Alzheimer's disease, diabetes type 1 or 2, or Huntington's disease may have prevalence for depression as high as 32%. Those with Parkinson's disease or multiple sclerosis have prevalence rates as high as 50%.

A family history of depression is the most widely recognized risk factor. An inherited depression may have an earlier age at onset and manifest recurrences.

Females are more at risk, which may be due to genetic influences. Other risk factors include impaired functional status, poor social support, uncontrolled pain, and external stressors.

Malignancies that have been linked to depression include retroperitoneal tumors (e.g., pancreatic cancer), primary brain tumors, and head and neck cancers.

Medications that increase the risk of depression include interferon, interleukin, intrathecal methotrexate, vincristine, β-blockers, and steroids. Drug withdrawal can also be a precipitating factor.

Diagnosis

Depressed mood is a complex and heterogeneous problem that has multiple manifestations and etiologies (see Box 8.1). The clinician should not fall under the illusion that all such patients will present alike.

According to *DSM-5* criteria, depression is classified as mild, moderate, or severe. An episode of psychotic features is sometimes associated with major depression, which is then classified as major depressive disorder with psychotic features. Other types include persistent depressive disorder (dysthymia) if the depressed mood persists for at least 2 years, substance/medication-induced depressive disorder, mood disorder due to another

---

Box 8.1 Features of Major Depression

Depressed mood
Diminished interest of pleasure (anhedonia) (one of the above must be present)
Weight loss or weight gain
Insomnia or hypersomnia
Psychomotor agitation or retardation
Fatigue or loss of energy
Feelings of worthlessness or excessive guilt
Diminished ability to think or concentrate, indecisiveness
Recurrent thoughts of death or suicide

medical condition, and premenstrual dysphoric disorder. Bipolar disorder is differentiated by an episode of mania.[3]

DSM-5 has categorized the conditions that do not meet the full definition of the syndrome under "other specified depressive disorder." These include recurrent brief depression, if symptoms persists 2–13 days at least once per month for at least 12 consecutive months; short duration depressive episode when clinically significant distress persists for 4–13 days (if depressed mood lasts 4–13 days); and depressive episode with insufficient symptoms when clinically significant distress is present for at least 2 weeks and does not meet the criteria for another depressive or bipolar disorder. In *DSM-5* bereavement is listed under "other specified trauma and stress-related disorder."

The diagnosis of major depressive disorder requires the presence of five or more of the nine symptoms occurring for 2 consecutive weeks, and one symptom is either depressed mood or loss of interest or pleasure (anhedonia). There must be a change from the patient's previous level of functioning. These symptoms must be present most of the day, nearly every day, during this period. The other symptoms include weight loss or gain, decrease or increase in appetite, insomnia or hypersomnia, psychomotor agitation or retardation, fatigue, feelings of worthlessness, inappropriate guilt, diminished concentration, indecisiveness, and thoughts of death or suicide.

However, many serious illnesses or their treatments can be the cause of some of these symptoms. One example of this would be cancer, which in many cases causes weight loss, fatigue, and anorexia.

One approach to the assessment of depression in cancer patients is to substitute the somatic symptoms that can be influenced by the cancer with other psychological symptoms (such as hopelessness, social withdrawal, brooding, pessimism, depressed appearance, tearfulness, and lack of reactivity).

A single screening question ("Are you depressed most of the time?") has been found to be a brief, reliable screen in terminally ill cancer patients. Asking about suicidal thoughts and plans for self-harm is important for any patient being screened for depression.

These questions have not been found to increase the risk of suicide, as some clinicians may fear, but rather greatly aid the detection of a patient at suicidal risk and enable interventions to minimize occurrences.

It is helpful to destigmatize the question posed to the patient. The question could be phrased as follows: "It would not be unusual for someone in your situation to have thoughts of harming themselves. Have you had thoughts like that?"

Depression may be associated with all serious illnesses. Short periods of sadness are expected when dealing with physical symptoms that accompany a medical illness, such as pain and fatigue. However, when a depressed mood persists and becomes pervasive, together with other symptoms of major depressive disorder, the diagnosis needs to be considered to direct effective management.

Treatment

Management of depression requires ongoing communication between the clinician and the patient. This helps the patient regain self-control over symptoms of depression, and is especially effective in mild to moderate depression. Managing major depressive disorder is a challenge that requires forming a therapeutic alliance through supportive therapy with frequent clinic visits, medications, and utilization of psychosocial resources.

Two main interventions are psychotherapy and antidepressant medication. While these may be used separately, their combined use may prove most effective.[1,2] Also, altering other factors that may be adversely affecting the patient, such as discontinuing highly toxic therapies, can markedly improve depression.

The vicious cycle of pain and depression is important to consider when caring for palliative patients. Recognizing that chronic pain can cause depression may lead to effective treatment by focusing on analgesic strategies. Also, recognizing the converse, that depression causes an increase in pain perception, is important.

Depression has been closely associated with somatization or "total pain." An important finding of a survey of palliative care patients was that fully 82.9% of participants with both depression and anxiety reported a moderate to extreme degree of global suffering resembling "total pain."

Supportive psychotherapy that allows expression of the patient's worries, fears, and concerns, as well as validating and supporting the patient, is the basis of psychotherapy for the seriously ill. Often it is the social worker, chaplain, or psychologist who is available and inclined to provide this. Mental health professionals may play a major role in the management of these patients. A "therapeutic relationship" is important for effective psychotherapy. The development of a good alliance between the two individuals is more likely to result in a successful outcome, regardless of the type of therapy employed.

Supportive psychotherapy helps patients in crisis. It enables them to move forward and make adjustments to adapt to the acute changes in health and life. An important aspect of counseling the very ill is re-establishing their autonomy through attempts to empower the individual. This is necessary, as the illness has often robbed the patient of basic abilities and freedom as well as privacy. Attempts to listen and provide information, while allowing patients as much control as possible over their treatment and care options, as well as their day-to-day living, are often very significant to the individual. Establishing what the patient's goals and priorities are and developing strategies to work toward achieving them often result in effective empowerment of the individual.

Other types of psychotherapy that have been recommended include individual and group, cognitive-behavioral, family, interpersonal, and mindfulness-based therapy.

Newer developments by experts in the field of psycho-oncology include the development of meaning-centered psychotherapy (developed by Breitbart) and dignity psychotherapy (developed by Chochinov).[4] These therapies are often directed to those who have expressed a desire for death or existential distress.

Meaning-centered group therapy is based on the principles of Viktor Frankl's logotherapy and deals with issues of sustaining meaning and hope in the context of illness and impending death.

Dignity psychotherapy focuses on bolstering the patient's sense of purpose, meaning, and worth. It also focuses on maintaining hopefulness, autonomy, and pride. The goal of dignity therapy is to maintain normalcy and to seek spiritual comfort at the end of life. The concern that nothing in one's life will transcend death is approached through a life-review process that is intended to develop a sense of legacy.

Therapy with antidepressant medication is the mainstay of treatment for major depressive disorder (see Table 8.1). The selective serotonin reuptake inhibitors (SSRIs), serotonin-norepinephrine reuptake inhibitors (SNRIs), and psychostimulants are most frequently used because of their more tolerable side-effect profiles.

Since few psychiatric studies have focused on the palliative population, studies involving the general population have been used as a basis for treating depression in palliative care. Historically, clinical trials have shown that virtually all antidepressant medications have similar efficacy in addressing major depression. Thus the choice of antidepressant is based on the drug's side-effect profile, the patient's history of antidepressant use in the past, and antidepressants with minimum risk of drug interactions.[4]

More recently, a large meta-analysis challenges this approach.[5] Although this study may not be generalizable to the palliative population, it reports that mirtazapine, escitalopram, venlafaxine, and sertraline were significantly more efficacious than duloxetine, fluoxetine, fluvoxamine, paroxetine, and reboxetine. Escitalopram and sertraline showed better acceptability, leading to fewer discontinuations than with duloxetine, fluvoxamine, paroxetine, reboxetine, and venlafaxine. The authors concluded that important differences exist among these antidepressants in terms of efficacy and acceptability, in favor of escitalopram and sertraline. Also of note is that both of

Table 8.1 Commonly Used Antidepressants

Generic (Trade Name)	Therapeutic Daily Dosage (mg)
Selective serotonin reuptake inhibitors (SSRIs)	
Citalopram (Celexa)	10–40
Escitalopram (Lexapro, Cipralex)	10–20
Fluvoxamine (Luvox)	50–300
Paroxetine (Paxil, Seroxat)	10–60
Sertraline (Zoloft, Lustral)	25–150
Combination agents (serontonin/noradrenergic)	
Mirtazapine (Remeron)	15–45
Venlafaxine (Effexor)	37.5–225
Duloxetine (Cymbalta)	40–60
Psychostimulants	
Methylphenidate (Ritalin)	5–30
Dextroamphetamine (Dexedrine)	5–30

these drugs have fewer drug interactions via the cytochrome P450 system than most other agents.

Side effects of the SSRIs are commonly nausea, sleep disturbance, headache, and sexual dysfunction. The SNRI venlafaxine has been reported to cause more nausea and vomiting than that with the SSRIs. Mirtazapine has been linked to weight gain; trazadone to somnolence; sertraline to diarrhea; paroxetine and venlafaxine to discontinuation syndrome; and paroxetine to more sexual dysfunction. Bupropion is an activating antidepressant that is sometimes used to counteract the sexual side effects of SSRIs. Fluoxetine is not favored because of its long half-life. The onset of antidepressant effect with these medications is often after a minimum of 2–3 weeks, with 4–6 weeks being a typical trial period.

Psychostimulants such as methylphenidate and dextroamphetamine have the benefit of a more rapid effect, which may be particularly important for patients with a short life expectancy. These agents are usually taken in the morning and mid-day so as to not interfere with sleep.[6]

Combining psychostimulants with an SSRI or other antidepressants may be indicated especially in severely depressed or suicidal patients. The best strategy in cancer patients is to "start low and go slow," especially considering the fragile nature of this patient population.[7]

For patients who are not improving despite a fair trial with antidepressant treatment, there are other options. Most important is to give at least a 6–8-week trial of an antidepressant with the FDA-approved maximum dosage. If this does not work, then augmentation with another drug is indicated. If this strategy fails, then switching to another drug or class of drug is worthwhile. Professional help from a psychiatrist is recommended while managing severely depressed patients. Patients who present serious suicidal risk require increased clinician diligence.

Collaborative Assessment and Management of Suicidality (CAMS) is a newer approach, which emphasizes a good-faith commitment between the patient and the clinician.[8] It is a therapeutic tool that engages both to work together to find suitable alternatives to deal with pain and suffering. In the CAMS approach, strong clinical alliance is the key, which optimizes the patient's motivation to find better coping strategies This strategy has shown better patient outcomes.

It is also judicious to ask family members to remove excess medications or weapons (e.g., a gun) that could be used for suicide. Again, expert psychiatric assistance is beneficial in these situations.

Bereavement and Complicated Grief

Family members and caregivers are at risk for bereavement throughout the illness but also especially following the patient's death. It is estimated that an average of five persons are left bereaved following each death.

Risk factors for a more difficult bereavement include a sudden or unexpected death, a perception of the patient suffering from pain or other symptoms, a stigmatized death (e.g., AIDS, suicide), substance abuse, psychiatric disorder, and dysfunction within the family. It is important to distinguish between bereavement and major depressive disorder. In bereavement the focus is on the loss, with a predominant feeling of emptiness. Symptoms last for 12 months or less. In major depressive disorder, there is persistent depressed mood, with loss of interest in any pleasurable activity.

Persistent complex bereavement disorder is a more serious condition that is prevalent in 2.4%–4.8% individuals. It is diagnosed when an adult has been grieving for more than 12 months after the death of a loved one. In the case of children, the time frame is 6 months. Symptoms usually begin within the first few months after the loss but may be delayed for 6 months or longer. Important features include (1) a sense of disbelief regarding the death; (2) anger and bitterness over the death; (3) recurrent pangs of painful emotions, with intense yearning and longing for the deceased; and (4) preoccupation with thoughts of the loved one, often including distressing intrusive thoughts related to the death.

Avoidance behaviors are often part of this condition. This disabling condition leaves individuals in a protracted difficult mourning, unable to lead a productive or enjoyable life. The diagnosis of persistent complex bereavement disorder can co-occur with major depressive disorder or post-traumatic stress disorder (PTSD). Studies show that persistent complex bereavement disorder may not respond to medications alone or in combination with interpersonal therapy, and requires psychotherapy specifically designed for this disorder.

Innovative research by Katherine Shear[9] has produced a therapy that borrows from cognitive behavioral therapy for trauma and PTSD. Similar to PTSD therapy, periods of re-experiencing the trauma of the loved one's death in a controlled way are an important part of the therapy. A randomized trial has shown that this complicated grief treatment produced higher response rates and faster times to response than the standard interpersonal psychotherapy.

Anxiety

Prevalence and Diagnosis

Anxiety is the most common psychiatric diagnosis reported in cancer patients. Anxiety level fluctuates during the course of the illness and is usually very high in newly diagnosed patients and understandably common in terminally ill patients. It is estimated that the prevalence of anxiety in the individual with cancer is in the range of 25%. High level of anxiety may interfere with the patients' understanding of the illness and treatment plan and may interfere with compliance. This will result in poor treatment response and compromised quality of life. Hence a thorough evaluation and management of anxiety are crucial to patients' well-being and outcome.

The most common presentation of anxiety seen in cancer patients is adjustment disorder with anxiety, commonly triggered by the breaking of bad news. Patients may have prior conditions, such as generalized anxiety disorder, panic disorder, or phobias, that increase their experience of anxiety during their illness. An example of this is claustrophobia, a common difficulty exacerbated by the requirements of MRI imaging or during radiation treatment in head and neck cancer patients.

Agitated depression can present with symptoms of anxiety. In cancer patients, a mix of anxiety and depressive symptoms is found to occur more frequently than anxiety alone. Not surprisingly, anxiety often increases with the progression of disease and the worsening of physical health.

Medical complications such as sepsis, pulmonary embolism, and other acute problems often induce apprehension. Poor control of pain or dyspnea, and drug withdrawal states also incur anxiety. Patients with agitated delirium may be misdiagnosed as having anxiety or pain if a careful assessment for cognitive dysfunction is not undertaken. Adverse drug reactions also need to be considered.

Severe anxiety is seen in patients with akathisia. Akathisia is a subjective feeling of muscular discomfort and inner restlessness associated with anxiety. This syndrome of extra-pyramidal side effects and anxiety is seen in patients who are taking dopamine antagonists. This is usually seen in cancer patients who are prescribed anti-emetic agents to control chemotherapy-induced nausea and vomiting. Metoclopramide seems to top the list of medications prone to induce akathisia in cancer patients. Other medications that may lead to akathisia are prochlorperazine and promethazine. This condition causes patients to feel as if they cannot sit still. The ambulatory patient is often seen pacing; bed-bound individuals are more difficult to diagnosis. Both can have their presentation misinterpreted as being due to emotional distress. A thorough evaluation of the symptoms, a good history, and review of all medications are necessary to make the diagnosis of akathisia.

More commonly, lucid individuals have normal fears and worries related to death or existential issues. Often the existential anxiety is about the loss of autonomy and meaning in life. Issues around death usually relate to concern about separation from family and the future well-being of family members.

Financial and legal issues can also be important at this time. Also, fear about worsening pain or other symptoms may preoccupy the patient. Over the course of a prolonged illness, individuals suffer multiple losses of their normal health. This may result in difficulty coping with their new restrictions and loss of the life they used to enjoy. Important questions to ask may include "What is your biggest fear?" or What things worry you now?"

Treatment

Determining the likely etiology of the patient's anxiety and addressing it are the most fruitful approach. Too often the reflex reaction of the clinician is to simply add an anti-anxiety medication without a careful evaluation of the underlying causes, which may result in poor response and in some cases needless side effects.

Excellent communication skills are needed to listen empathically to the patient's story and concerns. This is time well invested, as patients often feel that they have not had their concerns heard. Taking time to address issues and to answer questions may be all that is required. Effective communication is the first and most important step. A catharsis of emotion may be necessary for healing.

A team of skilled and trained staff, including social workers, chaplains, and therapists, is required to address any psychological or psychosocial issues that may arise and interfere with the treatment. Individuals skilled in relaxation techniques, behavioral modification, hypnosis, and guided imagery can help patients to handle stress and anxiety better. This may result in a better quality of life and a better patient outcome.

Family meetings are an important intervention, as the patient does not live in isolation but is usually closely connected to family members. Addressing openly the worries, concerns, and fears of the patient and family members helps to break down the "conspiracy of silence" that so often accompanies a family's adaptation to serious illness. More functional communication may result. Addressing the family members' anxiety may also result in a less anxious patient.

Pharmacological treatment of anxiety requires careful assessment of the symptoms and choice of medications.[7] Benzodiazepines may be necessary for patients who have profound symptoms related to anxiety, including pervasive worry, insomnia, and autonomic hyperactivity. However, the use of benzodiazepines in the frail terminally ill patient needs to be carefully assessed, as these medications may cause sedation, delirium, falls, and disturbance of normal sleep pattern, as well as inducing tolerance.

A careful assessment of the risks and benefits of such treatment is needed, as well as consideration for discontinuing the drug after a course of initial management. Shorter-acting benzodiazepines, such as lorazepam or alprazolam, are the most commonly prescribed benzodiazepines. In the general population, doses of lorazepam prescribed are 0.5–2.0 mg tid–qid PO or IV and doses of alprazolam prescribed are 0.25–2.0 mg tid–qid PO. In cancer patients, the smaller doses of benzodiazepines are used. A longer-acting benzodiazepine such as clonazepam may be useful to control the overall anxiety throughout the day, which may reduce the frequency of breakthrough anxiety attacks. The doses usually recommended are 0.5–1.0 mg PO bid–tid.

For patients with agitation related to delirium, management with a neuroleptic, such as haloperidol, quetiapine, olanzapine, or chlorpromazine, is preferable. These agents may also be preferred for individuals with anxiety who are deemed fragile and at risk for delirium secondary to administration of a benzodiazapine.

For patients with panic attacks that are frequent and severe, long-term management of anxiety or panic attacks is warranted. These patients are usually managed with SSRI along with benzodiazepine. Benzodiazapines are used to bridge the gap and to provide immediate control of the symptoms while waiting for the SSRI to become effective, which usually takes 2–3 weeks. Treatment of anxiety related to uncontrolled pain or dyspnea with a strong opioid is standard management.[7]

Clinical Pearls

- Asking about suicidal thoughts is an important part of assessing depression.
- Psychotherapy is an important modality for treating depression and adjustment reaction.
- Pain and depression can function in a vicious cycle, one causing the other.
- Complicated grief occurs in 10%–20% of bereaved individuals and requires specialized treatment.
- Excellent communication skills help in managing anxiety.

References

1. Skakum K, Chochinov HM (2005). Anxiety and depression. In: MacDonald N, Oneschuk D, Hagen N, Doyle D (eds.), *Palliative Medicine: A Case-Based Manual*. New York: Oxford University Press, pp. 97–110.
2. McClement SE, Chochinov HM (2009). Depression. In: Walsh D, Caraceni AT, Fainsinger R, Foley K, et al. (eds.), *Palliative Medicine*. Philadelphia: Saunders-Elsevier, pp. 865–70.
3. *Diagnostic and Statistical Manual of Mental Disorders*, 5th edition. (2013). Washington, DC: American Psychiatric Publishing.
4. Breitbart W, Chochinov HM, Passik D (2004). Psychiatric symptoms in palliative medicine. In: Doyle D, Hanks G, Cherny N, Calman K (eds.), *Oxford Textbook of Palliative Medicine*. New York: Oxford University Press, pp. 746–71.
5. Cipriani A, Furukawa TA, Salanti G, et al. (2009). Comparative efficacy and acceptability of 12 new-generation antidepressants: a multiple-treatments meta-analysis. *Lancet* 373:746–58.
6. Wilson KG, Chochinov HM, Skirko MG, et al. (2007). Depression and anxiety disorders in palliative cancer care. *J Pain Symptom Manage* 33(2):118–29.
7. Qaseem A, Snow V, Denberg TD, et al. (2008). Using second-generation antidepressants to treat depressive disorders: a clinical practice guideline from the American College of Physicians. *Ann Intern Med* 149:725–33.
8. Jobes DA, Shneidman ES. (2006). *Managing Suicidal Risk: A Collaborative Approach*, 1st ed. New York: Guilford Press.
9. Shear K, Frank E, Houck PR, et al. (2005). Treatment of complicated grief, a randomized controlled trial. *JAMA* 293(21):2601–8.

Sleep Disturbance

**Marvin Omar Delgado Guay
and Sriram Yennurajalingam**

Introduction

Sleep is a fundamental physiological process that performs a restorative function for the brain and body. It improves energy and the sense of well-being, and for persons living with cancer, sleep provides respite from physical discomfort and psychological stressors.[1-3] Disturbances in both sleep architecture and circadian factors account for the majority of sleep disturbances encountered in the context of cancer.[4]

Sleep disturbances constitute a significant source of distress for patients with cancer.[1-3] Sleep disturbance results in decline in cognitive function, inability to engage in work or recreational activities, and reduced quality of life.[1-4] It is extremely important to identify, recognize, and properly manage these sleep disturbances in order to reduce suffering and improve the quality of life of our patients (see Box 9.1).

This chapter focuses on the impact of sleep disturbances in patients with cancer and other life-limiting illness and on the appropriate assessment and management of these sleep disturbances.

Box 9.1 Assessment and Management of Sleep Disturbances in Patients with Advanced Cancer

Assess

a. Characterize the sleep complaint intensity using a scale from 0 to 10, and characterize the type and duration of the sleep disturbance with the use of sleep diaries and logs (e.g., difficulty initiating sleep, recurrent nocturnal awakenings).

b. Take a comprehensive history, perform an exam, and use objective measures such as actigraphy and polysomnography as indicated to rule out common causes:

1. Cancer-related symptoms, including pain, delirium, anxiety, depression, nausea and vomiting, and dyspnea

2. Side effects of medications, including corticosteroids; psychostimulants, such as modafinil methylphenidate (short and long acting), caffeine, and herbal remedies; antihypertensives, including diuretics and benzodiazepines; and medication withdrawal from alcohol, sedative hypnotics, or opioids

3. Issues affecting the sleep–wake cycle, such as polyuria, nocturia, and disruption in normal schedule (e.g., multiple hospital admissions, poor sleep hygiene)

4. Conditions affecting sleep: brain metastasis, sleep apnea, restless leg syndrome, heart failure, severe COPD

Treat Interdisciplinary Approach

a. Treat the underlying symptom and/or cause.

b. Symptom management, using a combination of pharmacological and nonpharmacological approaches, should be explored if the primary cause cannot be treated.

Pharmacological treatments

- Consider the use of hypnotics on an individual basis but only for short-term use.
- Consider issues such as drug interaction, drug pharmacokinetics and pharmacodynamics, drug side-effect profile, tolerance, addiction, and dependency.

Nonpharmacological treatments

- Sleep hygiene
- Cognitive behavioral therapy
- Muscle relaxation training
- Biofeedback
- Supportive brief psychotherapy.

Sleep Disturbance and Cancer Patients

Patients living with cancer can experience significant disruptions of the normal behaviors and physiology that lead to restful sleep.[1,4] Behaviors of cancer patients that disrupt the sleep cycle include spending more time in bed, reduced daytime activity, and mental stimulation.[1,5] Cancer patients also have a higher probability of being hospitalized or institutionalized, worsening the sleep disturbance.[6]

The prevalence of sleep disturbances in patients living with cancer ranges from 24% to 95%.[1,4,7] This wide range in percentages reflects the use of different definitions of *insomnia* in assessment tools.

According to the International Classification of Sleep Disorders[8] and the *Diagnostic and Statistical Manual of Mental Disorders*,[9] the diagnostic criteria for insomnia syndrome include difficulty initiating sleep (greater than 30 minutes to sleep onset) and/or difficulty maintaining sleep (greater than 30 minutes nocturnal waking time); the presence of sleep difficulty at least 3 nights per week; and sleep difficulty that causes significant impairment of daytime functioning.[4,7–9]

One of the major factors that affect sleep quality in patients living with cancer is the presence of poorly controlled symptoms, especially pain. Patients with pain can experience difficulty with sleep onset and sleep maintenance.[1,4,7] Psychosocial distress, such as depression[10] and anxiety,[11] also plays an important role in the development of sleep disturbances in patients with cancer.[1,4]

The most commonly reported sleep disturbance is frequent waking.[12,13] Of the patients surveyed, 44% reported trouble achieving sleep, and one-third of patients reported waking for extended periods of time (35%) or waking too early (33%).[14] More than half of patients (52%) attributed their sleep disturbance to "intrusive thoughts" and 45% attributed their sleep disturbance to physical discomfort.[1,14]

Silberfarb et al.[15] reported that patients with lung cancer stayed in bed significantly longer than other groups. These patients reported poorer sleep efficiency and more difficulty falling asleep and staying asleep than either patients with breast cancer or normal sleepers.

Women with breast cancer who have completed chemotherapy have lighter sleep, less deep sleep, less REM sleep, and lower sleep efficiency compared to normal sleepers.[4,16] In addition, the presence of hot flashes in breast cancer patients is associated with a higher percentage of wake time, lower percentage of stage 2 sleep, and less efficient sleep compared to nights with no hot flashes.[17]

When the patients receiving hospice care were queried, 70% reported difficultly sleeping, and frequent waking was the most common problem.[18] Interestingly, these patients receiving hospice care reported more than 60% of uncontrolled symptoms.

In another study, Mercadante et al.[19] showed that 30% of patients in an inpatient palliative care unit had insomnia (reported as less than 5 hours of sleep per night). These patients had difficulty with early waking, and waking and falling asleep were associated with fewer hours of sleep. In that study, the presence of depression and anxiety was also associated with insomnia.[19]

Sleep disturbance has a negative impact on quality of life.[20] The presence of sleep deprivation heightens the physical, psychological, social, and existential suffering of cancer patients.[20]

It also contributes to diminished coping capacity and exacerbates symptoms, such as pain and discomfort, and increases the perception of illness severity. Furthermore, the patient's family members also experience these symptoms of distress.

Recent evidence suggests the role of inflammatory mediators such as IL-RA, IL-6, TNF-α, and other inflammatory cytokines, which deregulate the circadian rhythm and hypothalamic pituitary axis, resulting in persistent symptoms such as chronic insomnia, fatigue, and depression in cancer patients; however, the exact mediating mechanisms underlying the pathobiology of sleep disturbances in advanced cancer are unclear.[21]

Assessment of Sleep Disturbances

Insomnia is underreported; Engstrom et al.[22] showed that only 16% of cancer patients with sleep disturbances reported their problem to healthcare providers. Thus, objective measures of sleep disturbance and enhanced questioning by caregivers are necessary.

Assessment Tools

It is important to assess sleep disturbances and to identify related factors and symptoms associated with them. There are several tools used to evaluate sleep disturbances, one being the Edmonton Symptom Assessment System (ESAS),[4,23] which assesses multiple symptoms. The ESAS has been widely used in the clinical setting[23] and has been validated for use in patients with advanced cancer.[24] It consists of 10 questions, rated on a scale of 0 to 10, that evaluate a mix of psychological and physical symptoms, which may include sleep disturbance as an "other symptom."

In addition to the ESAS, it is also very important to evaluate for the presence of delirium, which can be related to insomnia in patients with advanced illnesses.[1]

One of the most frequently used tools to evaluate sleep disturbances is the Pittsburgh Sleep Quality Index (PSQI).[25] It is an effective instrument to measure the quality and patterns of sleep. This instrument enables differentiation of "poor" from "good" sleep through measurement of seven areas: subjective sleep quality, sleep latency, sleep duration, habitual sleep efficiency, sleep disturbances, use of sleeping medication, and daytime dysfunction over the last month. The patient self-rates each of the seven areas of sleep.

The scoring of the answers is based on a 0 to 3 scale, and the seven component scores are added to obtain a global score ranging from 0 to 21. A global sum of 5 or greater indicates a "poor" sleeper.

The PSQI can be used for both an initial assessment and ongoing comparative measurements across all healthcare settings. The PSQI has an internal consistency and a reliability coefficient (Cronbach's alpha) of 0.83 for its seven components.[25] However, because of its length and its relatively complex scoring, it may be difficult to use the PSQI in the clinical setting, particularly in palliative care patients who also require frequent assessments of many other symptoms such as pain, delirium, dyspnea, and fatigue.

Another method for measuring sleep disturbances is an actigraph. It is a simple, noninvasive device approximately the size of a watch that is worn on the wrist. It is used to measure levels of daytime and nighttime activity and can be used to accurately estimate the duration of both daytime and nighttime sleep. Activity data are stored to memory, typically in 30- to 60-second epochs for 24-hour intervals. These data provide diurnal activity counts, nocturnal activity counts, and the means by which to infer sleep continuity parameters, for example, time in bed (sleep period), time awake after sleep onset, total sleep time, and, potentially, sleep latency.

Once uncontrolled symptoms are identified, it is important to treat them properly to reduce suffering in these distressed patients. We will address several methods for treating sleep disturbances in cancer patients in the next section.

Management of Sleep Disturbances

The management of sleep disturbances, as in the case of fatigue, requires a multimodal approach, including pharmacological (Table 9.1) and nonpharmacological interventions. However, research on the efficacy of any specific modality in patients at the end of life is limited.

Pharmacologic Management

Benzodiazepines

Benzodiazepines are used because of their sedative properties to reduce the time to sleep onset and to improve sleep efficiency. Unfortunately, tolerance to these medications occurs rapidly, and their prolonged use can

Table 9.1 Pharmacological Management of Sleep Disturbances in Patients with Advanced Illnesses

Activity	Initial Dose	Considerations
Ultra-short acting		
Zaleplon	5–10 mg	Little to no anxiolytic effect; costly
Short-onset, brief duration		
Triazolam	0.125 mg	Rapid sleep induction; limited effect on
Alprazolam	0.5–1 mg	sleep maintenance
Short-onset, intermediate duration of action		
Zolpidem	5–10 mg	No clear advantage over
Zopiclone	5–7.5 mg	benzodiazepines; costly; minimal
Eszopiclone	3 mg	anxiolytic effect
Intermediate onset, duration		
Lorazepam	0.5–4 mg	Adequate effect on sleep induction
Temazepam	7.5–15 mg	and maintenance; risk of daytime drowsiness
Longer latency to onset, prolonged activity (half-life, metabolites)		
Clonazepam	0.5–2 mg	Slow sleep induction with increased
Chlordiazepoxide	50–100 mg	risk of accumulation of metabolites;
Diazepam	5–10 mg	high risk of daytime sedation
Longer latency to onset, prolonged activity (off-label treatment for insomnia)		
Amitryptilene	25–100 mg	Increased risk of daytime
Imipramine	25–100 mg	sedation, confusion, constipation,
Doxepin	25–100 mg	and cardiac conduction
Trazodone	25–100 mg	abnormalities. Start with 15 mg
Mirtazapine	15–30 mg	at bedtime.
Variable activity (off-label treatment for insomnia)		
Haloperidol	0.5–5 mg	Used mainly in sleep disturbance
Risperidone	0.5–1 mg	related to delirium or psychosis
Olanzapine	5–10 mg	
Quetiapine	25 mg	

cause sleep disturbances, such as fragmented sleep and dependence on medication for sleep onset.[26]

Despite their effect on sleep patterns and architecture, agents acting on the gamma-amino-butyric acid/benzodiazepine receptor, such as zaleplon and zolpidem, do not have a clear clinical advantage for cancer patients with sleep disturbances.[27]

In addition, several side effects have been observed with benzodiazepines, such as daytime sedation, delirium, and fatigue, particularly in the elderly and in those with impaired processing of the medications.[26,27] Furthermore, benzodiazepines have the potential to exacerbate respiratory suppression when combined with opioids, as has been described with methadone, even at a low dose.[28]

Antidepressants

Antidepressants are the first choice if the patient presents with major depression complicated by insomnia. It is important to mention, however, that data on the use of most of these antidepressant agents for primary insomnia are not compelling.[29]

Some antidepressants, especially tricyclics, have been used in persons with neuropathic pain or headache disorders with insomnia.[30] Antidepressant medications can produce desirable side effects, such as sedation, but can also produce undesirable side effects, such as orthostasis, constipation, and anticholinergic activity. In addition, tricyclic antidepressants are associated with the development of cardiac arrhythmias.[29]

Data on the use of antidepressants for sleep disorders are described later in this section.

Selective serotonin reuptake inhibitors (SSRIs) do not have a role in the treatment of insomnia other than depression-related insomnia, because of their very low sedating effects.[1]

The serotonergic antidepressant trazodone has been used for insomnia related to depression because of its sedative and hypnotic effects. However, there are no conclusive data evaluating the minimum effective dose for treating sleep disorder.[31]

Mirtazapine, another antidepressant, acts on different receptors, including serotonin and histamine receptors. It is sedating, can stimulate appetite, and is less toxic than other antidepressants.[32]

Antihistamines do not have a role in the treatment of insomnia associated with cancer because of their side-effect profile, which includes cognitive impairment, delirium, and constipation.[1]

There are limited data regarding the safety and efficacy of alternative or complementary agents, such as valerian root, kava, and melatonin. Melatonin and its agonists have some usefulness in primary insomnia in persons with sleep disturbances secondary to a "phase-shift" disruption of the sleep cycle,[1] although this has not been studied in advanced cancer patients with insomnia.[1,33]

Paltiel et al.[34] reported that cancer patients with sleep disturbances taking tranquilizers and sleeping pills had poorer quality of life and increased severity of physical symptoms when compared with cancer patients who were not taking those medications.

Antipsychotic medications have an important role in managing insomnia in patients with delirium,[35] a common and distressing disorder that affects the advanced-cancer population.[1]

Nonpharmacological Management

Nonpharmacological interventions, such as *cognitive behavioral therapies, sleep hygiene,* and *muscle relaxation,* have been demonstrated to be effective in the treatment of primary insomnia.[35–37] Recent evidence suggests significant benefit in cancer patients.[38] However, cognitive behavioral therapy can be challenging to patients with advanced cancer due to cost, time, limited availability of counselors, and symptom burden; therefore it needs to be customized to a given patient and can be provided by telephone or Internet if the patient is unable to attend the sessions in person. However, further studies in its use in patients with advanced cancer are needed.

Another promising method used in the treatment of sleep disturbances in advanced cancer patients is bright light therapy.[39] Patients with advanced illnesses not only have disruption in the architecture of sleep but also alterations in the circadian rhythm, causing sleep disturbances. Thus, a light, which is the main stimulus for coordinating the circadian system with the external environment, may improve sleep disturbances in these patients.

Ancoli-Israel et al.[39] presented a preliminary report about the effect of bright light on sleep in 11 breast cancer patients receiving chemotherapy, concluding that bright white light may increase the number of hours of sleep in women undergoing chemotherapy, as well as decrease sleep latency and improve sleep quality. No side effects were reported in that study.

Bright light therapy also has been effective in sleep disturbances among demented nursing home patients. Light therapy has also been used for the treatment of seasonal affective disorder and has some effect in nonseasonal depression.[40]

Recent studies also suggest the role of mindfulness-based stress reduction and yoga.[41,42] However, there are limited studies in advanced cancer.

Nonpharmacological therapies demonstrate some advantages over pharmacological interventions in patients with sleep disturbances, including persistent efficacy and no risk of drug interactions or severe adverse effects, although behavioral treatments may have limited application in patients with advanced disease because of the time and energy required to acquire new skills.

Clinical Pearls

- Sleep disturbance is underreported and undertreated. Sleep disturbance affects the quality of life of patients with advanced illnesses and their caregivers and family members.
- A comprehensive evaluation of all symptoms related to sleep disturbances is extremely important.
- In the setting of sleep disturbances in advanced illnesses, always evaluate for the presence of delirium.
- When treating patients with sleep disturbances, it is very important to use a multimodal approach that includes both pharmacological and nonpharmacological interventions.

References

1. Mystakidou K, Parpa E, Tsilika E, et al. (2007). Sleep quality in advanced cancer patients. *J Psychosom Res* 62:527–33.
2. Zisapel N (2007). Sleep and sleep disturbances: biological basis and clinical implications. *Cell Mol Life Sci* 64:1174–86.
3. Maquet P (2001). The role of sleep in learning and memory. *Science* 294:1048–52.
4. Yennurajalingam S, Chisholm G, Palla SL, et al. (2015). Self-reported sleep disturbance in patients with advanced cancer: frequency, intensity, and factors associated with response to outpatient supportive care consultation—a preliminary report. *Palliat Support Care* 13(2):135–43.
5. Morgan K (2003). Daytime activity and risk factors for late-life insomnia. *J Sleep Res* 12:231–8.
6. Sheely L (1996). Sleep disturbances in hospitalized patients with cancer. *Oncol Nurs Forum* 23:109–11.
7. Fiorentino L, Ancoli-Israel S (2006). Insomnia and its treatment in women with breast cancer. *Sleep Med Rev* 10:419–29.
8. *The International Classification of Sleep Disorders*. (1997). Rochester, MN: American Sleep Disorders Association.
9. American Psychiatric Association (1994). *Diagnostic and Statistical Manual of Mental Disorders*, 4th ed. Washington, DC: American Psychiatric Association.
10. Shuster JL Jr, Breitbart W, Chochinov HM (1999). Psychiatric aspects of excellent end-of-life care. Ad hoc committee of end-of-life care. The Academy of Psychosomatic Medicine. *Psychosomatics* 40:1–4.
11. Davis MP, Goforth HW. (2014). Long-term and short-term effects of insomnia in cancer and effective interventions. *Cancer J* 20(5):330–44.
12. Koopman C, Nouriani B, Erickson V, et al. (2002). Sleep disturbances in women with metastatic breast cancer. *Breast J* 8:362–70.
13. Savard J, Simard S, Blanchet J, Ivers H, Morin CM (2001). Prevalence, clinical characteristics, and risk factors for insomnia in the context of breast cancer. *Sleep* 24:583–90.
14. Davidson J, MacLean A, Brundage M, Schulze K (2002). Sleep disturbance in cancer patients. *Soc Sci Med* 54:1309–21.
15. Silberfarb P, Hauri P, Oxman T, Schnurr P (1993). Assessment of sleep in patients with lung cancer and breast cancer. *J Clin Oncol* 11:997–1004.
16. Fiorentino L, Mason W, Parker B, Johnson S, Amador X, Ancoli-Israel S (2005). Sleep disruption in breast cancer patients post-chemotherapy. *Sleep* 28:A294.
17. Savard J, Davidson J, Ivers H, et al. (2004). The association between nocturnal hot flashes and sleep in breast cancer survivors. *J Pain Symptom Manage* 27:513–22.
18. Hugel H, Ellershaw J, Cook L, Skinner J, Irvine C (2004). The prevalence, key causes, and management of insomnia in palliative care patients. *J Pain Symptom Manage* 27:316–21.
19. Mercadante S, Girelli D. Casuccio A (2004). Sleep disorders in advanced cancer patients: prevalence and factors associated. *Support Care Cancer* 12:355–9.
20. Fortner B, Stepanski E, Wang S, et al. (2002). Sleep and quality of life in breast cancer patients. *J Pain Symptom Manage* 24:471–80.
21. Bower JE, Ganz PA, Irwin MR, Kwan L, Breen EC, Cole SW (2011). Inflammation and behavioral symptoms after breast cancer treatment: do fatigue, depression, and sleep disturbance share a common underlying mechanism? *J Clin Oncol* 29(26):3517–22.

22. Engstrom C, Strohl R, Rose L, Lewandowski L, Stefanek M (1999). Sleep alterations in cancer patients. *Cancer Nurs* 22:143–8.

23. Bruera E, Kuehn N, Miller MJ, Selmser P, Macmillan K (1991). The Edmonton Symptom Assessment System (ESAS): a simple method for the assessment of palliative care patients. *J Palliat Care* 7:6–9.

24. Chang VT, Hwang SS, Feuerman M (2000). Validation of the Edmonton Symptom Assessment Scale. *Cancer* 88:2164–71.

25. Buysee DJ, Reynolds CF, Monk TH, Berman SR, Kupfer DJ (1989). The Pittsburgh Sleep Quality Index: a new instrument for psychiatric practice and research. *Psychiatry Res* 28:193–13.

26. Ohayon M, Lader M (2002). Use of psychotropic medication in the general population of France, Germany, Italy, and the United Kingdom. *J Clin Psychiatry* 63:817–25.

27. Drover D (2004). Comparative pharmacokinetics and pharmacodynamics of short-acting hypnosedadives: zaleplon, zolpidem, and zopiclone. *Clin Pharmacokinet* 43:227–38.

28. Corkery J, Schifano F, Ghodse A, Oyefeso A (2004). The effects of methadone and its role in fatalities. *Hum Psychopharmacol* 19:565–76.

29. Fava M, Hoog S, Judge R, Kopp J, Nilson M, Gonzalez J (2002). Acute efficacy of fluoxetine versus sertraline and paroxetine in major depressive disorder including effects of baseline insomnia. *J Clin Psychopharmacol* 22:137–47.

30. Sindrup S, Jensen T (1999). Efficacy of pharmacological treatments of neuropathic pain: an update and effect related to mechanism of drug action. *Pain* 83:389–400.

31. Saletu-Zyhlarz G, Abu-Bakr M, Anderer P, et al. (2002). Insomnia in depression: differences in objective and subjective sleep and awakening quality to normal controls and acute effects of trazodone. *Prog Neuropsychopharmacol Biol Psychiatry* 26:249–60.

32. Theobald D, Kirsh K, Holtsclaw E, Donaghy K, Passik S (2002). An open-label, crossover trial of mirtazapine (15 to 30 mg) in cancer patients with pain and other distressing symptoms. *J Pain Symptom Manage* 23:442–7.

33. Kuriyama A, Honda M, Hayashino Y (2014). Ramelteon for the treatment of insomnia in adults: a systematic review and meta-analysis. *Sleep Med* 15(4):385–92.

34. Paltiel O, Marzec-Boguslawska A, Soskolne V, et al. (2004). Use of tranquilizers and sleeping pills among cancer patients is associated with a poorer quality of life. *Qual Life Res* 13:1699–1706.

35. Morin C, Colecci C, Stone J, Sood R, Brink D (1999). Behavioral and pharmacological therapies for late-life insomnia. *JAMA* 281:991–9.

36. Quesnel C, Savard J, Simard S, Ivers H, Morin CM (2003). Efficacy of cognitive-behavioral therapy for insomnia in women treated for nonmetastatic breast cancer. *J Consult Clin Psychol* 71:189–200.

37. Chesson A, Anderson W, Littner M (1999). Practice parameter for the non-pharmacologic treatment of chronic insomnia. *Sleep* 22:1128–33.

38. Roscoe JA, Garland SN, Heckler CE, Perlis ML, Peoples AR, Shayne M, Savard J, Daniels NP, Morrow GR (2015). Randomized placebo-controlled trial of cognitive behavioral therapy and armodafinil for insomnia after cancer treatment. *J Clin Oncol* 33(2):165–71.

39. Ancoli-Israel S, Rissling M, Trofimenko V, Parker A (2007). Preliminary effects of bright light on sleep in women with breast cancer. *J Clin Oncol ASCO Annual Meeting Proc Suppl*, p. 9094.

40. Eagles J (2006). Light therapy and seasonal affective disorder. *Psychiatry* 5:199–203.

41. Garland SN, Carlson LE, Stephens AJ, Antle MC, Samuels C, Campbell TS (2014). Mindfulness-based stress reduction compared with cognitive behavioral therapy for the treatment of insomnia comorbid with cancer: a randomized, partially blinded, noninferiority trial. *J Clin Oncol* 10:32(5):449–57.

42. Mustian KM, Sprod LK, Janelsins M, Peppone LJ, Palesh OG, Chandwani K, Reddy PS, Melnik MK, Heckler C, Morrow GR (2012). Multicenter, randomized controlled trial of yoga for sleep quality among cancer survivors. *J Clin Oncol* 31(26):3233–41.

Chronic Nausea and Vomiting

Shalini Dalal

Definition and Prevalence

Chronic nausea and vomiting are common symptoms in patients with advanced-stage disease, and these symptoms significantly impact patients' quality of life.[1] In advanced cancers, the reported prevalence is between 40% and 70%, depending on the patient characteristics and assessment methods used.

There is no standardized definition for chronic nausea. For research purposes it is often defined as nausea lasting more than 4 weeks. In the terminally ill, however, the presence of nausea for more than 1 week, in the absence of a well-identified, self-limiting cause (e.g., chemotherapy or radiotherapy), is used.

Pathophysiology

The pathophysiology of chronic nausea and vomiting is complex. In the palliative care population, multiple mechanisms may be simultaneously involved in the generation of symptoms. Figure 10.1 illustrates the various pathways and centers known to be involved in the emetic pathway. These are briefly described in this section.

Two areas in the brainstem (medulla) are critical for the control of emesis: the vomiting center (VC) and the chemoreceptor trigger zone (CTZ). The VC, located in the lateral reticular formation of the medulla, is the physiological control center. It is not a discrete anatomic site, but represents interrelated neuronal networks, including the nucleus tractus solitarius (NTS) and the dorsal motor nucleus of the vagus (DMV).[2]

The NTS receives various afferent neuronal pathways, which include (1) cortical pathways from higher cortical centers, which respond to increased intracranial pressures, sensory (pain, sight, smell) and psychogenic

Figure 10.1. Pathophysiology of nausea and vomiting.

CTZ = chemoreceptor trigger zone; ICP = intracranial pressure; 5-HT3 = serotonin; D2 = dopamine; M = muscarinic/cholinergic; NK-1 = neurokinin-1; H-1 = histamine.

(memory, conditioning, fear) stimuli; (2) vestibular pathways, which respond to vertigo and visuospatial disorientation; (3) peripheral pathways (via the vagus and splanchnic nerves) from the gastrointestinal (GI) tract, visceral capsules, and the parietal serosal surfaces; and (4) neuronal connections from the CTZ.

The CTZ, located in the area postrema of the medulla, also receives afferent input from the GI tract via the vagus and splanchnic nerves. Unlike the VC, the CTZ is functionally located outside the blood–brain barrier and is therefore able to sample emetogenic toxins, metabolic abnormalities, such as uremia or hypercalcemia, or drugs in the blood and spinal fluid. It cannot, however, initiate emesis independently and does so only via stimulation of the NTS.

Once the vomiting center (NTS) receives signals from the various afferent sources mentioned in the preceding paragraphs, the information is processed and the DMV puts out an appropriate vasomotor efferent response (respiratory, salivatory, gut, diaphragm, and abdominal muscles), inducing nausea, retching, or vomiting, depending on the intensity and duration of received signals.

Etiology

Chronic nausea has many etiologies. Some of the more common ones are illustrated in Figure 10.2. In many patients, the underlying cause(s) may be difficult to determine.

Opioids are one of the most common causes of chronic nausea in terminally ill patients. Although opioid-induced nausea is usually transient and responds well to anti-emetics, some patients, particularly those receiving high doses of opioids, may continue to experience chronic and severe

Figure 10.2. Etiology of chronic nausea and vomiting.

nausea. Other medications causing nausea include nonsteroidal anti-inflammatory drugs (NSAIDs) and antibiotics.

Delayed chemotherapy-induced nausea and vomiting (CINV) refers to symptoms that occur 24 hours after chemotherapy administration, which may last for as many as 6–7 days.

Patients with HIV may have nausea, which is a side effect of all the drugs of the antiretroviral therapy (ART) regimen.

Constipation is a common complication in terminally ill patients and may cause or aggravate nausea. Factors that predispose to the development of constipation include opioid analgesics, immobility, poor oral intake and dehydration, autonomic failure, and other medications.

The etiology of nausea may be related to the underlying disease. For instance, in cancer patients, nausea is often present in association with intra-abdominal disease, such as liver metastasis, bowel obstruction from mechanical compression by tumor, or peritoneal carcinomatosis.

The stomach and duodenum can be compressed, causing the "squashed-stomach syndrome." Nausea may be present secondary to primary or metastatic brain involvement by tumor or leptomeningeal disease. Radiation therapy to the spine or abdomen may be followed by nausea and vomiting.

Assessment

As nausea is a subjective symptom, its expression varies from patient to patient. From a practical point of view, this occasionally leads to a lack of correlation between the observed expression of nausea and the presumed pathophysiology of the underlying condition.

It is also important to note that the term *nausea* may mean different things to different people and may be used by some patients to describe other symptoms, including abdominal discomfort, pain, distention, or early satiety.

There are a number of ways to assess nausea intensity, such as visual analog scales, numerical scales, and verbal descriptors, but there is no gold standard for nausea assessment. Because the causes of chronic nausea and vomiting are often multifactorial, the assessment needs to be multidimensional, with awareness that these symptoms are dynamic processes and may frequently change in intensity.

Further, it is important to assess the symptom of nausea in the context of other commonly experienced symptoms, such as pain, appetite, fatigue, depression, and anxiety. This multidimensional assessment allows formulation of an overall therapeutic strategy. An example of a validated multidimensional assessment tool is the Edmonton Symptom Assessment System (ESAS).[3]

A detailed history and physical examination are essential and may provide clues to the underlying etiology of symptoms (see Table 10.1). Intensity, frequency, exacerbating and relieving factors, onset, and duration of nausea should be documented. If there is coexistent vomiting, the nature and volume of vomiting can give a clue to the etiology.

Large-volume emesis may indicate gastric outflow obstruction, whereas small-volume emesis may indicate gastric stasis. The extent to which emesis interferes with oral intake should be noted, as large and frequent volume vomiting puts the patient at risk of dehydration. A history of syncopal episodes or early satiety should alert the physician of the possibility of autonomic insufficiency.

Investigations to exclude renal impairment, hepatic failure, and other metabolic abnormalities such as hypercalcemia, hypokalemia, and hyponatremia should be undertaken.

A computed tomography scan of the brain may be indicated when brain metastases are suspected. Abdominal X-rays may be useful in assessing nausea. A supine X-ray may indicate the presence of stool and fecal impaction. Erect or decubitus views may show air and fluid levels in the bowel, which is typical of bowel obstruction.

Table 10.1 Clues from History and Physical Examination to the Etiology of Chronic Nausea and Vomiting

Findings on History and Physical Examination	Possible Etiology
Pattern of infrequent large-volume vomitus that relieves nausea	Bowel obstruction—partial or complete
	Gastric outlet obstruction
Symptoms of nausea or vomiting related to movements	Vestibular dysfunction; mesenteric traction
History of polyuria and polydipsia	Hyperglycemia
	Hypercalcemia
Associated changes in mental status	Brain metastasis, metabolic abnormalities (examples: hyperglycemia, hypercalcemia, hyponatremia, renal failure, liver failure [elevated ammonia levels])
Papilledema	Raised intracranial pressure as with brain metastasis
Orthostatic blood pressures, absence of heart rate variability with valsalva, syncopal episodes	Autonomic insufficiency
Decreased frequency of bowel movements	Constipation
History of a mood disorder or anxiety	Anxiety
Medication/treatment history	Treatment-specific syndromes (delayed chemotherapy-induced nausea and vomiting [CINV])
Chemotherapy or radiation	
Antibiotics; HIV medications	
Epigastric pain, anemia; melena	Peptic ulcer disease (use of NSAIDs or corticosteroids)
Use of NSAIDs	
Distended abdomen, shifting dullness, fluid wave	Ascites
Distended abdomen, absent bowel sounds	Bowel obstruction

Management

Appropriate management of chronic nausea and vomiting depends on a detailed assessment. General supportive measures should be instituted in all patients. These include maintenance of good oral hygiene (poor oral hygiene can contribute to nausea), the creation of a comfortable environment for the patient, regular baths to prevent unpleasant body odors, and attention to diet.

Small volumes of food at regular intervals should be considered for patients with early satiety associated with nausea.

Specific Interventions

When an underlying cause or causes of nausea and vomiting have been identified, there should be an attempt to correct these (Table 10.2). Metabolic abnormalities should be corrected if this is possible and appropriate for the clinic setting.

In situations where opioid toxicity is suspected, a change of opioids using equianalgesic doses can be expected to improve symptoms of nausea while maintaining pain control. Unnecessary medications should be discontinued.

Aggressive bowel care, including cleansing enemas and regular laxatives, should be instituted when constipation or stool impaction is suspected.

In some cases, such as in patients with brain metastases, symptom control may be attempted with radiation therapy or corticosteroids. If peptic ulcer disease is suspected, appropriate treatment should be instituted.

Pharmacological Interventions

Given the lack of well-designed relevant studies, there are no convincing data for the best pharmacological strategy for treatment of nausea and vomiting. Current management is based on expert opinion rather than on evidence. Both mechanistic-based and empiric regimens have been used with no head-to-head comparisons of these approaches.

The various classes of anti-emetics and their site of receptor action, if known, are presented in Table 10.3 and are briefly discussed further. Important considerations in choosing an anti-emetic should be likely etiology and severity of symptoms, the drug's potential adverse effect, available routes of administration, and cost.

Table 10.2 Examples of Specific Interventions When the Etiology of Nausea and Vomiting Is Known or Suspected

Etiology	Intervention
Hypercalcemia	Hydration, bisphosphonates
Opioid toxicity	Opioid rotation or decrease dose
Constipation	Aggressive bowel regimen. Consider X-rays
Gastric ulceration	Proton pump inhibitors (PPIs), H2-antagonists
Infection	Antibiotics
Tense ascites	Paracentesis, consider intraperitoneal (IP) catheter
Anxiety	Counseling, anxiolytics
Brain metastases	Radiation therapy, steroids
Bowel obstruction	Conservative versus surgical procedures (e.g., resection, bypassing, or stenting, venting gastrostomy)

Table 10.3 Anti-Emetic Agents

Class	Examples
Dopamine antagonists	Metoclopramide, haloperidol, prochlorperazine, chlorpromazine
Prokinetic agent	Metoclopramide
Antihistaminics	Diphenhydramine, meclizine, hydroxyzine, promethazine
Anticholinergics	Scopolamine (transdermal), hyoscyamine, glycopyrrolate
Serotonin antagonists	Ondansetron, granisetron, dolasetron
Cannabinoids	Dronabinol, nabilone
Corticosteroids	Dexamethasone, methylprednisolone
Other useful agents	Lorazepam, octreotide

Dopamine Antagonists

Agents from this group exert their anti-emetic effects centrally (predominantly CTZ) by antagonizing dopamine (D2) receptors. These agents do not increase GI motility and so are useful in patients presenting with bowel obstruction. Drugs in this group differ on the basis of their additional activities.

Haloperidol is a narrow-spectrum agent, with mainly D2 antagonistic activity with negligible anticholinergic or antihistaminic effects. Its oral bioavailability is approximately 65%. It is highly protein bound and is not cleared by the kidney, making it safe in the presence of renal failure.

Initial doses range from 0.5 to 2 mg/mL, which can be given orally or parenterally at 4-hour intervals. When used subcutaneously, it is recommended that the concentration of haloperidol be kept below 1.5 mg/mL to avoid precipitation of haloperidol crystals.[4]

The broader-spectrum agents include chlorpromazine, prochlorperazine, and promethazine, and have dopaminergic, cholinergic, and histamine receptor antagonism. Side effects may include extrapyramidal reactions, hypotension, urinary retention, constipation, dry mouth, and sedation.

Prochlorperazine has a low oral absorption (14%) and is usually administered via the rectal or parenteral routes. Promethazine has a slightly better oral bioavailability (25%) than that of prochlorperazine.

Prokinetic Agents

Metoclopramide hydrochloride, a substituted benzamide, has a dual mechanism of action. It is predominantly a dopaminergic antagonist but also has prokinetic effects via the cholinergic system in the myenteric plexus. Local acetylcholine release, mediated by the 5-HT4 receptor, appears to play an important role in reversing gastroparesis and bringing about normal peristalsis in the upper GI tract.

Because of its short half-life (3 hours), metoclopramide requires frequent administration via oral or parenteral routes. Continuous infusion of metoclopramide can be given when intermittent doses fail to control nausea.

Side effects include akathisia and extrapyramidal reactions (more likely in younger patients), which may not be dose dependent. Anticholinergic medications, including tricyclic antidepressants (TCAs), antagonize the prokinetic effect so should not be co-administered.

Antihistaminics

Antihistaminics, such as cyclizine, promethazine, and dimenhydrinate, are useful anti-emetics, particularly if a vestibular component to the nausea is identified. Drowsiness is a major side effect.

Antimuscarinic/Anticholinergic Agents

This group includes tertiary and quaternary ammonium derivatives. Tertiary compounds such as atropine and scopolamine are lipophilic, cross the blood–brain barrier, and frequently cause sedation and confusion.

Glycopyrrolate, a quarternary compound, has little CNS penetration and is therefore preferred. Anticholinergics have been used to reduce symptoms of nausea and abdominal colic when they are associated with mechanical bowel obstruction.

Serotonin Antagonists

These agents are widely used and effective in the management of chemotherapy- and radiotherapy-induced nausea and vomiting. In addition, they may also have a role in other situations, such as for refractory nausea in the palliative care setting, although more research is needed.

Trials comparing serotonin antagonists and metoclopramide have either had methodological problems or used inadequate doses of metoclopramide (e.g., 10 mg three times per day). There have been some reports of its effectiveness in treating patients' refractory nausea.

Neurokinin-1 Receptor Antagonists

In clinical studies, neurokinin-1 (NK-1) receptor antagonists have shown efficacy in reducing both acute and delayed CINV when added to other anti-emetics.[5] The potential role of NK-1-receptor antagonists in the treatment of chronic nausea and vomiting in advanced cancer or other palliative care population is currently unknown.

Cannabinoids

The proposed mechanism of action of dronabinol is through brainstem cannabinoid receptors. Several studies have demonstrated its efficacy as an anti-emetic agent for the treatment of CINV.

In a study of patients with AIDS-related cachexia, dronabinol showed significant improvement in nausea, appetite, and mood, without weight gain.[6] Side effects, such as somnolence, confusion, and perceptual disturbance, are common, particularly in the elderly. Euphoria is more common than dysphoria in younger patients.

Larger studies are needed to assess the value of cannabinoids as anti-emetics in patients with advanced disease.

Corticosteroids

Corticosteroids have powerful nonspecific anti-emetic effects that are not well understood. They may act by modulation of prostaglandin release. They can decrease peritumoral edema, thus reducing intracranial pressure, a known cause of nausea.

Corticosteroids are beneficial in combination with other anti-emetic agents such as 5-HT3 antagonists or metoclopramide in the prevention and management of acute and delayed chemotherapy-induced emesis.[7] Corticosteroids are also useful in the management of other symptoms that may coexist with nausea in the palliative care population, such as pain, anorexia, and asthenia.

Nonpharmacologic Interventions

Behavioral and Complementary Therapies

Much of the research on psychological and nonpharmacological interventions has been conducted in chemotherapy or postoperative patients.

Acupuncture and acupressure have been shown to augment the effect of anti-emetics during chemotherapy and to reduce postoperative nausea and vomiting.

Transcutaneous electrical nerve stimulation (TENS) has also been shown to enhance the effect of anti-emetic drugs. Its effects may be mediated by endogenous opioid peptides.

A meta-analysis of 19 randomized trials found equivalent benefit of non-pharmacological treatment of nausea in postsurgical patients compared to traditional therapy.[8] This benefit was not found in children. The modalities studied were acupuncture, electroacupuncture, TENS, acupoint stimulation, and acupressure.

Similar analysis has not been performed in patients with advanced disease. Other studies have included progressive muscle relaxation and guided mental imagery during periods of chemotherapy and have shown beneficial effects.

Cognitive therapy has been found to be effective in providing relief of psychological morbidity associated with physical symptoms in advanced cancer.[9] The adaptation of these techniques to palliative care patients with nausea warrants research.

Surgical Interventions

In patients with nausea or emesis caused by mechanical obstruction, surgical procedures such as percutaneous gastrostomy for gastric outlet obstruction, colostomy, intestinal bypass, or laparotomy for obstruction (such as secondary to tumors or adhesions) may be considered for symptom control and to improve life expectancy and quality of life. This is provided the patient's general physical condition suggests a life expectancy long enough to result in benefit from surgery.

Based on current evidence, there is no consensus on the indications for conservative versus surgical treatment of patients with advanced cancer. Thus, consideration for surgical interventions should be individualized, weighing the risks and benefits of the procedure.

Even when patients appear to be candidates for surgical procedures, these procedures are associated with complications and may not be successful in relieving symptoms.[10] Published data show operative mortality ranging from 9% to 40% and complication rates from 9% to 90%.

Newer endoscopically placed stents for gastric outlet obstruction offer the advantage of lower cost, the possibility of an outpatient procedure, and low risk of complications. Abdominal paracentesis or a permanent intraperitoneal catheter may be helpful in the patient with nausea and ascites who does not respond to conventional therapy.

Conclusion

Chronic nausea and vomiting are common and distressing symptoms in patients with terminal cancer. These symptoms are likely to be due to several factors, including autonomic failure, opioid analgesics, metabolic abnormalities, constipation, and cachexia.

Promotility agents (sometimes in combination with corticosteroids) are in most cases the drug of choice for management of chronic nausea and vomiting. Pharmacological agents, such as progestational drugs and thalidomide, need further evaluation of their potential beneficial effects in patients with chronic nausea.

Despite significant ongoing research of acute chemotherapy-induced and postoperative emesis, research is lacking for treatment of chronic nausea. Drugs that have been found to be effective in acute vomiting, such as serotonin and neurokinin-1 (NK-1) receptor antagonists, require further evaluation in advanced-cancer patients with chronic nausea.

References

1. Portenoy RK, Thaler HT, Kornblith AB, et al. (1994). Symptom prevalence, characteristics and distress in a cancer population. *Qual Life Res* 3:183–9.
2. Carpenter DO (1990). Neural mechanisms of emesis. *Can J Physiol Pharmacol* 68:230–6.
3. Bruera E, Kuehn N, Miller MJ, et al. (1991). The Edmonton Symptom Assessment System (ESAS): a simple method for the assessment of palliative care patients. *J Palliat Care* 7:6–9.
4. Storey P, Hill HH, St Louis RH, et al. (1990). Subcutaneous infusions for control of cancer symptoms. *J Pain Symptom Manage* 5:33–41.
5. Glare P, Miller J, Nikolova T, et al. (2011). Treating nausea and vomiting in palliative care: a review.
6. Beal JE, Olson R, Lefkowitz L, et al. (1997). Long-term efficacy and safety of dronabinol for acquired immunodeficiency syndrome-associated anorexia. *J Pain Symptom Manage* 14:7–14.
7. Ioannidis, JPA, Hesketh, PJ, Lau J (2000). Contribution of dexamethasone to control of chemotherapy-induced nausea and vomiting: a meta-analysis of randomized evidence. *J Clin Oncol* 18:3409–22.
8. Lee A, Done ML (1999). The use of nonpharmacologic techniques to prevent postoperative nausea and vomiting: a meta-analysis. *Anesth Analg* 88:1362–9.
9. Greer S, Moorey S, Baruch JD, et al. (1992). Adjuvant psychological therapy for patients with cancer in a prospective randomized trial. *BMJ* 304:675–80.
10. Ripamonti C, Conno FD, Ventafridda V, et al. (1993). Management of bowel obstruction in advanced and terminal cancer patients. *Ann Oncol* 4:15–21.

Constipation and Bowel Obstruction

Joseph A. Arthur

Bowel Obstruction

Definition and Prevalence

Bowel obstruction is a common and distressing complication of intra-abdominal cancer.[1] Impairment to the aboral passage of intestinal contents may result from either mechanical obstruction or failure of normal intestinal motility in the absence of an obstructing lesion (ileus).

Intestinal obstruction may be categorized according to the degree of obstruction to the flow of intestinal contents (partial or complete), the absence or presence of intestinal ischemia (simple or strangulated), and the site of obstruction (small intestinal or colonic).

The three most common causes of small bowel obstruction (SBO) are postoperative intra-abdominal adhesions, hernias, and neoplasms. In the palliative care setting, cancer is usually the underlying cause. Bowel obstruction is particularly common in patients with intra-abdominal malignancies.[1]

Malignant bowel obstruction (MBO) can lead to multiple distressing symptoms that require urgent palliative interventions. In a consecutive series of 163 patients referred with malignant ovarian tumors, 24 (14.7%) patients developed major bowel complications. In terminal patients with recurrent ovarian cancer, the incidence is estimated to be around 42%. Once an MBO occurs, median survival is approximately 3 months.[2]

Causes

Malignant bowel obstruction is an odious complication of numerous malignancies, most notably ovarian and colorectal cancers. The two most common primary malignancies causing SBO in a series of 32 patients were colorectal (41%) and ovarian adenocarcinoma (28%).

Hematogenous metastases from breast adenocarcinoma, melanoma, or Kaposi sarcoma also may involve the intestine and can cause MBO.

Primary neoplasms of the small bowel are the cause of SBO in less than 3% of cases. Both carcinoid tumors and adenocarcinoma have been reported as the most common malignancies of the small intestine to cause symptoms of obstruction.

Mechanisms of bowel obstruction in malignancy are illustrated in Figure 11.1.

Pathophysiology

Bowel obstruction results in an accumulation of gastric, pancreatic, and biliary secretions that are a potent stimulus for further intestinal secretions, reduced absorption of water and sodium from the intestinal lumen, and an increase in water and sodium secretion because of increased gastric distension. Depletion of water and salt in the lumen is considered the most important toxic factor in bowel obstruction.[3]

Impaired water and electrolyte absorption and enhanced secretion cause the net movement of isotonic fluid from the intravascular space into the intestinal lumen. The accumulation of swallowed air and, to a lesser extent, hydrogen, carbon dioxide, and methane generated by bacterial overgrowth within the obstructed bowel contribute to intestinal dilatation.

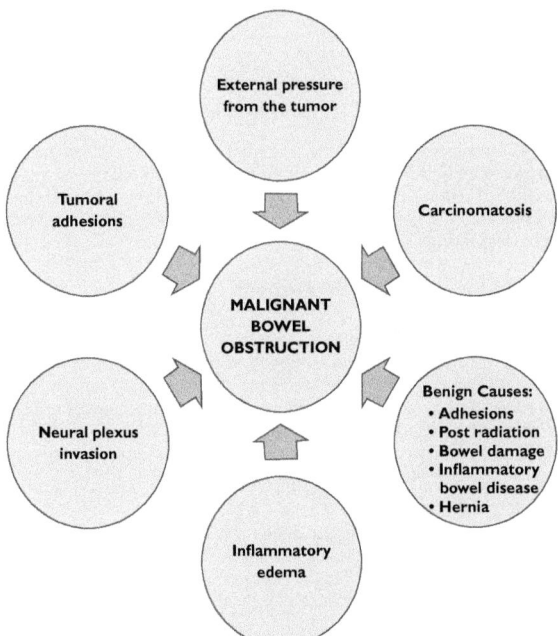

Figure 11.1. Common causes of malignant bowel obstruction.

The failure of normal intestinal motility with SBO allows the overgrowth of bacteria within the small intestine and loss of the normally increasing concentration gradient of bacteria from the jejunum to the ileum.

In one study using a porcine model of ileal obstruction, there was a 10,000-fold increase in the concentration of *Escherichia coli* in the ileum and a 40 million–fold increase in the jejunum over counts in normal controls. Data in humans and in animals suggest that the overgrowth of enteric bacterial flora occurs within a few hours of obstruction and is maximal by 24 hours.

Clinical Presentation

The clinical picture of MBO can vary greatly from patient to patient, depending on the location of the obstruction, the number of obstruction points (single or multiple), the mechanism of obstruction, exacerbating medications, and the extent and sites of tumor recurrence.[4]

The symptoms, which are almost always present, include nausea and vomiting, intestinal colic, and continuous abdominal pain. Vomiting generally develops early in high intestinal-tract occlusion (gastric or duodenal and small bowel), whereas it occurs later in patients with large-bowel obstruction.

Abdominal colic is present in 72%–76% of cases with advanced ovarian cancer and bowel involvement, and it this is usually due to bowel distension. Continuous abdominal pain is experienced by more than 90% of these patients.[2]

The absence of stool and flatus passage is a common symptom reported by patients, especially those with complete bowel obstruction. Patients with bowel obstruction can also suffer from diarrhea, which is caused by bacterial liquefaction. In palliative care patients, management of these symptoms can be challenging.

Diagnosis and Clinical Assessment

History and Physical Exam

The diagnosis of SBO requires a thorough assessment. It is usually established on clinical grounds and is supported or confirmed by radiographic testing. A history of previous episodes and intra-abdominal surgery is highly suggestive of obstruction. The abdomen should be inspected for any surgical scars and the degree of distention.

Auscultation may reveal high-pitched or hypoactive bowel sounds and is therefore not very helpful in making a diagnosis.

Laboratory and Imaging Data

Laboratory investigations have a limited role in the diagnosis of SBO but can be of help in the determination and management of metabolic and electrolyte abnormalities. Radiological examinations include an upright chest film to rule out the presence of free air, as well as supine and upright abdominal films.

Contrast X-rays may help in defining the site and the extent of the obstruction, including the accompanying dysmotility. Barium provides excellent radiological definition, but it is not absorbed and may interfere with subsequent endoscopic procedures or cause severe impaction.

Gastrografin is preferable because it offers similar radiological definition. In some circumstances, it is useful in restoring the intestinal transit in reversible obstruction.

An abdominal CT scan is useful in evaluating the global extent of malignancy and aids in making therapeutic decisions regarding further treatment. CT findings of obstruction are similar to traditional radiographic findings: disparate dilation of proximal bowel loops compared with more distal ones.

Comparative studies have shown that CT is superior to plain-film radiography in detecting intestinal obstruction and in determining the cause of obstruction. Studies have shown CT sensitivities ranging from 90% to 95% in detecting obstruction, with no false-positive examinations.

Differential Diagnoses

The differential diagnoses include the possibility of other causes of nausea and vomiting, constipation, and abdominal pain of other causes, including progressive intra-abdominal malignancy.

It is important to assess the possibility of metabolic abnormalities such as hypercalcemia or hypokalemia, the type and dosage of different medications that could have effects on intestinal motility, and nutritional and hydration status.[3]

Management

Symptom relief is the main goal of palliative care for these patients, although management of this situation is not well defined.

Surgical Approach

Surgical palliation is a complex issue in patients with advanced cancer. The decision to proceed with a surgical approach should be individualized to the disease stage, the patient's condition, and the possibility of future antineoplastic therapy. Patients with a life expectancy of > 2 months are more likely to benefit from surgery. Surgery should not be routinely undertaken in patients with advanced and end-stage cancer who do not have a benign cause of occlusion. It will only benefit select patients with mechanical obstruction and/or limited tumor or a single site of obstruction and those with a reasonable chance of further response to antineoplastic therapy.

Nonsurgical Approach

In inoperable patients, the usual treatment consists of drainage with a nasogastric tube associated with parenteral hydration. This treatment can cause great discomfort and a number of complications to the patient. Therefore, it should be considered a temporary measure to reduce the gastric distension while pharmacological treatment is initiated to control the amount of secretion and vomiting. If continued drainage is required, a gastrostomy is much more tolerable for medium- and long-term decompression of the GI tract.

In patients with single-site colonic obstruction, the use of endoscopically inserted, self-expanding metallic stents is a rapid and effective nonsurgical means of relieving left-sided colonic obstruction.

Pharmacological Measures

Several drugs have proved useful in controlling symptoms and avoiding use of a nasogastric tube, which can lead to several complications such as nasal cartilage erosion, aspiration pneumonia, otitis, esophagitis, and bleeding.

The main drugs used are analgesics, anti-emetics, and drugs to decrease bowel secretions. Other agents commonly used include steroids, smooth muscle relaxants, and anticholinergic drugs like atropine, scopolamine, and its analogs.[4]

Most patients with MBO cannot tolerate the oral route, so alternative routes should be considered for drug administration.

Opioids

Opioids are the most effective drugs for the management of abdominal pain associated with bowel obstruction. These drugs can be administered subcutaneously, transdermally, or intravenously.

Anticholinergic Drugs

Anticholinergic drugs such as hyoscine in the form of either butylbromide or hydrobromide, and glycopyrrolate can be added to opioids for colicky pain if the opioids alone are not effective.

Hyoscine butylbromide and glycopyrrolate have less penetration to the blood– brain barrier and thus have much fewer CNS side effects than hyoscine hydrobromide. Both hyoscine hydrobromide and butylbromide can be given intravenously, intramuscularly, or subcutaneously. Hyoscine hydrobromide can also be delivered transdermally (scopolamine patch). Glycopyrrolate is given intravenously or intramuscularly.

Corticosteroids

Corticosteroids are used commonly in the medical management of MBO. They exert their effect by reducing intestinal and tumor-associated edema.

A recent systematic review of the role of corticosteroids in management of MBO in patients with ovarian and colorectal cancer showed evidence that corticosteroids in the dose range of 6–16 mg dexamethasone given intravenously may resolve bowel obstruction.[5]

Metoclopramide

Metoclopramide is the first-line anti-emetic for patients with partial bowel obstruction in the absence of colicky pain. It is contraindicated in patients with complete obstruction because it might produce vomiting and pain due to its prokinetic activities.

Other Pharmacological Agents and Anti-Emetics

Other pharmacological agents and anti-emetics include neuroleptics such as haloperidol or prochlorperazine, or antihistamines such as dimenhydrinate or cyclizine. Haloperidol is considered the first-line anti-emetic because it can be added to morphine and to scopolamine butylbromide or octreotide in the same subcutaneous (SC) infusion.

Somatostatin and Its Analogs (Octreotide and Vapreotide)

Somatostatin and its analogs have been used either alone or in combination to alleviate symptoms from an MBO in ovarian cancer and other malignancies. Somatostatin inhibits hormones such as glucagon and insulin, reduces acid secretion, slows intestinal mobility, decreases bile flow, and reduces splanchnic blood flow.

Among the antisecretory drugs, octreotide has been shown to reduce nausea and vomiting in bowel-obstructed patients through a reduction of gastrointestinal (GI) secretions, thus allowing removal of the nasogastric tube and alleviation of associated distress in most patients.

Octreotide exerts actions similar to those of somatostatin, but it has a longer half-life and more potently inhibits growth hormone, glucagon, and insulin. Octreotide suppresses luteinizing hormone (LH) response to gonadotropin-releasing hormone (GnRH) and inhibits the release of gastrin, secretin, vasoactive intestinal peptide (VIP), motilin, and pancreatic polypeptide. Its duration of action is 8–12 hours and it has been used successfully for management of MBO.

Octreotide can be administered by SC or IV infusion, or by bolus parenteral injection with duration of approximately 12 hours.

In a recent study of octreotide (300 mcg/day) used for bowel obstruction in 43 evaluable terminally ill cancer patients, the symptom score as evaluated by the M. D. Anderson Symptom Inventory improved in 59%–72% of patients and overall quality of life improved in 56% of patients.[4]

Summary

Bowel obstruction is a distressing condition in palliative care patients. Malignant bowel obstruction is the most common type. Symptom relief should be the fundamental focus of management in these patients. Surgical approaches have limited benefit in patients with MBO.

Pharmacological decompression is the mainstay of management. Some patients may require a temporary nasogastric tube or a long-term gastrostomy tube for decompression. Common pharmacological agents used include opioids, anticholinergics, steroids, and somatostatin analogues.

Constipation

Definition and Prevalence

Constipation is a clinical syndrome, rather than a symptom. It is defined as the passage of small, usually hard feces, infrequently and with difficulty.[6,7]

Constipation is one of the most common complaints in the general population, the prevalence ranging from 1.9% to 27.2% (an average of 15% has been described in most studies). It is more common in women than in men and also more common in terminally ill people with cancer than in those with other terminal diseases. Constipation affects more than 50% of patients in a palliative care unit or hospice. This might actually underestimate the problem, since many of these patients are already on stool softeners and/or laxatives.

The Rome criteria are often used to define constipation for research or drug regulatory purposes: the presence of two or more of the following symptoms for at least 3 months:

- Straining at least 25% of the time
- Hard stools at least 25% of the time
- Incomplete evacuation at least 25% of the time
- Two or fewer bowel movements per week.

Practically, these criteria might be difficult to apply in palliative care patients. There is a wide interindividual variability in normal bowel patterns. Therefore, constipation in an individual patient should be defined according to that patient's experience.

Causes of Constipation in Palliative Care Patients

In the palliative care population, the etiology of constipation can be related to the primary illness or secondary associated factors such as autonomic failure, drugs (especially opioids), dehydration, and electrolyte abnormalities.

Figure 11.2 illustrates the most common causes contributing to constipation in palliative care patients.

Primary Causes

- Intestinal abnormality
- Tumor compression
- Neural plexus invasion
- Idiopathic constipation
- Slow-transition constipation
- Dyssynergic defecation

Secondary Causes

Electrolyte Imbalance
- Hypercalcemia
- Hyperkalemia

Endocrine Abnormality
- Hypothyroidism
- Diabetes mellitus

Neurogenic Disorders
- Multiple sclerosis
- Spinal cord injury

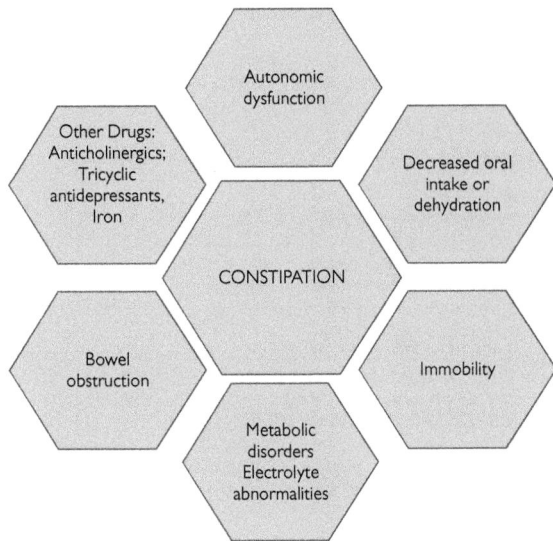

Figure 11.2. Common causes of constipation in palliative care patients.

Drugs
- Analgesics (mainly opioids)
- Anticholinergic drugs (antidepressants, antispasmodics, antipsychotics)
- Chemotherapeutic agents

Other Causes
- Dehydration
- Immobility
- Decreased oral intake

Pathophysiology
In palliative care patients, disturbance in normal bowel habits can be multi-factorial, and pathologies at different levels can contribute to altered bowel function. These include dysmotility syndromes secondary to central and autonomic dyssynergy between neurohormonal and myogenic pathways and fluid and electrolyte imbalance.

Normal bowel function requires the coordination of motility, mucosal transport, and defecation reflexes. Motility of the small intestine, colon, and sphincteric regions is controlled by myogenic characteristics, central nervous system mechanisms, activity of the peripheral autonomic nervous system, and circulating GI hormones.

The autonomic nervous system regulates colonic movements through both of its divisions: the sympathetic and parasympathetic nervous systems.

Constipation, as a sign of peripheral nerve damage, is seen in generalized as well as localized autonomic dysfunction. The most frequently observed condition is diabetic autonomic neuropathy.

Histopathological studies of the vagus nerve in patients with diabetes and GI manifestations have shown reductions in the number of unmyelinated fibers, indicating a role for autonomic dysfunction (AD) in these symptoms.

Clinical Assessment

History and Physical

Initial management includes a thorough history of the individual's previous normal bowel habits. Recent variation and change in the pattern in bowel habits need to be defined in terms of the amount, frequency, consistency, straining, drug history, and associated symptoms. Since it is mainly the patient's perception, in certain cases, obtaining a diary of bowel habits can be useful.

Subjective measures of constipation, such as questionnaires or visual analog (VAS) or adjectival scales, are easy to use and are valid. One less time-consuming questionnaire, the Constipation Assessment Scale (CAS) designed by McMillan and Williams, determines constipation severity.

Physical examination includes abdominal auscultation for quality of bowel sounds, inspection, palpation, and percussion. Digital rectal exam is an important component of assessment to rule out fecal impaction and obstruction.

Diagnostic Tests

Check for reversible causes such as electrolyte imbalance or endocrine disorders. Sometimes the history and physical examination may not be very reliable in palliative care patients, and an objective study is required to assess constipation.

Although a static tool, Bruera et al. showed that radiographic studies provide good correlation with fecal load in the palliative care population.[8]

Management

Management of constipation can be divided into preventive measures and therapeutic measures. Figure 11.3 illustrates general guidelines for the assessment and management of constipation.

Preventive Measures

- Patient education
- Increase dietary and fluid intake
- Prophylactic laxatives when initiating the patient on opioids
- Encourage patients to increase mobility
- Providing a comfortable environment for defecation

Therapeutic Measures

Therapeutic modalities to treat existing constipation can also be divided into general interventions and pharmacological treatment.

Pharmacological Approaches

Oral laxatives include emollients, bulk-forming agents, osmotic (saline) agents, hyperosmolar agents, contact cathartics, prokinetic drugs, and opioid antagonists (Table 11.1). Bulk-forming agents like psyllium and

Figure 11.3. General guidelines for the assessment and management of constipation. Opioid antagonists are approved only for treatment of opioid-induced constipation.

methylcellulose require at least 300–500 mL of water ingestion, otherwise fecal impaction may occur. Hence their use is discouraged in palliative care patients who usually tend to have decreased oral intake. Rectal preparations include suppositories and enemas (Table 11.1). The rectal route may be very unpleasant for sick patients, but the quick satisfactory results in most cases make them an acute short-term choice of treatment for intractable constipation. Apart from their specific mechanisms of action, rectal agents act by stimulating the ano-colonic reflex to induce defecation. They are contraindicated in patients with thrombocytopenia and neutropenia.

Several forms of lubricant, osmotic, surfactant, and polyphenolics laxatives are available as rectal preparations, including suppository and enemas, but the latter form is reserved for constipation unrelieved by suppository.

Investigational and New Approaches

In recent years, new pharmacological agents have been studied that have shown promising results. These include opiate antagonists, chloride channel activators, neurotrophins, and serotonergic enterokinetic agents.

Opioid Antagonists

Opioid-induced constipation (OIC) is mediated by mu receptors in the GI system. Medications that act on the mu opioid receptor to selectively antagonize the GI effects of opioids, particularly constipation, have been studied in several studies.[9,10] Examples include methylnaltrexone, naloxone, and alvimopan.

Methylnaltrexone, a quaternary derivative of naltrexone, has restricted ability to cross the blood–brain barrier and therefore does not affect opioid analgesic effects or induce opioid withdrawal symptoms. It has been approved for the treatment of OIC in patients with advanced illness.[11]

Table 11.1 Commonly Used Laxatives for Treatment of Constipation

Laxatives	Mechanism	Recommended Doses	Onset of Action	Comments
Emollients Docusate Mineral oil	Act as detergents and help lower surface tension	Start 300 mg/day. Maximum 800 mg/day 15–45 mL/day	1–3 days Oral: 6–8 hours Rectal: 2–15 minutes	Ensure adequate fluid intake Lipid pneumonitis with aspiration
Bulk forming Psyllium Methylcellulose	Natural or synthetic, act by absorbing water in the intestine, increasing stool bulk, thereby promoting peristalsis and reducing transit time	Start 5–7 g/day Start 4–7 g/day	12–72 hours 12–72 hours	Requires at least 300–500 mL of water ingestion, otherwise impaction may occur
Hyperosmolar agents Lactulose Polyethylene glycol Sorbitol	These laxatives are undigestible, unabsorbable compounds that remain within the colon and retain the water that already is in the colon. The result is softening of the stool.	Start: 15–30 mL/day Max: 60 mL/day in 1–2 divided doses 17–34 g/day 30–150 mL (as 70% solution)	24–48 hours 48–96 hours 24–48 hours	Abdominal bloating, colic, and flatulence Urticaria Pulmonary edema and hyperglycemia
Stimulants Bisacodyl Senna	Stimulate peristalsis by directly irritating smooth muscle of the intestine, possibly the colonic intramural plexus; alter water and electrolyte secretion, producing net intestinal fluid accumulation and laxation	Start: 5 mg/day Max: 30 mg/day Start 15 mg/day Max 70–100 mg/day	6–10 hours 6–12 hours	Electrolyte and fluid imbalance Nausea, vomiting, melanosis coli

Prokinetic agents Metoclopramide	Promote colonic transit by increasing colonic motor activity	40–120 mg/day 30–80 mg/day	Variable Variable	Extrapyramidal symptoms Results are not impressive. Consider for refractory constipation. Avoid in cardiac patients.
Opioid antagonists Methylnaltrexone	Mu-receptor antagonist	38 ≤62 kg: 8 mg 62–114 kg: 12 mg > 114 kg: 0.15 mg/kg (round dose up to nearest 0.1 mL of volume)	30–60 minutes	Only approved for opioid-induced constipation
Rectal preparation Sorbitol Lactulose enemas	Hyperosmolar agent	120 mL of sorbitol 25%–30% solution 200–300 mL of lactulose solution should be mixed with 700 mL of water or saline and retained for 30 to 60 minutes.	0.5–3 hours	Also used for hepatic encephalopathy
Saline enemas Glycerine suppository Bisacodyl suppository	Saline enemas cause water to be drawn into the colon. Glycerin suppositories act by irritating the rectum Bisacodyl act as a stimulant laxative	Dose varies by the type of saline laxative Single dose 2–3 g/day 10 mg daily	0.5–6 hours 0.5–3 hours Less than 1 hour	Repeated enemas may result in electrolyte disturbances May cause local irritation

A systematic review and meta-analysis randomized controlled trials looking at the efficacy of these agents demonstrated that they are more effective than placebo for the treatment of OIC. The number needed to treat (NNT) with methylnaltrexone, naloxone, and alvimopan in order to prevent one patient with OIC failing to respond to therapy were 3, 4, and 5, respectively.[12] There was no significant increase in likelihood of reversal of analgesia with these medications. The most common side effect was diarrhea.

Chloride Channel Activator

Chloride channel activators enhance chloride-rich intestinal fluid secretion and increase intestinal motility.

Lubiprostone has been approved on the basis of two placebo-controlled trials in which it achieved significant results to relieve constipation and abdominal symptoms in patients with chronic idiopathic constipation. The most common adverse effect observed was nausea, which was dose related. The approved dose is 24 mcg twice a day with food.

Neurotrophins

The neurotrophic factor involved in the development of the nervous system has been studied in a phase II, randomized, double-blind trial. Subcutaneous neurotrophin-3, three times per week, significantly increased the frequency of bowel movements and improved other measures of constipation.

Serotonergic Enterokinetic Agents

Serotonin is involved in regulating gut motility, visceral sensitivity, and intestinal secretion through serotonin 5-HT4 receptors, which are expressed mainly by enteric nervous system interneurons. Serotonergic enterokinetic agents stimulate 5-HT4 receptors on these enteric nervous system interneurons to enhance the peristaltic reflex and have shown efficacy for the treatment of chronic constipation. An example is prucalopride, a selective 5-HT4 receptor agonist.

Nonpharmacological Approaches

The nonpharmacological measures used in prevention can also be incorporated into the treatment of constipation.

Biofeedback has proved to be beneficial in patients with dyssynergic defecation but has not shown any significant improvement in patients with slow-transit constipation.

In a Cochrane database review, aromatherapy and massage were not found to be effective for the treatment of constipation in cancer patients.

Summary

Constipation is a common symptom in patients with advanced illnesses that is underestimated even by palliative care physicians. The focus of treatment should start with proactive interventions. Disease processes should be taken into account for individualized management to effectively treat this debilitating complaint.

A lack of evidence-based clinical research leaves us with little guidance as to which laxative regimen to choose over another. Convenience of use, cost, tolerance, and effectiveness of the particular agent should be taken into consideration when managing constipation in palliative care patients.

Clinical Pearls

Bowel Obstruction

- Once MBO is diagnosed, median survival is 3 months.
- Surgery has little or no role in the management of MBO.
- Metoclopramide and other prokinetics are contraindicated in patients with complete MBO.
- Octreotide can be beneficial in reducing intestinal secretions and motility.

Constipation

- Constipation can present as pseudo-diarrhea.
- Always perform a thorough medication history and discontinue constipating drugs when possible.
- Bulk-forming agents should be discouraged in palliative care patients.
- When in doubt, a plain abdominal X-ray can confirm the diagnosis of constipation.
- Opioid antagonists can be beneficial in patients with opioid-induced constipation.

Reference

1. Mangili G, Aletti G, Frigerio L, et al. (2005). Palliative care for intestinal obstruction in recurrent ovarian cancer: a multivariate analysis. *Int J Gynecol Cancer* 15(5):830–835.
2. Baines M, Oliver DJ, Carter RL (1985). Medical management of intestinal obstruction in patients with advanced malignant disease. A clinical and pathological study. *Lancet* 2(8462): 990–993.
3. Ripamonti C, Bruera E (2002). Palliative management of malignant bowel obstruction. *Int J Gynecol Cancer* 12(2):135–143.
4. Hisanaga T, Shinjo T, Morita T, Nakajima N, et al. (2010). Multicenter prospective study on efficacy and safety of octreotide for inoperable malignant bowel obstruction. *Jpn J Clin Oncol* 40(8):739–745.
5. Feuer DJ, Broadley KE (2000). Corticosteroids for the resolution of malignant bowel obstruction in advanced gynaecological and gastrointestinal cancer. *Cochrane Database Syst Rev* 2000(2):CD001219.
6. Bruera E, Fadul N (2004). Constipation and diarrhea. In *Oxford Textbook of Palliative Medicine*. Oxford, UK: Oxford University Press.
7. Sykes, N (2010). Constipation and diarrhea. In *Oxford Textbook of Palliative Medicine*. Oxford, UK: Oxford University Press.
8. Bruera E, Suarez-Almazor M, Velasco A, et al. The assessment of constipation in terminal cancer patients admitted to a palliative care unit: a retrospective review. *J Pain Symptom Manage* 9(8):515–519.
9. Thomas J, Karver S, Cooney GA, et al. (2008). Methylnaltrexone for opioid-induced constipation in advanced illness. *N Engl J Med* 358(22):2332–2343.
10. Michna E, Blonsky ER, Schulman S, et al. (2011). Subcutaneous methylnaltrexone for treatment of opioid-induced constipation in patients with chronic, nonmalignant pain: a randomized controlled study. *J Pain: Official Journal of the American Pain Society* 12(5):554–562.
11. Jansen JP, Lorch D, Langan J, et al. (2011). A randomized, placebo-controlled phase 3 trial (Study SB-767905/012) of alvimopan for opioid-induced bowel dysfunction in patients with non-cancer pain. *J Pain: Official Journal of the American Pain Society* 12(2):185–193.
12. Ford AC, Brenner DM, Schoenfeld PS (2013). Efficacy of pharmacological therapies for the treatment of opioid-induced constipation: systematic review and meta-analysis. *Am J Gastroent* 108(10):1566–1574; quiz 1575.

Delirium

Shirley H. Bush

Definition and Prevalence

Delirium is a complex multifactorial syndrome that results from global organic cerebral dysfunction. It is a severe neuropsychiatric syndrome that is frequently overlooked or misdiagnosed by healthcare professionals. Hence some prodromal delirium symptoms such as anxiety, insomnia (resulting from sleep–wake cycle disturbance), and mood changes may be treated with anxiolytics, benzodiazepines, and antidepressants, which may inadvertently worsen the delirium episode.

Delirium prevalence ranges from 26% to 62% of patients during admission to an inpatient palliative care setting, and increases up to 88% in the last weeks and hours before death.[1]

Delirium causes significant distress to patients, their families, and caregivers.[2] Distress was rated as "severe" in 80% of hospitalized cancer patients who recalled their delirium experience.[3] Delirium impairs patient communication, thus making the assessment of pain and other symptoms challenging.

Agitated delirium and accompanying disinhibition may be misinterpreted as increased pain intensity, with the resulting increased opioid administration exacerbating the delirium severity. Delirium also causes significant morbidity and prognosticates an increased likelihood of death.

Pathophysiology

This is highly complex, and many neurotransmitter disturbances are thought to be involved in the pathogenesis of delirium.[4] In addition to the dopamine excess and acetylcholine deficiency theories, circulating cytokines, other neuroinflammatory mediators, and increased microglial activity have also been implicated.

Causes

The etiology of delirium is usually multifactorial (Figure 12.1), with a median of 3 (range 1–6) precipitants per delirium episode. Causes of delirium can be categorized into potential predisposing and potential precipitating factors, but often a specific cause remains unidentified.

Predisposing factors increase a patient's baseline susceptibility for developing delirium—for example, preexisting cognitive impairment and reduced sensory input with poor vision or deafness.

Precipitating factors are the actual causative triggers for the delirium episode—for example, electrolyte disturbance, infection or sepsis, and psychoactive medications.

Urinary retention and constipation are factors that are capable of aggravating agitation, especially in the elderly.

Medication-Induced Delirium

Many psychoactive drugs can cause a patient to become acutely confused. Commonly implicated medications are opioids, benzodiazepines, corticosteroids, and anticholinergics. Other causative drugs include antidepressants, antihistamines, antipsychotics, certain anti-emetics and antivirals, antibiotics (quinolones), cimetidine and ranitidine, anticonvulsants, and chemotherapeutic agents.

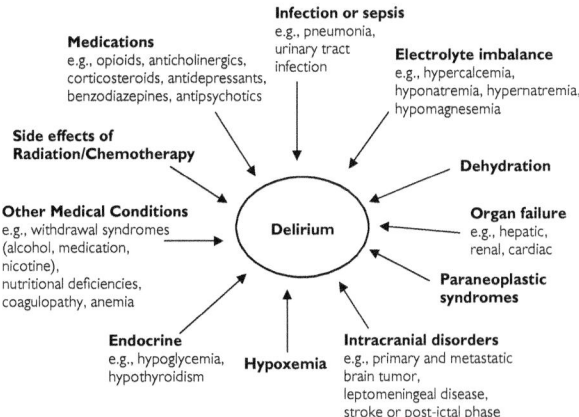

Figure 12.1. Potential precipitating factors contributing to delirium in cancer patients.

Opioid-induced neurotoxicity (OIN) is a syndrome of neuropsychiatric side effects seen with opioid therapy. The components of OIN are severe sedation, hallucinations, cognitive impairment or delirium, myoclonus and seizures, allodynia (pain associated with a nonpainful stimulus, like light touch), and hyperalgesia (increased response to a painful stimulus). There is no specific order of development of these symptoms—they may occur as a single feature or in any combination.

The healthcare professional must remain vigilant, as any patient prescribed opioids is at potential risk of OIN with the accumulation of toxic opioid metabolites (see Chapter 4 on pain management with opioids).

Presentation and Diagnosis

Early identification is important and enables earlier treatment of delirium and education. An essential feature for the clinical diagnosis of delirium (Criteria A) from the *Diagnostic and Statistical Manual of Mental Disorders*, 5th edition (*DSM-5*) is a disturbance in attention and awareness (reduced orientation to the environment).[5] Other *DSM-5* diagnostic criteria for delirium include development over a short period of time (usually hours to a few days) and fluctuation in severity during the course of a day (Criteria B), as well as an additional disturbance in cognition, such as memory deficit, disorientation, language, visuospatial ability, or perception (Criteria C). Specifically, the disturbances in Criteria A and C do not occur in the context of a severely reduced level of arousal, such as coma.

Non-core clinical features of delirium include sleep–wake cycle disturbance, altered psychomotor activity, delusions, and emotional lability.

Three clinical subtypes of delirium have been described according to the type of psychomotor activity:

- *Hyperactive*: impaired cognition + agitation ± hallucinations ± delusions ± myoclonus ± hyperalgesia (may be mistaken for anxiety or extrapyramidal side effects, such as akathisia)
- *Hypoactive*: impaired cognition + somnolence ± withdrawal (may simulate depression)
- *Mixed*: alternating symptoms of both hyperactive and hypoactive delirium.

The majority of delirium episodes in palliative care patients are either of the hypoactive or mixed subtype. Hyperactive and mixed subtypes are highly associated with drug-induced delirium. Predominantly hypoactive delirium is associated with dehydration and encephalopathies.

Differential Diagnosis

Dementia

- Change in cognition with little or no clouding of consciousness, insidious onset over months.

Lewy Body Dementia

- Fluctuating symptom severity: cognitive impairment, visual hallucinations, delusions, and parkinsonism.

Depression

- Hypoactive delirium in particular may be misdiagnosed as depression.

Screening and Diagnostic Tools

Multiple validated delirium-specific assessment tools are available.[6] For the purposes of this chapter, a few will be detailed. The Mini-Mental State Examination (MMSE)[7] and Blessed or Short Orientation Memory and Concentration Test (SOMCT)[8] are cognitive screening tools that can assess cognitive impairment but not necessarily diagnose delirium.

Delirium Screening Tools

These should be used in all patients, even with no overt signs of delirium, to enable early diagnosis and treatment.

The Confusion Assessment Method (CAM)[9] is a brief, easy-to-use, four-item diagnostic algorithm based on the *DSM-III-R* criteria. It is a widely used screening tool that requires a brief assessment of cognition or attention but does not measure delirium severity. It has been validated in the palliative care setting and requires a moderate level of training.

The Nursing Delirium Screening Scale (Nu-DESC)[10] is an observational five-item scale (possible range 0–10) that includes the four items of the Confusion Rating Scale (CRS) and an additional assessment of psychomotor retardation. It is a low-burden tool that takes less than 2 minutes to complete for each nursing shift. It is used for delirium screening and may potentially be used to monitor delirium severity.

The Delirium Observation Screening (DOS) Scale is also a nurse-rated observational tool (13-item) that has recently been validated in a palliative care unit.[11]

Delirium Severity Rating Tools

The Memorial Delirium Assessment Scale (MDAS)[12] is a 10-item, 4-point, clinician-rated instrument (possible range 0–30). It was originally designed to measure delirium severity, but has diagnostic potential. A cutoff total MDAS score of 13/30 was used for delirium diagnosis in the original validation study, but a subsequent validation study used a cutoff score of 7 (with scores ≥ 7/30 indicating the presence of delirium).[13]

The Revised Delirium Rating Scale (DRS-R-98)[14] is a 16-item, clinician-rated scale. It has three diagnostic items (temporal onset of symptoms, fluctuation of symptom severity, and physical disorder) and 13 severity-related items. Items are rated on a scale of 0 to 2 or 3, with a maximum total score of 46. The 13-item severity section can be used as a separate scale. Training in the use of the DRS-R-98 is necessary.

Clinical Assessment and Investigations

▶ Fifty percent of delirium episodes in advanced-cancer patients are reversible. If consistent with the patient's goals of care, reversible causes should be identified and treated as appropriate.

Clinical History

In addition to a comprehensive medical history (including a history of alcohol or substance abuse, and multidimensional symptom assessment), ask the patient specifically about hallucinations (they are more often tactile than visual) and delusional thoughts, as patients frequently do not volunteer these symptoms. Medication history (new and continuing drugs) should also be reviewed.

It may be necessary to obtain a surrogate history from a family member or caregiver, and to ascertain the patient's baseline mental status.

Physical Examination

Look for clinical signs of sepsis, OIN (including myoclonus), other medication side effects, dehydration, metabolic abnormalities, and other potential causes of delirium (see Figure 12.1). Abnormal movements such as asterixis and signs of bifrontal dysfunction (e.g., palmo-mental, snout, and grasp reflexes) may be present.

Investigations

Order investigations as appropriate to the patient's goals of care and illness trajectory, such as CBC, electrolytes, calcium (with albumin), renal and liver function, magnesium, random blood glucose, urinalysis +/− urine culture, and O_2 saturation. Other tests may be indicated, such as chest X-ray, ammonia levels if severe liver impairment is suspected, and radiological imaging of the brain with CT or MRI scan (see Figure 12.2).

Figure 12.2. Delirium assessment and treatment algorithm.

CAM = Confusion Assessment Method; AP = antipsychotic; EOL = end of life.

Management

Comprehensive management should involve the multidisciplinary team.

Treatment of Underlying Causes

For patients who are at the end of life, treatment strategies should be individualized according to the patient and family's goals of care. Reversibility correlates with the precipitating factor(s).

- *Opioid-induced neurotoxicity (OIN)*: Rotate or switch opioids. The equianalgesic dose of the new opioid should be reduced by 30%–50% (see Chapter 4 on pain management and opioid rotation).
- *Other medications*: Dose taper all deliriogenic medications and discontinue where possible.
- *Infection or sepsis*: Start appropriate antibiotics if this is the agreed-upon management approach after discussing goals of care and treatment options with the patient and the patient's family.
- *Dehydration*: Start IV hydration if a line is already established. Alternatively, start hypodermoclysis (HDC) with normal saline at 40–80 mL/hour, or alternatively give subcutaneous (SC) boluses of 250 cc administered over 1 hour, three or four times daily.
- *Hypercalcemia*: Treat with hydration, using saline, and bisphosphonates. Denosumab has been used in the management of refractory hypercalcemia.
- *Hypoxia*: Treat the underlying cause and administer oxygen.
- *Brain tumor or metastasis*: Consider high-dose corticosteroids (e.g., dexamethasone 8–16 mg daily, in divided doses).

Pharmacological Treatment of Distressing Delirium Symptoms

Antipsychotics are considered to be first-line agents. Haloperidol is the most commonly used (see Table 12.1). Titrate the antipsychotic dose to delirium severity, as long as there are no rate-limiting side effects. Once symptoms are under control, start reducing the antipsychotic dose to the minimal effective dose as soon as possible. If the delirium episode resolves, discontinuation of the antipsychotic should be trialed.

Low-dose haloperidol has also been used by some specialists for the management of hypoactive delirium.

More sedating antipsychotics, such as chlorpromazine and levomepromazine (methotrimeprazine) (not available in the United States), may be helpful for patients with severe agitation.

- ► Dose reduction of antipsychotics and slower titration are often needed for the elderly.
- ► Exercise caution when using benzodiazepines, as they can worsen the delirium. They should not be used as single agents. For acutely disturbed patients, lorazepam has been used in conjunction with haloperidol, as has midazolam.
- ► Antipsychotics can reduce the seizure threshold, thereby potentially increasing the risk of seizures in susceptible patients.
- ► QTc interval prolongation can occur with many antipsychotics, including atypical antipsychotics (also see Table 12.2).

Table 12.1 Guide to Commonly Used Antipsychotics for Symptomatic Treatment of Delirium in Palliative Care

Drug (Generic) Name	Route	Commonly Used Starting Doses (Reduce in Elderly)	Other Comments
Conventional Antipsychotics			
Haloperidol	PO (tablet and oral solution), SC, IV, IM	0.5–2 mg every 6–12 hours and 0.5–2 mg every 1–4 hours as needed For severe agitation: ↑ to 1–2 mg SC/IV every 30 minutes as needed during first hour, then every hour as needed	Average oral bioavailability of haloperidol is 60%; thus parenteral doses are approximately twice as potent as oral Need ECG monitoring when IV route used
Chlorpromazine	PO, IV, IM	12.5–25 mg every 4–12 hours	More sedating than haloperidol Adverse effect of orthostatic hypotension
Levomepromazine (methotrimeprazine) Not available in US	PO, SC, IV, IM	12.5–25 mg every 4–12 hours	More sedating than haloperidol Adverse effect of orthostatic hypotension
Atypical Antipsychotics			
Risperidone	PO (tablet & oral solution), ODT	0.25–1 mg every 12–24 hours	
Olanzapine	PO, ODT, IM	2.5–5 mg every 12–24 hours	Sedating Metabolic syndrome can occur, but significance is not clear as usually only used for short time period in delirium
Quetiapine	PO	12.5–25 mg every 12–24 hours	Sedating Less likely to cause EPS

EPS = extrapyramidal side effects; ODT = orally disintegrating tablet.

Table 12.2 Adverse Effects of Haloperidol*

Extrapyramidal Side Effects (EPS)	Comments	Management
Acute dystonias (typically within days) *Acute akathisia* (typically within weeks) *Antipsychotic-induced parkinsonism* (usually after several weeks) Triad: bradykinesia, tremor, rigidity *Tardive dyskinesia* (usually after months of treatment)	↓ with parenteral administration ↓ with coadministration of anticholinergic ↑ with CYP2D6 substrate slow metabolizers	*Acute dystonias/akathisia:* If possible, reduce or cease causative drug. Prescribe an oral anticholinergic drug, such as benzatropine. Prescribe an antihistaminic antimuscarinic drug, such as diphenhydramine. Consider switching to an atypical antipsychotic. *Antipsychotic-induced parkinsonism:* If possible, reduce or cease causative drug. Prescribe an oral anticholinergic drug. Consider switching to an atypical antipsychotic. *Tardive dyskinesia:* Often poor response to drug treatment. Withdrawal of causative drug may lead to slow improvement, but sometimes irreversible. May be worsened by oral anticholinergic drugs.

(continued)

Table 12.2 (Continued)

Extrapyramidal Side Effects (EPS)	Comments	Management
QTc Interval Prolongation	**Risk Factors**	1. Review and correct electrolyte levels if low ($\downarrow$ K, $\downarrow$ Mg, $\downarrow$ Ca).
With any prolongation of QTc interval, especially > 500 msec, patient is at risk of developing torsades de pointes (polymorphic ventricular tachycardia), with the threat of sudden cardiac death in the absence of medical intervention.	High-dose haloperidol (any route) IV haloperidol Congenital long QT syndrome Electrolyte abnormalities ($\downarrow$ K, $\downarrow$ Mg, $\downarrow$ Ca) $\uparrow$ Age (> 65 years) Female Cardiac disease Bradycardia Hypothyroidism Concomitant administration of other drugs associated with QTc interval prolongation	2. Review other administered drugs that also have the potential to $\uparrow$ QTc interval.
		3. May require dose reduction or discontinuation of haloperidol (and other contributory medications) if QTc > 450 msec for males and > 470 msec for females, or increases > 25% from baseline. APA guidelines (1999).[†]
FDA alert (September 2007): Recommends ECG monitoring if haloperidol given by IV route		4. Consider pharmacy and cardiology consultations.
Sedation	Rare	Cease causative drug
Neuroleptic (Antipsychotic) Malignant Syndrome Severe muscle rigidity Hyperthermia Altered mental status Autonomic dysfunction	Infrequent and idiosyncratic Potentially fatal	General supportive care Benzodiazepines may help muscle rigidity. In severe cases, consider bromocriptine (IV dantrolene has been used in acute medical settings).

* Note: There is often marked variation in patient sensitivity.

† Practice guideline for the treatment of patients with delirium. *Am J Psychiatry* 1999;156(5 Suppl):1–20.

► Although extrapyramidal side effects (EPS) are less likely with atypical antipsychotics, they can occur at higher doses, especially risperidone > 6 mg/day.

⚠ Caution using antipsychotics in patients with Lewy body dementia, Parkinson dementia, and Parkinson disease because of the risk of EPS.

⚠ The use of typical and atypical antipsychotics in the elderly has been associated with an increased risk of cerebrovascular events and mortality, especially in patients with dementia taking antipsychotics for a median of 2–4 months.

⚠ The US Food and Drug Administration (FDA) has previously released Public Health Advisories and alerts for conventional and atypical antipsychotics. See www.fda.gov for current information.

Psychostimulants, such as methylphenidate, have been used in the management of hypoactive delirium. They may exacerbate or cause agitation and may cause hallucinations, restlessness, insomnia, and cardiovascular effects. In the absence of RCT evidence, they are not currently recommended.[15]

Nonpharmacological Approaches

Simple environmental measures are extremely important but often underutilized.

- Ensure a physically safe environment and minimize noise and excessive light.
- Normalize sleep–wake cycle (open blinds during day, minimize background noise at night, and discourage excessive daytime napping where possible).
- Ensure the presence of familiar objects, and a visible clock and calendar.
- Enlist family members to assist with reorientation; use orientation board.
- Use clear and simple communication (do not forget the importance of glasses, hearing aids, dentures).

Psychosocial Support and Education

Hypoactive delirium is just as distressing for patients as hyperactive delirium. Patients who have recovered from an episode of delirium may need debriefing. Delirium also causes significant family distress. Emotional and informational support should be proactively provided.

Confusion and agitation are expressions of brain malfunction and not necessarily of discomfort or suffering. Disinhibition is one of the main components of delirium that must be appropriately explained to families and, at times, to other healthcare professionals.

Refractory Agitated Delirium

This will often necessitate the use of more sedative medications for patient symptomatic relief and comfort when other interventions have failed (see Chapter 13 regarding palliative sedation at the end of life).

Clinical Pearls

- To avoid missing the diagnosis of delirium, screen regularly using a validated delirium-specific assessment tool.
- Approximately 50% of delirium episodes in patients with advanced cancer are reversible.
- Review for contributing factors, especially opioids and psychoactive medications, as well as other potentially reversible causes if consistent with goals of care.
- Agitated delirium and accompanying disinhibition with grimacing and moaning may be incorrectly interpreted as pain, with the resulting inappropriately increased opioid administration worsening the agitated delirium, thus creating a vicious cycle.
- Providing psychosocial support and education may help to reduce the distress of patients, families, and professional caregivers.

References

1. Hosie A, Davidson PM, Agar M, Sanderson CR, Phillips J (2013). Delirium prevalence, incidence, and implications for screening in specialist palliative care inpatient settings: a systematic review. *Palliat Med* 27(6):486–98.
2. Lawlor PG, Bush SH (2015). Delirium in patients with cancer: assessment, impact, mechanisms and management. *Nature Rev Clin Oncol.*12(2):77–92.
3. Breitbart W, Gibson C, Tremblay A (2002). The delirium experience: delirium recall and delirium-related distress in hospitalized patients with cancer, their spouses/caregivers, and their nurses. *Psychosomatics* 43(3):183–94.
4. Maldonado JR (2013). Neuropathogenesis of delirium: review of current etiologic theories and common pathways. *Am J Geriatr Psychiatry* 21(12):1190–222.
5. American Psychiatric Association. (2013). *Diagnostic and Statistical Manual of Mental Disorders*, 5th edition. Arlington, VA: American Psychiatric Association.
6. Leonard MM, Nekolaichuk C, Meagher DJ, et al. (2014). Practical assessment of delirium in palliative care. *J Pain Symptom Manage* 48(2):176–90.
7. Folstein MF, Folstein SE, McHugh PR (1975). "Mini-mental state": a practical method for grading the cognitive state of patients for the clinician. *J Psychiatr Res* 12(3):189–98.
8. Katzman R, Brown T, Fuld P, Peck A, Schechter R, Schimmel H (1983). Validation of a short orientation-memory-concentration test of cognitive impairment. *Am J Psychiatry* 140(6):734–9.
9. Inouye SK, van Dyck CH, Alessi CA, Balkin S, Siegal AP, Horwitz RI (1990). Clarifying confusion: the Confusion Assessment Method. A new method for detection of delirium. *Ann Intern Med* 113(12):941–8.
10. Gaudreau JD, Gagnon P, Harel F, Tremblay A, Roy MA (2005). Fast, systematic, and continuous delirium assessment in hospitalized patients: the Nursing Delirium Screening Scale. *J Pain Symptom Manage* 29(4):368–75.
11. Detroyer E, Clement PM, Baeten N, et al. (2014). Detection of delirium in palliative care unit patients: a prospective descriptive study of the Delirium Observation Screening Scale administered by bedside nurses. *Palliat Med* 28(1):79–86.
12. Breitbart W, Rosenfeld B, Roth A, Smith MJ, Cohen K, Passik S (1997). The Memorial Delirium Assessment Scale. *J Pain Symptom Manage* 13(3):128–37.
13. Lawlor PG, Nekolaichuk C, Gagnon B, Mancini IL, Pereira JL, Bruera ED (2000). Clinical utility, factor analysis, and further validation of the memorial delirium assessment scale in patients with advanced cancer: assessing delirium in advanced cancer. *Cancer* 88(12):2859–67.
14. Trzepacz PT, Mittal D, Torres R, Kanary K, Norton J, Jimerson N (2001). Validation of the Delirium Rating Scale-revised-98: comparison with the delirium rating scale and the cognitive test for delirium. *J Neuropsychiatry Clin Neurosci* 13(2):229–42.
15. Breitbart W, Alici Y (2012). Evidence-based treatment of delirium in patients with cancer. *J Clin Oncol* 30(11):1206–14.

Clinical Issues Related to Palliative Sedation

Shirley H. Bush

Definition

Palliative sedation (PS), or deep and continuous sedation, is the monitored use of *proportionate* sedative medication to reduce a patient's awareness of intractable and refractory symptoms near the end of life when other interventions have failed to control them.[1–3]

Consultation with a palliative care specialist is strongly recommended before initiating PS (see Box 13.1).

Appropriately titrated PS to relieve intractable distress at the end of life (i.e., last hours, days, or 1–2 weeks of life) is an ethically and legally accepted intervention (see Chapter 24 on the ethics of palliative sedation).

PS is distinct from euthanasia, as the aim of PS is to relieve suffering by controlling distressing symptoms, not to shorten life. The use of proportionate sedation is not associated with hastening death.[4] During PS it may

---

Box 13.1 Checklist for Palliative Sedation

⚠ Consultation with a palliative care specialist is advisable before initiating PS.

1. Establish that symptom(s) are severe, intractable, and refractory to treatment.
2. A symptom is *refractory* when all possible interventions known to control that symptom (including consultation with other providers) have been exhausted and failed, "or it is estimated that no methods are available for palliation within the time frame and the risk–benefit ratio that the patient can tolerate."[1]
3. Confirm that the patient is in the terminal phase of illness or close to death.
4. Discuss reasons and goals of palliative sedation with the patient (if possible) and/or family, and other members of the interprofessional healthcare team (including primary team, if applicable). Reinforce that the goal is to relieve refractory symptoms, not to shorten life.
5. Document these discussions in the medical record, with confirmation of informed consent of the patient or substitute decision maker.
6. Select the appropriate sedative medication and use the smallest effective dose to achieve symptom relief, as guided by a validated monitoring tool.
7. Only increase the medication dose (in appropriate increments) if lower doses have been ineffective, and document the indication for the dose increase.
8. Continue other ongoing symptom control management (e.g., opioid for pain and/or dyspnea, antipsychotics for delirium, and other comfort measures).
9. Continue to provide emotional support to the family and healthcare team.
10. Regularly re-evaluate the need to continue PS. It may be possible to reduce or discontinue sedative medications if the indication for PS has improved.

be possible to maintain patient consciousness if lower doses of sedative medication are sufficient to control the refractory symptom(s).

Refractory agitated delirium is the most common indication for PS.[4] Other indications include refractory dyspnea, terminal hemorrhage, intractable seizures, and uncontrolled pain.

The American Academy of Hospice and Palliative Medicine (AAHPM) 2006 position statement on PS is available at http://www.aahpm.org/positions/default/sedation.html (see Chapter 24 for more discussion of the AAHPM position statement). The European Association for Palliative Care (EAPC) published a framework for PS in 2009.[5]

Medications Used

Midazolam is the most commonly used medication for PS.[4] It has a rapid onset of action, short half-life, and dose-dependent sedative effect. Use the lowest dose possible to provide comfort, for example, commence a continuous SC or IV infusion of midazolam at 1 mg/hour (with additional PRN bolus doses available) and titrate according to clinical response.

Other medications that have been used for refractory delirium and PS include lorazepam, phenobarbital (phenobarbitone), propofol, chlorpromazine, and levomepromazine (methotrimeprazine; not available in the US).

• Phenobarbital usual dosing: 50–100 mg SC bolus stat, then 200–800 mg/24 hours by continuous SC infusion. Occasionally, higher doses are needed. Phenobarbital needs to be administered as a separate infusion, as it is not compatible with most other drugs.

• Propofol is an ultrafast-acting IV anesthetic agent. Use requires specialist input.

Monitoring Palliative Sedation

Standardized instruments should be used to ensure best practice in monitoring the level of sedation and the efficacy of sedative medications, enhancing documentation and ensuring patient safety.[5,6] Tools should measure levels of distress in patients receiving PS in addition to sedation levels.

The EAPC Expert Working Group on PS recommended using the Richmond Agitation-Sedation Scale (RASS) or a similar instrument to monitor PS.[5] The RASS is a simple and brief observational tool that was developed and validated in adult ICU patients.[7] The RASS-PAL is a modified version of the RASS that was validated in palliative care inpatients.[8] Like the RASS, the RASS-PAL scores range from +4 to −5. Thus titrating sedation to a "RASS-PAL score of −3" would indicate moderate sedation, with the patient demonstrating any eye or body movement or eye opening (but no eye contact) to verbal stimulation.

Clinical Pearls

- Consultation with a palliative care specialist is advisable before initiating PS.
- Establish that symptom(s) are severe, intractable, and refractory to treatment and confirm that the patient is in the terminal phase of illness.
- Discuss, and document, the indications and goals for initiation of PS with the patient (if possible), family, and healthcare team.
- Commence with the lowest effective dose of sedative medication and then appropriately titrate according to clinical response, using a validated PS monitoring instrument.
- Provide support and frequent information to the family and healthcare team.

References

1. de Graeff A, Dean M (2007). Palliative sedation therapy in the last weeks of life: a literature review and recommendations for standards. *J Palliat Med* 10(1):67–85.
2. Elsayem A, Curry Iii E, Boohene J, et al. (2009). Use of palliative sedation for intractable symptoms in the palliative care unit of a comprehensive cancer center. *Support Care Cancer* 17(1):53–9.
3. Lo B, Rubenfeld G (2005). Palliative sedation in dying patients: "we turn to it when everything else hasn't worked." *JAMA* 294(14):1810–6.
4. Maltoni M, Scarpi E, Rosati M, et al. (2012). Palliative sedation in end-of-life care and survival: a systematic review. *J Clin Oncol* 30(12):1378–83.
5. Cherny NI, Radbruch L (2009). European Association for Palliative Care (EAPC) recommended framework for the use of sedation in palliative care. *Palliat Med* 23(7):581–93.
6. Brinkkemper T, van Norel AM, Szadek KM, Loer SA, Zuurmond WW, Perez RS (2013). The use of observational scales to monitor symptom control and depth of sedation in patients requiring palliative sedation: a systematic review. *Palliat Med* 27(1):54–7.
7. Sessler CN, Gosnell MS, Grap MJ, et al. (2002). The Richmond Agitation-Sedation Scale: validity and reliability in adult intensive care unit patients. *Am J Respir Crit Care Med* 166(10):1338–44.
8. Bush SH, Grassau PA, Yarmo MN, Zhang T, Zinkie SJ, Pereira JL (2014). The Richmond Agitation-Sedation Scale modified for palliative care inpatients (RASS-PAL): a pilot study exploring validity and feasibility in clinical practice. *BMC Palliat Care* 13(1):17.

Breathlessness

Jeff Myers and Deborah Dudgeon

Definition and Epidemiology

Breathlessness is a distressing symptom experienced commonly by patients with advanced disease. The most widely cited definition continues to be the 2001 American Thoracic Society consensus statement, which outlines breathlessness as "a subjective experience of breathing discomfort that consists of qualitatively distinct sensations that vary in intensity. The experience derives from interaction among multiple physiologic, psychological, social, and environmental factors, and may induce secondary physiologic and behavioral responses."[1]

Breathlessness can be either continuous or episodic. Despite optimal treatment of the underlying chronic cause(s), a number of conditions leave people with continuous breathlessness at rest or with minimal exertion. This is termed *chronic refractory breathlessness* and is a distinct entity, rather than simply being a failure to treat the underlying condition(s). *Chronic* is often defined by a time frame such as 8 weeks or 3 months; however, in practice, breathlessness that persists despite maximal treatment of an underlying irreversible cause should be considered chronic.[2]

Episodic breathlessness is characterized by a severe worsening of breathlessness beyond usual fluctuations and can be in the presence or absence of underlying continuous breathlessness. Episodes are time limited (seconds to hours), occur intermittently, and may be either unpredictable or predictable if trigger(s) can be identified. Four broad categories of triggers include exertion, emotions, comorbidities, or external environment. Although a number of specific types of episodic breathlessness are described, the two most important elements are specific triggers and whether or not an episode is predictable.[3]

Reported prevalence of breathlessness varies and is dependent on the underlying diagnosis and the extent and stage of disease, as well as choice of both assessment tool and the words or phrases used by investigators. At least 60% and 90% of patients with advanced heart disease and advanced chronic obstructive pulmonary disease (COPD), respectively, will report feeling breathless.[3] Among patients over the age of 65, breathlessness is the second most common reason for presentation to the emergency department. In the cancer population, breathlessness prevalence is dependent on the primary tumor site (46%, advanced lung cancer; 7%, advanced gastric cancer) and stage of disease.[3] In the final 6 weeks of life, 70% of all patients with cancer will experience breathlessness.

Patient Experience and Pathophysiology

Although the neural pathways influencing the perception of breathlessness are not fully understood, Figure 14.1 outlines the current understanding of the contributing pathophysiological mechanisms.

Sensory input is composed of a combination of multiple afferent impulses that influence both the brainstem respiratory network (medulla and pons) and the higher brain centers located in the somatosensory and association cortices. The following outlines four main categories of sensory input.

Biochemical

- Central and peripheral chemoreceptors (detect changes in pH, pCO_2, and pO_2) via the vagus nerve

Vascular

- Baroreceptors (stretch sensitive mechanoreceptors) in the carotid and aortic bodies via the vagus nerve

Mechanical

Sensory input is via receptors in the following:
- *Nasopharynx*: (cold, air flow) via trigeminal nerve
- *Airway*: rapidly adapting receptors within epithelium from trachea to bronchioles (lung irritants); slow-adapting receptors close to smooth muscle of extra- and intrathoracic lower airway (airway wall tension); *bronchial C* fibers (irritants). All are via the vagus nerve.
- *Lung parenchyma*: pulmonary C-fibers within alveolar wall (pulmonary congestion, embolism, infection, chemicals) via vagus nerve
- *Muscles*: Golgi tendons (tension), intercostal muscles (length), diaphragm via spinal and supraspinal reflexes

Psychogenic

- An affective state (i.e., distress) can elicit changes in ventilation and sensation

The control of respiratory motor activity resides in the brainstem (medulla and pons), and efferent impulses from here produce voluntary and involuntary contraction of the muscles in both the chest wall and the diaphragm.

Central modulation of breathlessness appears to occur via two distinct pathways, one for perceived intensity level (i.e., severity) and one for the affective component of unpleasantness that is associated with the breathlessness. Functional MRI imaging has confirmed that awareness of intensity is mediated by peripheral chemo-mechanical receptors projecting to the brainstem medulla and somatosensory cortex.[3] Awareness of unpleasantness involves pathways of the limbic system. To date, endogenous opioids are the only neurotransmitters shown to modulate breathlessness, as they reduce both the intensity and the unpleasantness observed when breathlessness is induced in a controlled setting.[3]

In summary, breathlessness is the conscious representation of a mismatch between the central ventilatory drive (the demand to breathe) and the responding respiratory output (the ability to breathe). The intensity and the unpleasantness of the experience are perceived separately.

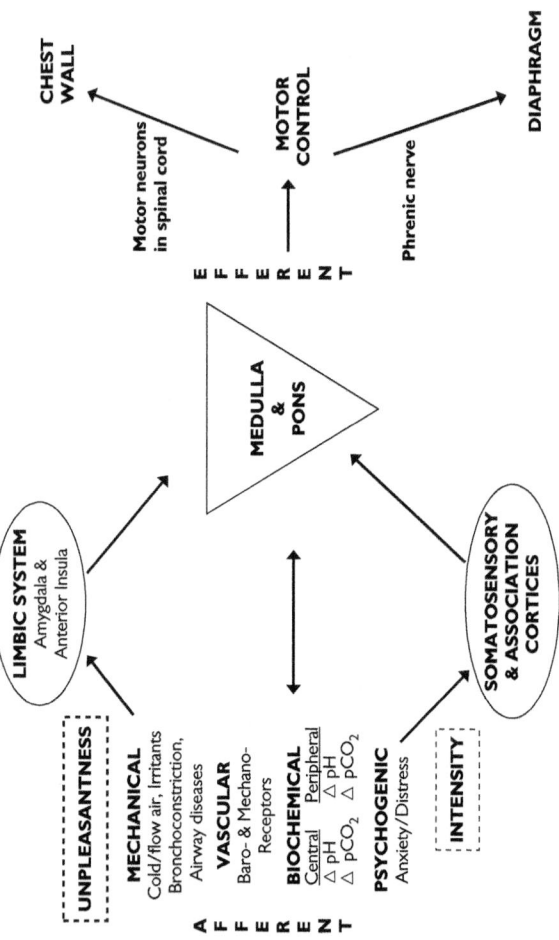

Figure 14.1. Overview of breathlessness pathophysiology.

Etiology

In the setting of advanced disease, breathlessness may be multifactorial in etiology and can be categorized on the basis of both underlying disease and acuity of onset.

Malignant

Acute (Within Minutes)

- Pulmonary embolism
- Pneumothorax
- Aspiration
- Anxiety

Subacute (Within Hours to Days)

- Pneumonia
- Pleural effusion (can also be chronic)
- Pericardial effusion
- Superior vena cava obstruction
- Anemia
- Radiation-induced pneumonitis (can also be chronic)
- Progressive metastatic disease (can also be chronic)

Chronic (Within Days to Weeks)

- Radiation-induced pneumonitis/fibrosis
- Progressive metastatic disease
- Chemotherapy-induced (pulmonary fibrosis, cardiomyopathy)
- Contributing factors may include cachexia, ascites, and/or hepatomegaly

Nonmalignant

Acute (Within Minutes)

Pulmonary

- Pneumothorax
- Pulmonary embolism
- Bronchospasm
- Acute bronchitis
- Asthma (with previous history)

Cardiac

- Acute myocardial ischemia or infarction
- Anxiety disorder

Subacute (Within Hours to Days)

- Pneumonia
- CHF exacerbation
- Anemia

Chronic (Within Days to Weeks)

Pulmonary
- Obstructive lung disease
- Restrictive lung disease
- Interstitial lung disease
- Pleural effusion

Other
- CHF or ventricular dysfunction
- Neuromuscular disease
- Renal disease

Clinical Evaluation

Given its multifactorial nature, the assessment of breathlessness should include physical, psychosocial, and spiritual domains of the experience. All reversible factors should be identified, even where there appears to be a single dominant explanation for the symptom.

History: Key Questions

- Acuity? (Onset and course)
- Severity? (Use VAS or NRS; see following discussion)
- Pattern?
- Triggering factors?
- Effect on activities of daily living?
- Mood and psychological state? (Mental status, current or history of anxiety, current or history of depression)
- Meaning? (Is patient fearful of dying?)
- Current and previous medications?
- Underlying or concurrent diagnosis?
- Associated symptoms: cough, sputum production/color fever/chills, sweats, chest pain, wheeze, chest tightness, hemoptysis, hoarseness, edema, weight loss/gain
- Advance directives and substitute decision-maker?

Clinical Pearls

- The patient's opinion of the severity of the symptoms is the gold standard for symptom assessment.
- Often patients with advanced disease will have previously expressed or discussed their goals of care. This can provide clear guidance when formulating a plan for further assessment and management.

A visual analog scale (VAS) is a tool for assessing symptom severity, which uses a vertical or horizontal line. Word anchors at each end could indicate either severity (i.e. "no breathlessness" to the "worst intensity of breathless") or level of the affective component (i.e., "no breathlessness" to the "most unpleasant breathlessness").

An example of a numerical rating scale (NRS) is the Edmonton Symptom Assessment System (ESAS), which is a valid and reliable assessment tool to assist in the assessment of nine common symptoms experienced by patients with advanced disease.[4] The severity at the time of assessment of each symptom is rated from 0 to 10 on an NRS, 0 meaning that the symptom is absent and 10 that it is of the worst possible severity.

Several scales have been developed specifically for dyspnea; however, as yet, no one scale can accurately reflect breathlessness for all patients with advanced disease. Alternatively, if overall quality of life is the emphasis, then a multidimensional tool is preferable. A unidimensional scale (e.g., VAS or NRS) should be combined with a disease-specific scale (if available) or a multidimensional scale in conjunction with other methods (such as qualitative techniques) to gauge distress level for the assessment of breathlessness in advanced disease.

Physical Exam

In the setting of advanced disease, the physical exam should be focused and guided by history and underlying illness.

Vital Signs

- Heart (HR) and respiratory rate (RR), BP, O_2 saturation, walking oximetry

Observe

- Overall level of distress
- Use of accessory muscles
- Elevated jugular venous pressure
- Pursed lips
- Cyanosis
- Ability to speak

Palpate

- Presence of dullness to percussion
- Decreased tactile fremitus

Auscultate

- Absent breath sounds?
- Adventitious breath sounds?
- Audible third heart sound (S3) or distant heart sounds?
- Wheeze?
- Pulses paradoxus?

Clinical Pearls

- Tachypnea does not equate with breathlessness.
- Superior vena cava obstruction (SVCO) causes acute breathlessness and is a medical emergency characterized by swelling and redness of face, distension of superficial and deep neck and upper arm vasculature, and cough.

Laboratory Investigations and Imaging

In patients with advanced disease, the appropriateness of an investigation will depend on the stage of disease and the goals of care. It is important to consider the burden of procedures and weigh this against the risk.

Investigations may contribute meaningful information in the assessment of breathlessness for patients; however, the results may not impact the options for treatment. The choice of an appropriate test (or tests) will be guided by history, physical exam, and clinical scenario.

Investigations to consider may include the following:
- CBC, serum K^+, PO_4, Mg
- Chest X-ray
- Blood gas
- Pulmonary function test
- CT
- Echocardiogram

Many clinicians make the mistake of equating breathlessness with hypoxemia; however, studies show very poor correlation between patient reports of breathlessness and oxygen levels or abnormalities in pulmonary function. In addition, patients may not show signs of hypoxia but report high levels of breathlessness. Oximetry (in particular, walking oximetry) may unmask the etiology for the breathlessness.

Management

The mainstay of management of breathlessness is, whenever possible, to identify any underlying cause that is potentially reversible, to begin appropriate and targeted treatment or intervention, to evaluate the effectiveness of the treatment or intervention, and to ensure that the symptom of breathlessness is well managed throughout.

An example is breathlessness resulting from malignant pleural effusions. For appropriate patients, thoracentesis, pleurodesis, and/or ongoing drainage procedures should be offered, and if effective can both reverse the immediate cause and effectively manage the symptom.

Basic nonpharmacological and pharmacological interventions for breathlessness, based on severity, are summarized in Table 14.1.[5]

Clinical Pearl

- When available, opioids can and should be administered subcutaneously, particularly if breathlessness is severe; ½ of the PO dose is equivalent to the SC dose and can be safely offered q30min prn.

Nonpharmacological Interventions

Based on a meta-analysis of randomized controlled trials, strong evidence now exists in support of interventions that reverse deconditioning and optimize the efficiency of skeletal muscle. The strongest evidence exists for the two such strategies, *transcutaneous quadriceps muscle stimulation* and *chest wall vibration*. In addition, studies demonstrate a moderate level of benefit with the use of *walking aids* to improve performance status. Studies in patients with COPD show that structured cognitive-behavioral and self-management strategies improve both health service utilization and depression.[6]

Opioids

For the management of chronic refractory breathlessness, there is now Level 1 evidence that regularly monitored, low-dose, sustained-release morphine is effective and well tolerated. For both cancer and noncancer populations, along with this is confirmation of the usefulness of oral and/ or parenteral opioids in providing significant clinical benefit in the setting of acute, subacute, and chronic breathlessness.

It is suggested that when using opioids, only oral and systemic routes be considered. There is no evidence that nebulized opioids have any greater benefit than systemic opioids in reducing breathlessness.[6]

Respiratory depression is a commonly feared side effect of opioids. Although some studies showed a decrease in respiratory rate with the use of opioids, this was not found to be clinically significant, as neither hypercapnia nor hypoxygenation resulted.

Nonopioid Medications

Although it may seem counterintuitive, evidence does not support the use of benzodiazepines in the direct management of breathlessness.[6] Given the distinct psychogenic role in the severity of breathlessness, however,

Table 14.1 General Features and Quick Reference Management of Breathlessness

	Mild (VAS/ESAS 1-3)	Moderate (VAS/ESAS 4-6)	Severe (VAS/ESAS 7-10)
Clinical Features	Usually can sit/lie quietly	Usually persistent	Often acute on chronic
	Intermittent or persistent	May be new or chronic	Has worsened over days to weeks
	Increase with exertion	Settles partially with rest	Anxiety present
	No or mild anxiety	Patient pauses while talking every 30 seconds	Patient pauses while talking every 5–15 seconds
	Patient does not appear uncomfortable	Breathing appears mildly labored	Patient appears uncomfortable
Management Strategies	Consider oxygen (if hypoxemic or deemed helpful by patient)	Start oxygen (if hypoxemic or deemed helpful by patient)	Start oxygen (up to 6L/min by NP or higher with mask)
	If opioid naïve, consider low dose routine or prn opioid (morphine 2.5–5.0 mg or hydromorphone 0.5–1.0mg)	If opioid naïve, consider low dose routine or prn opioid (morphine 2.5–5.0 mg or hydromorphone 0.5–1.0mg)	Use only short-acting opioids to titrate
	If on opioids, increase by 25%	If on opioids, increase by 25%	If opioid naïve, begin either morphine PO 5–10 mg q4h and 5 mg q1h prn or hydromorphone 1–2 mg q4h and 1 mg q1h prn
	Ensure breakthrough avail q2h	Ensure breakthrough avail q1h prn	Titrate opioid dose by 25% every 1–2 doses until relief

(continued)

Table 14.1 (Continued)

Mild (VAS/ESAS 1–3)	Moderate (VAS/ESAS 4–6)	Severe (VAS/ESAS 7–10)
Titrate short-acting opioid by 25% every 3 to 5 hours until relief	Titrate opioid dose by 25% every 2–3 doses until relief	Consider adjuvant (midazolam, promethazine)
Consider oxygen (if hypoxemic or deemed helpful by patient)	Start oxygen (if hypoxemic or deemed helpful by patient)	Start oxygen (up to 6 L/min by NP or higher with mask)

For all:

- Ensure access to fresh air or fan directing air on the face.
- Open door, window(s), curtain(s).
- Encourage rest as needed.
- When laying—elevate head of bed.
- When sitting—use reclining chair and footrest.
- When moving—use assistive devices (walker, wheelchair).

aggressively managing comorbid psychiatric conditions (anxiety and/or depression) warrants consideration.

Other medications with limited evidence but potential benefit include nebulized furosemide (for its bronchodilator effects), selective serotonin reuptake inhibitors (SSRIs), and promethazine.[6] Well-designed and adequately powered trials are necessary before recommendations can be made about any of these.

There are no randomized controlled trials of corticosteroids to manage breathlessness, regardless of setting.[7] Anecdotal reports suggest a role for corticosteroids when targeting specific cancer-related conditions:

- Obstruction (SVCO and/or airway)
- Lymphangitic carcinomatosis
- Radiation pneumonitis

Oxygen

A consistent beneficial effect of oxygen has not been shown for patients with advanced cancer or advanced heart disease, or in patients with advanced lung disease among those found to be ineligible for long-term oxygen. New findings from a meta-analysis suggest a possible role in all patients with advanced lung disease; however, this requires confirmation by an adequately powered study.[3]

Summary

Breathlessness is a common and distressing symptom for patients with advanced disease. Assessment and management plans should be targeted to the individual patient. Reversible conditions contributing to breathlessness should be addressed, and patient self-report should be used in determining severity of the symptom and efficacy of a management plan. No single therapy is likely to resolve chronic breathlessness, but combinations of strategies is likely to improve the burden and impact of breathlessness.

References

1. American Thoracic Society (2001). Dyspnea: mechanisms, assessment, and management: a consensus statement. *Am J Respir Crit Care Med* 163:951–7.
2. Simon S, Weingartner V, Higginson IJ, Voltz R, Bausewein C (2014). Definition, categorization, and terminology of episodic breathlessness: consensus by an International Delphi Survey. *J Pain Symptom Manage* 47(5):828–38.
3. Currow D, Higginson IJ, Johnson M (2013). Breathlessness—current and emerging mechanisms, measurement and management: a discussion from an European Association of Palliative Care workshop. *Palliat Med* 27(10) 932–8.
4. Bruera E, Kuehn N, Miller MJ, Selmser P, Macmillan K. (1991). The Edmonton Symptom Assessment System (ESAS): a simple method for the assessment of palliative care patients. *J Palliat Care* 7(2):6–9.
5. Dyspnea management guidelines for palliative care (2003). In *Kingston, Frontenac, Lennox and Addington (KFL and A) Palliative Care Integration Project: Symptom Management Guidelines*, pp. 26–36.
6. Currow D, Johnson M, White P, Abernethy A (2013). Evidence-based intervention for chronic refractory breathlessness: practical therapies that make a difference. *Brit J Gen Pract* 63: 609–10.
7. Viola R, Kiteley C, Lloyd NS, Mackay JA, Wilson J, Wong RKS (2008). The management of dyspnea in cancer patients: a systematic review. *Support Care Cancer* 16:329–37.

Chapter 15

Emergencies in Palliative Care

Meiko Kuriya and Rony Dev

Hypercalcemia

Introduction

Approximately 10%–30% percent of patients with cancer have complications of hypercalcemia at some time during the course of their illness.[1] Hypercalcemia is responsible for a significant number of hospitalizations and results in distressing symptoms in patients with cancer. Hypercalcemia is also an indicator of poor prognosis; however, treatment with bisphosphonates may be decreasing the incidence and outcome for cancer patients.

Clinical Presentation

Hypercalemia results in nonspecific clinical symptoms: "bones, stones, abdominal groans, and psychic moans."

Symptoms include
- Anorexia
- Nausea
- Abdominal pain
- Muscle weakness and fatigue
- Nephrolithiasis
- Dehydration
- Bony tenderness

Complications of severe hypercalcemia
- Acute pancreatitis
- Hypercalemia
- Acute renal failure
- Altered mental status and coma
- Pathogenesis

Hypercalcemia associated with cancer can be classified into four types (Table 15.1).

Management

Hydration with intravenous saline is essential to reverse decreased glomerular filtration rate and impaired renal calcium excretion. Furosemide can also promote calcium excretion by inhibiting Na/K/Cl transporter in the loop of Henle; however, diuretics are not recommended in cancer patients, who are often volume depleted.

Bisphosphonates are first-line medical therapy; they work by blocking osteoclastic bone resorption and include pamidronate and zolendronate.[2] Bisphosphonates should be given intravenously since they are poorly absorbed when given orally. Common adverse effects include fever, nausea, vomiting, renal toxicity, and osteonecrosis of the jaw.

Second-line medications include glucocorticoids (useful in lymphoma patients with elevated 1,25(OH)2 vitamin D) and calcitonin, which results in rapid transient reduction in calcium levels.

Supportive care measures include the removal of calcium in vitamin supplementations and from parenteral feeding solutions, discontinuation of medications that may lead to hypercalcemia (e.g., calcitriol, vitamin D, lithium, and thiazides), and replacement of phosphorous orally if serum phosphorous is less than 3 mg/dl. IV phosphorous replacement should be avoided unless phosphorous is critically low (< 1.5 mg/dl) since it can cause seizures, hypocalcemia, renal failure, and arrythmias.

Table 15.1 Types of Hypercalcemia Associated with Cancer

Type	Frequency (%)	Bone Metastasis	Causal Agent	Typical Tumors
Local osteolytic hypercalcemia	20	Common, extensive	Cytokines, chemokines, PTHrP	Breast cancer, multiple myeloma, lymphoma
Humoral hypercalcemia of malignancy	80	Minimal or absent	PTHrP	Squamous cell cancer (e.g., of head and neck, esophagus, cervix, or lung), renal cancer, ovarian cancer, endometrial cancer; HTLV-associated lymphoma, breast cancer
1,25 (OH)2D-secreting lymphomas	< 1	Variable	1,25(OH)2D	Lymphoma (all types)
Ectopic hyper-parathyroidism	< 1	Variable	PTH	Variable

PTH = parathyroid hormone; PTHrP = PTH-related protein; 1,25(OH)2D = 1,25-dihydroxyvitamin D; HTLV = human T-cell lymphotrophic virus.

Bleeding

Mild to severe bleeding is an emergent complication that occurs in approximately 6%–10% of cancer patients and 1.5% of patients receiving palliative care. Active bleeding can be very distressing for patients, families, and healthcare providers. For patients with a poor prognosis, advanced care planning is critical in order to anticipate possible catastrophic bleeding.

Etiology

1. *Tumor invasion*: Cancer infiltration of both small and large vessels and factors secreted by tumors that promote angiogenesis predispose patients to bleeding. Past radiation exposure can often weaken vessels, resulting in bleeding complications. Head and neck tumors, lung, gastrointestinal, and gynecologic malignancies are often associated with tumor destruction of small and large vessels. Hepatocellular carcinoma may be complicated by bloody ascites and is a poor prognostic indicator. Vascular tumors, including renal cell carcinoma, choriocarcinoma, and melanoma, are also prone to bleeding.
2. *Treatment side effects*: Mucositis secondary to chemotherapy or radiation treatment and the complication of graft versus host disease can increase the risk for bleeding.
3. *Thrombocytopenia*: Bone marrow suppression, bone marrow invasion of the cancer, disseminated intravascular coagulation (DIC), or splenomegaly secondary to portal hypertension from hepatocelluar carcinoma can result in thrombocytopenia.
4. *Nutritional deficiencies*: Vitamin K, zinc, folate, and vitamin B_{12} deficiencies can also promote bleeding.
5. *Drugs*: Coumadin, heparin products, and COX-inhibitors can potentiate bleeding.
6. *Coagulation abnormalities*: DIC, primary fibrinolysis, and liver disease can result in coagulopathy, contributing to increased bleeding risk.

Presentation

Bleeding could happen in several ways: oozing from the tumor, intracranial hemorrhage, epistaxis, hemoptysis, hematemesis, melena, hematochezia, hematuria, and vaginal bleeding.

Workup

In cases of non-catastrophic bleeding, it is important to detect any reversible causes while initiating measures to control bleeding and anxiety in patients and families associated with visible blood loss. Labs should include complete blood count, platelet count, activated partial thromboplastin time (PTT), and international normalization ratio (INR). Liver function test could be included if liver dysfunction is suspected. In cases of catastrophic bleeding, controlling the bleeding and associated symptoms takes priority over reversing underlying factors.

Management

Interventions should be consistent with a patient's goals of care and are formulated based on overall prognosis, performance status, and previous therapies. The most important point is to make the patient and family aware and prepared for the possibility of visible bleeding. If catastrophic bleeding is anticipated, dark colored (preferably the color red) linen, towels, and basins should be available at bedside to make bleeding less obvious. For control of anxiety, IV or SC midazolam should be available and family members should be trained in administration.

Local measures to control bleeding include the following:

- Packing
  - Nose, rectum, vagina
- Compressive dressings
  - Transparent films, hydrogel dressings, hydrocolloid dressing
- Topical hemostatics
  - Fibrin sealants
- Proper positioning
  - Lateral decubitus on the side of bleeding for patients with hemoptysis or hematemesis
- Astringents
  - Silver nitrate, aluminum ammonium sulphate, or aluminum potassium sulphate

Treatment modalities for bleeding include the following:

- Radiation therapy
  - Gynecologic, lung, and superficial skin tumors
- Palliative transcatheter chemo-embolization
- Endoscopy
  - Injection of sclerosing agents
  - Ligation
  - Laser coagulation

Systemic measures include the following:

- Vitamin K
- Vassopresin
- Antifibrinolytic agents
  - Transexaminic acid
  - Aminocaproic Acid
- Octreotide for GI bleeding from varacies
- Platelet transfusion
  - Thrombocytopenia
  - Platelet dysfunction
- Fresh frozen plasma
  - Coagulopathies

When bleeding is catastrophic, palliative sedation for the patient should be provided in conjunction with psychosocial support for the family.

Superior Vena Cava Syndrome

Superior vena cava (SVC) syndrome results from the impairment of blood flow through the SVC. It is usually caused by malignancies, the majority of which are due to non-small-cell lung cancer. Other etiologies include small-cell lung cancer, germ cell tumors, lymphoma, thymoma, esophageal cancer, mediastinal or lung metastasis from other tumors. Recently, nonmalignant conditions resulting in SVC syndrome have arisen secondary to the increased use of intravascular devices.

Clinical Presentation

Increased venous pressure secondary to SVC syndrome may result in symptoms of edema of the head, neck, and arms, which often develop over a period of 2 weeks. Clinical features may include cyanosis and distended subcutaneous vessels of the neck. Cough, hoarseness, stridor, and dysphagia may occur secondary to edema occluding the airways or esophagus. Cerebral edema may result in head discomfort, confusion, and coma, which can be fatal. In severe cases, hemodynamic compromise can occur. In addition, pleural effusions are common in cancer patients with SVC syndrome.

Diagnosis

When SVC syndrome is suspected based on clinical signs and symptoms, CT scan with contrast and MRI, for patients allergic to contrast, are the most useful imaging studies. Once SVC syndrome has been confirmed by imaging, obtaining a tissue diagnosis is critical in patients with suspected malignancies to guide future treatment. Patients with pleural effusion, consideration for thoracentesis with cytologic analysis should be considered. Bronchoscopy, transthoracic needle-aspiration biopsy, mediastinoscopy, or mediastinotomy is used to obtain a tissue diagnosis.

Management

The management of SVC syndrome depends on the etiology, severity of symptoms, and the patient's goal of therapy. When there is enough collateral blood flow with minimal symptoms, the patient might not require further treatment. Systemic chemotherapy could be the initial treatment of choice for sensitive tumors such as lung cancer (small cell and non-small cell), lymphoma, and germ cell tumors. When SVC syndrome is caused by a tumor that is refractory to chemotherapy, radiation therapy could be considered.

Percutaneous placement of an intravascular stent is another possible intervention. Stent placement can be done before a tissue diagnosis has been obtained, and it is a useful procedure for patients with severe symptoms such as dyspnea. In addition, stent placement should also be considered for patients with mesothelioma, which tends to be refractory to chemotherapy and radiation therapy. Complications of stent placement for treatment of SVC syndrome include infection, pulmonary embolus, stent migration, hematoma formation at the insertion site, perforation, bleeding, and rarely death. Anticoagulation is often recommended after stent placement.

A multidisciplinary approach to treatment planning should be considered. The presence of SVC syndrome often does not affect the prognosis, which is directly related to the tumor type and stage of the cancer.

Spinal Cord Compression

Introduction

Cancer patients may develop spinal cord compression, which can result in pain, incontinence of bowel or bladder, and paraparesis or paralysis. Breast, prostate, and lung cancer account for the majority of spinal cord compression cases. Breast and lung cancers cause thoracic lesions while colon and pelvic malignancies involve the lumbosacral spine.

Clinical Presentation

The most common clinical presentation of spinal cord compression is back pain, which can be localized, referred, and/or radicular in nature. Complications of cauda equina syndrome results in decreased sensation over the buttocks, thighs, and perineal region and may result in decreased sphincter tone, urinary retention, and overflow incontinence. Spinal cord compression presents with radiculopathy, sensory changes, weakness, autonomic dysfunction (i.e., urinary retention), and loss of sphincter tone, resulting in stool incontinence.

Diagnosis

Delay in the diagnosis of spinal cord compression can lead to increased morbidity and mortality. When spinal cord compression is suspected, gadolinium-enhanced MRI of the whole spine should be urgently obtained and is considered the gold standard.

Management

A multidisciplinary team approach is critical to formulate the treatment for patients with spinal cord compression and includes a surgical team, radiation oncologist, rehabilitation practitioner, and a palliative medicine consultant. Treatment should be customized according to the patient's disease status, prognosis, performance status, comorbidities, and the severity of symptoms.

Glucocorticoid Therapy

The general consensus is that glucocorticoid therapy is beneficial. Optimal dose of steroid therapy is unknown, but an initial bolus of dexamethasone 10 mg IV, followed by a scheduled dose of 6–10 mg every 6 hours, is commonly initiated. After completion of radiation therapy, it is recommended to taper the least effective dose that maintains neurological benefits while minimizing side effects. For patients who need prolonged glucocorticoid therapy, consideration for prophylaxis to prevent Candida and Pneumocystis jiroveci infections should be considered.

Radiation Therapy

Cancer metastasis to the vertebral column can be painful and may result in various degrees of spinal cord compression. Radiation therapy has been shown to provide pain relief and to preserve the ability to ambulate and maintain sphincter function. Serious complications that may occur include myelosuppression and radiation myelopathy. Longer courses of radiation therapy have not been shown to be superior to a short course, but patients receiving a shorter course have been reported to have increased recurrence. High-precision radiotherapy techniques have been developed, which are being used for primary treatment and for recurrence of disease while minimizing radiation exposure to surrounding tissue. Depending on the prognosis, the radiation oncologist can formulate a treatment regimen that is consistent with the patient's goals of care.

Surgery

Surgical decompression with reconstruction can provide benefit, including pain control and preserving neurological function for patients with spinal cord compressions. Currently, the optimal treatment with surgical decompression and reconstruction followed by radiation therapy versus radiotherapy alone is unclear. Surgery for patients with progressive neurological deficits, vertebral column instability, radio-resistant tumors, and patients with persistent pain despite radiotherapy has been recommended. Most surgeons agree that a patient's life expectancy should be greater than 3 months prior to undergoing any invasive surgical procedures.

Rehabilitation

Rehabilitation has been shown in observational studies to improve quality of life, to improve mood, and to provide better pain control in patients with spinal cord compressions. Paraplegic patients are taught how to manage bowel or bladder incontinence and to transfer safely, and ambulatory patients receive assistance with their strength and mobility. In addition, family support is incorporated into a debilitated patient's bowel and bladder care, nutritional needs, and daily hygiene regimens.

Palliative Care

Regardless of whether radiation or surgery is offered for treatment of spinal cord compression, patients should be provided medical treatment and psychosocial support to assist with coping with the loss of independence or function. For patients with a poor prognosis, palliative care consultants can assist with transition from disease-orientated therapy to treatment focused on symptom control and improving quality of life.

Seizures

Introduction

Seizures in the palliative care setting may be seen in patients with a primary brain tumor, a metastatic brain lesion, metabolic abnormalities, a CNS (central nervous system) infection, or drug toxicity or withdrawal.

Presentation

Seizures can be either focal or generalized; not all seizures present with convulsions, but can also present with altered mental status. Focal seizures can develop into a generalized seizure. Status epilepticus is an emergent condition and is defined as a single seizure activity lasting for more than 5 minutes or repeated seizures over a period of time of more than 30 minutes without full recovery of neurological function in between.

Workup

Electroencephalography (EEG) may be useful if the diagnosis is in doubt (e.g., nonconvulsive seizure), but is not routinely needed for patients who give a clear history of seizures or for those without suggestive symptoms.

Management

The management of seizures in palliative care setting is similar to that in noncancer patients.

Benzodiazepines

The most commonly used benzodiazepine for seizures is lorazepam. The mean time of lorazepam to achieve clinical effect is 3 minutes and the half-life is 10–15 hours; 2 mg should be given intravenously and can be repeated up to total dose of 0.1 mg/kg. It should be infused no faster than 2 mg/minutes.

Because of its high lipid solubility, diazepam enters the brain rapidly, but its half-life is 15–30 minutes; therefore, its anticonvulsant effect is very brief and a second dose may be necessary after only 20–30 minutes. The recommended dose is 10 mg in adults.

Phenytoin/Fosphenytoin

Traditionally, treatment with benzodiazepine is followed by phenytoin therapy. Recommended dosage is 15–20 mg/kg, not more than 50 mg/minute. The advantage of phenytoin therapy is that it is non-sedating.

Fosphenytoin is metabolized into phenytoin by the liver. Initial dose is the same as phenytoin, although it can be given faster than phenytoin at 100–150 mg/minute.

Valproic Acid

Valproic acid can be used as an alternate of phenytoin or fosphenytoin. The dose is 6 mg/kg/minute up to a total dose of 30 mg/kg followed by a maintenance dose of 1–2 mg/kg/hour.

Newer Agents

In order to avoid interactions with other medications such as chemotherapy agents or antibiotics, newer agents such levatiracetem, pregabalin, lamotrigine, and toprimate are known to not induce hepatic cytochrome P450 enzymes. These agents could be used as a maintenance agent once seizure is under control.

Clinical Pearls

- A high index of suspicion for hypercalcemia is necessary since symptoms are nonspecific.
- Screen for hypercalemia by checking ionized calcium level since formulas to correct serum calcium levels are not reliable.
- Hydration and bisphosphonates are the main treatment of hypercalcemia.
- Anticipation of bleeding catastrophes in cancer patients is critical to minimize distress for patients and their family.
- A CT scan of the chest or an MRI is indicated to diagnose SVC syndrome.
- A gadolinium enhanced MRI of the whole spine is the gold standard test to diagnose spinal cord compression.
- Cancer patients may have nonconvulsive epilepsy when having altered mental status without convulsions.

Further Reading

1. Stewart AF. Hypercalcemia Associated with Cancer (2005). *New Engl J Med* 352:373–9.
2. Sanders Y, Ross JR, Bradly KE, et al. (2004). Systematic review of bisphosphonates for hypercalcemia. *Palliat Med*18:418–31.
3. Gagnon B, Mancini I, Pereira J, Bruera E (1998). Palliative management of bleeding events in advanced cancer patients. *J Palliat Care* 14:50–4.
4. Prommer E (2005). Management of bleeding the terminally ill patient. *Hematology* 10:167–75.
5. Wilson L, Detterbeck F, Yahalom J (2007). Superior vena cava syndrome with malignant causes. *N Engl J Med* 356:1862–9.
6. Abrahm J, Banffy M, Harris M (2008). Spinal cord compression in patients with ad-vanced meta-static cancer: "All I care about is walking and living my life." *JAMA* 299:937–46.
7. Knake S, Hamer H, Rosenow F (2009). Statue epilepticus: a critical review. *Epilepsy Behav* 15:10–4.

Other Symptoms: Xerostomia, Hiccups, Pruritis, Pressure Ulcers and Wound Care, Lymphedema, and Myoclonus

Paul W. Walker

Introduction

This chapter includes "orphan" symptoms that usually receive less attention than do more common symptoms such as pain or nausea. These symptoms may have multiple etiologies and often have a long list of possible remedies or limited options, reflecting our lack of understanding and our limitation in management.

Xerostomia

The complaint of dry mouth, or xerostomia, is a common one in palliative care but is often perceived by clinicians as less serious than pain or other symptoms. It is important not to make light of its impact on the patient, as xerostomia can result in difficulty in mastication and swallowing and with speech. Also, there is increased risk of dental caries, periodontal disease, candidiasis, and changes in taste sensation.

In patients with advanced cancer, the prevalence of xerostomia is reported at 30%–97%.[1] The two main mechanisms underlying most cases include indirect alteration in the nervous tone supplying the salivary glands (e.g., as caused by medication) or destruction of the salivary tissue (e.g., by radiotherapy). Causes of this condition are many, but for the most part can be divided into three groups: medications, radiotherapy, and systemic diseases that cause decreased salivary flow.

Drug classes that can cause this problem include anticholinergics and antihistamines (e.g., scopolamine, diphenhydramine, oxybutynin, meclizine), psychotropics (e.g., amitiptyline, desipramine, lorazepam, hydroxyine, trazadone), opioids (e.g., codeine, fentanyl, tramadol, oxymorphone, hydromorphone), cardiovascular medications (e.g., hydrochlorothiazide, metoprolol, doxazosin, fosinopril, felodipine), and sympathetic agonists (e.g., albuterol, meta-proterenol, carbidopa-levodopa, selegiline).

Radiotherapy treatments for head and neck cancers commonly result in prolonged xerostomia.[4] The list of medical conditions that can produce dry mouth is long but includes rheumatic disorders such as Sjogren's syndrome, sarcoidosis, diabetes mellitus, graft-versus-host disease, and anxiety or depression. Dehydration can cause dry mouth, as can mouth breathing that occurs in the terminal phase of illness.

Management consists of evaluating for reversible causes, which includes a careful evaluation of the patient's drug regimen for medications that can be contributing to dry mouth and determining if they can be changed or the dose reduced.

Providing careful medical management for systemic conditions that can cause xerostomia (e.g., diabetes mellitus or chronic inflammatory rheumatic disorders) is prudent. Regular oral hygiene is important, and use of a fluoride-containing toothpaste and regular dental brushing help reduce caries, periodontal disease, and halitosis.

What remains are strategies for improving oral moisture.[2,3] These include frequent sips of fluid, ice, or popsicles; water spray; use of saliva substitutes; chewing sugarless gum; or sucking on sugar-free candy. Maintaining room humidity may also be helpful. Mealtime strategies aimed at providing moist and soft foods and avoiding dry foods are advised.

Pilocarpine is a muscarinic agonist with effects on the beta-adrenergic receptors of the sweat and salivary glands. It has been studied for the treatment of radiation and drug-induced xerostomia with positive results. Pilocarpine must be used with caution, as glaucoma and cardiac disturbances can occur. The most common side effect with this agent is sweating, but also lacrimation and dizziness. The usual dose of pilocarpine for this indication is 5 mg PO tid. Recently, cevimeline 30 mg tid has been shown to produce similar effects on salivary secretion, as pilocarpine with a side-effect profile that is comparable.[5]

Some studies report effective use of acupuncture and hypnosis.

Hiccup

Hiccup, or singultus, is an infrequent but troublesome symptom for which there are few research studies. It is defined as repeated, involuntary, spasmodic, diaphragmatic, and inspiratory intercostal muscle contrations with early glottic closure terminating inspiration.

Presently there is no known physiological function of the hiccup in the adult, and its existence is ascribed to coordination of fetal respiration or some persistent evolutionary reflex. Its neural mechanism is attributed to an afferent limb consisting of the phrenic and vagus nerves and the sympathetic chain (T6–T12), a central mediator between the cervical spine (C3–5) and the brainstem, and an efferent limb consisting mainly of the phrenic nerve.

The pathophysiology of the hiccup reflex is poorly understood. Pathological presentations are attributed to disturbances affecting one of the components of this reflex.

Although the list of conditions that have been associated with hiccup is extensive, they may be grouped into four categories: (1) disturbances affecting the phrenic or vagus nerve, (2) disturbances of central neurological control, (3) those produced by toxic and metabolic disturbances or drugs, and (4) psychogenic causes.

The perceived most frequent cause is gastroesophageal reflux disease (GERD) and gastric distention. Corticosteroids and benzodiazepines are the two drugs most associated with causing hiccup.

Males may be afflicted with hiccup up to 5 times more than women.

Persistent or recurrent hiccups lasting up to 48 hours are considered *acute*, those lasting longer than 48 hours are termed *persistent*, and those lasting longer than 2 months are *intractable*. The adverse effects can be multiple, including fatigue, significant discomfort, insomnia, depression, difficulty with speech and oral intake, weight loss, and decrease in quality of life.

Management is first directed at evaluating the possible underlying cause and taking corrective action, if possible.[6,7] To this end, the history and physical examination are important, and investigations such as laboratory, imaging, and endoscopic studies need to be considered.

Decreasing or discontinuing corticosteroids and benzodiazapines can be an important intervention.

Often the cause is unknown or cannot be rectified. In these cases, there is little from research studies to direct management; most guidelines suggest empiric management based on case studies or postulated mechanisms of action.

Traditional folk remedies may be tried and have little harm, but are unlikely to improve persistent hiccups. Such maneuvers include pharyngeal and gag reflex stimulation, vagal maneuvers, and breath-holding, among a long list of many others reported throughout history.

Drug treatments are many and varied. An "add-on therapy" approach is recommended given the likelihood of multiple etiologies and the difficulty of this clinical situation.[8] The commonly suggested approach is to start with metoclopramide (10 mg q4h IV or SC) and a proton pump inhibitor (PPI), because GERD plays an important role in many patients.

If this is not effective and renal function is adequate, baclofen (5 mg tid, increased by 5 mg/dose every 3 days to a maximum of 80 mg/day) may be added and titrated upward, while watching for the side effects of sedation, vertigo, ataxia, slurred speech, and weakness.[8] This agent is an analog of gamma-aminobutyric acid (GABA) and is inhibitory at the spinal level. It has been used successfully in the palliative care population for this indication, with many case studies and a small randomized, double-blind, placebo-controlled crossover study to support its use.

Gabapentin (100–300 mg tid starting dose) may be the next agent to consider adding, again considering renal function.

Chlorpromazine (25 mg PO tid) or haloperidol (3–5 mg PO/SC tid) are the next-considered agents to add on.

Nifedipine (30–60 mg/day) or sertraline may also be considered.

Acupuncture and vagal nerve stimulation are final options to consider. Phrenic nerve ablation is the treatment of last resort because of the risk to pulmonary function.

Pruritis

Pruritis is an unpleasant sensation that elicits a desire to scratch or itch. When experienced chronically, pruritis becomes a severely distressing and troublesome symptom.

Histamine appears to be an important mediator of itch in many conditions. Also, centrally acting mu-opioid agonists can mediate pruritis.[9] Unfortunately, there is a paucity of research into this complex symptom. Treatments based on randomized controlled trials are rare.

A large number of diseases may present with itch as an important symptom. It is often helpful to think of these in four broad groups, with some examples listed in the following sections.

Dermatological Diseases

These include common conditions such as dry skin (xerosis). Examples of other skin conditions include scabies, urticaria, atopic dermatitis, dermatitis herpetiformis, bullous pemphigoid, miliari, and pediculosis, among many others.

Systemic Conditions

This is a large group including malignancy, drug reactions, hepatic disorders, renal disorders, autoimmune diseases, endocrine, and hematopoietic and infectious diseases, including HIV disease.

Disorders of the Central or Peripheral Nervous System

These include peripheral neuropathy, depression, multiple sclerosis, and brain tumor.

Psychogenic Disorders

Psychogenic disorders in which pruritis can occur include delusions of parasitosis, neurodermatitis, and anxiety.

Evaluation of the patient who presents with pruritis should include a careful history, probing for use of topical or ingested agents that could induce pruritis. Ask about new drugs or therapies instituted in the weeks prior to the itch. Determine whether there is a history of excessive bathing, other family members with itch, or symptoms of neurological or psychiatric diseases.

A physical examination with careful attention to inspection of the skin can reveal a classic dermatological diagnosis, such as xerosis or urticaria. Dermatological consultation is often helpful if lesions are hard to classify. This may result in recommendations for skin biopsies or special examinations for fungal infections or scabies.

Laboratory investigations screening for systemic conditions that cause pruritis are useful if no etiology is apparent after the history-taking and the physical examination. It is important to screen for hepatogenic and nephrogenic pruritis, as these make up a large proportion of cases of systemic pruritis.

Treatment is most effective when a specific cause is diagnosed and an effective treatment is available.[10,11] Any new medication likely to cause pruritis should be stopped, if possible.

General measures are appropriate in most cases. These include avoiding topical products with fragrance or alcohol and limiting bathing to once per day as a gentle wash with a non-soap, low-pH cleanser. Emollients should be applied in most cases after bathing and frequently throughout the day to improve the skin barrier.

The list of possible systemic treatments for pruritis is extensive. The rationale for using a particular therapy should relate to the etiology involved.[12,13] While the many choices of agents may seem baffling, there are some recommended drug choices:

- Hepatogenic pruritis: mirtazapine (15–30 mg/day), butorphanol (1–4 mg intranasally every day)
- Nephrogenic pruritis: ultraviolet B (UVB) phototherapy (3 times per week), mirtazapine.
- Dermatological pruritis: hydroxyzine (25–100 mg q8h), doxepin (10–50 mg hs).
- Psychogenic pruritis: mirtazapine, paroxetine (20–50 mg every day).

Other agents that may be useful for hepatic or nephrogenic pruritis include cholestyramine, ondansetron, and naltrexone. Thalidomide (HIV, uremia), gabapentin (neurological), charcoal (uremia), and rifampin (hepatic) have been reported to be helpful as well.

Pressure Ulcers and Wound Care

Wounds presenting in the severely ill patient need to be evaluated for the underlying cause in order to direct management properly. Wounds in this population are commonly due to pressure ulceration, malignancy, venous stasis, arterial insufficiency, infection, or surgical dehiscence.

In the terminally ill, goals of care need to be established, as healing of the wound may not always be realistic. The goals of providing comfort and improving quality of life, promoting healing, and limiting wound progression, as well as preventing further wound development, may be appropriate for many patients.

Pressure ulcers are caused by compression of cutaneous and subcutaneous tissue between a bony prominence and a support surface. This results in ischemia and tissue necrosis.[14,15] Other forces that can traumatize these tissues include friction and shearing of the skin along the bed sheets or other surfaces.

Factors that cause immobility are important in the development of these wounds. It is common to find patients at higher risk for these lesions as their illness progresses and they become less mobile.

Typical areas for the development of pressure ulcer are the sacrum, trochanter, ischial tuberosity, posterior heel, elbow, scapula, and occipital region. These areas deserve careful inspection in the routine care of the severely ill patient.

If a wound is evident, strategies for treating the lesion need to be instituted, including increasing the patient's mobility with frequent position changes and turning the patient. It is sometimes helpful to determine what the patient's position was that caused a lesion in a particular area and to inform the patient and caregiver of this, as well as to consider alternative positioning strategies. The assessment of a physical or occupational therapist can greatly assist with this process.

It is important to remember that unrelieved pressure on the area is the cause of a pressure ulcer.[16] The single most important strategy is the relief of that pressure.[17] Special pressure-reducing mattresses or wheelchair cushions (e.g., Roho) can be helpful in relieving pressure in vulnerable areas.

Attention to dressings is also important. Consultation with a wound-ostomy care (WOC) nurse is useful, as these practitioners are familiar with the variety of dressings and their uses.

The principle of moist wound healing, one of the prime functions of an appropriate dressing, is important in treating this condition. The wound should not be allowed to become dry. Excess exudates can be managed with special dressings such as alginate, hydrofiber, or foam dressings.

It is important to protect the wound and normal skin from the maceration caused by incontinence. Cleansing the wound with a noncytotoxic cleaner such as normal saline, Ringer's lactate, or sterile water between dressing changes is recommended.

Assessment of the wound for infection by observing for inflammation, purulent discharge, and odor can result in effective treatment with antimicrobials, either topically or systemically.

In patients whose wound healing is possible, nutrition should be optimized. Nutritional strategies are feasible, and a dietician's expertise can be useful in developing these for individual patients.

Debridement improves healing and reduces infection. Surgical, enzymatic, and hydrotherapy techniques for debridement should be considered. For difficult situations, vacuum-assisted closure or surgical closure with a flap may be warranted.

General wound management includes consideration of radiotherapy for managing malignant wounds.

Topical sprinkling of crushed metronidazole tablets can decrease wound odor resulting from anaerobic bacteria. Lidocaine gel and compounded morphine gel are topical agents that may be considered when addressing local wound pain.

Lymphedema, Edema, and Anasarca

Lymphedema is swelling caused by failure of the lymphatic system to adequately drain lymph fluid.[18-20] This occurs secondary to disease (e.g., cancer) or as a result of surgery or radiotherapy of the draining lymph system. The involved limb is at risk for cellulitis because of the accumulation of protein-rich interstitial fluid. Chronic lymphedema results in inflammation that produces fibrosis and sclerosis.

Treatment for breast cancer with surgery and radiotherapy is a common cause of upper limb lymphedema. Surgery or involvement of the inguinal or pelvic lymph nodes with cancer often results in lower-extremity lymphedema.

Symptoms of limb heaviness, discomfort, decreased range of motion, body image concerns, and decreased quality of life are common. The presentation of an acute unilateral limb swelling requires the exclusion of deep venous thrombosis and cellulitis.

The management of lymphedema is optimized by using the skills of a lympedema therapist, who is usually a physiotherapist, nurse, or kinesiologist who has undergone special training.[21,22] These therapists use a combination of skin care, manual lymph drainage (specialized massage), compression bandaging, pneumatic compression with electric pumps, education, and exercise, termed *combined/complex decongestive therapy* (CDT).

Compression garments are fitted to the limb for maintenance of the reduction in swelling.

Pharmacological therapy has not been effective. Diuretics are ineffective and place the patient at risk for electrolyte imbalance and hypotension. Placement of an IV or SC site in the affected limb is best avoided because of the risk of infection.

Previously, exercise was thought to worsen this condition, but recent evidence shows that even vigorous exercise does not worsen swelling.

Surgery may be an option early in the development of lymphedema. Procedures such as liposuction, lymphovenous anastomoses, and lymph node transplantation are reported to produce improvements.

Edema refers to excess fluid in body tissue. *Anasarca* describes generalized edema. Both conditions occur commonly in the terminally ill, with lower extremity edema being very frequent in advanced-cancer patients. In these cases, other factors in addition to impaired lymphatic drainage occur, such as hypo-albuminemia or obstruction of the inferior vena cava.

Therapy with diuretics rarely results in significant reduction in swelling and is troublesome due to the complications of these drugs. Elevation of the affected limb, massage drainage, and compression bandaging remain the most effective strategies.

Body-image concerns of the patient and caregivers' distress are often addressed to the clinician and require appropriate discussion and reassurance.

External lymph drainage, a technique developed by Lawrence Clein, is[19] an exciting new development for symptomatic management at the end of life that requires further study, as it is supported by only a small number of case reports at present.

Scrotal edema can be very uncomfortable and can be reduced by scrotal elevation (a small towel or face cloth placed under the scrotum), a customized scrotal support, or bicycle shorts.

Myoclonus

Myoclonus is defined as sudden, brief, involuntary contractions of a muscle or a muscle group.[23] Progression to seizure can occur if the condition escalates. The complete pathophysiological mechanism has not been determined.

It is usually classified as physiological, essential, epileptic, or symptomatic. The latter category is of most concern in palliative care.

Toxic-metabolic syndromes such as renal and hepatic disease are etiologies, as are neurodegenerative disorders such as Parkinson's disease, Alzheimer's disease, Huntington's disease, and Lewy body dementia. Posthypoxic syndromes and drug-induced myoclonus also occur.

Medications associated with myoclonus include opioids, antipsychotics, antidepressants (TCAs and SSRIs), anticonvulsants, antibiotics, calcium channel blockers, and anti-arrhythmics.

Opioid-induced neurotoxicity (OIN) is a syndrome that occurs frequently in the palliative setting, where opioids are regularly administered.[24] Myoclonus is one of the most common manifestations of OIN and can alert the clinician to this syndrome. Accumulation of opioid metabolites is the perceived mechanism causing OIN.

Management is directed at reversing this mechanism by decreasing the opioid dose, or by opioid rotation to an alternative opioid. Clonazepam (starting at 0.5 mg twice daily) and midazolam are agents that can reduce myoclonus if opioid reduction or rotation is ineffective.

For other conditions causing myoclonus, management consists of treating the underlying disorder or augmenting the GABAergic deficiency. Agents often used include clonazepam (often the drug of choice), valproic acid, and barbiturates.[25,26]

Clinical Pearls

- Eliminating the causative drug(s) may reduce xerostomia.
- Many patients presenting with hiccup benefit from treatment of GERD.
- In the workup of pruritis, it is important to screen for hepatic and renal disease.
- The most important strategy in the management of pressure ulcers is the relief of pressure on the wound.
- Do not use diuretics to manage lymphedema.
- Consider opioid-induced neurotoxicity as a common cause of myoclonus.

References

1. Dion D, Lapointe B (2005). Mouth care. In: MacDonald N, Oneschuk D, Hagen N, Doyle D (eds.), *Palliative Medicine: A Case-Based Manual*, 2nd ed. Oxford: Oxford University Press, pp. 317–31.
2. Fusco F (2006). Mouth care. In: Bruera E, Higginson IJ, Ripamonti C, von Gunten C (eds.), *Textbook of Palliative Medicine*. Oxford: Hodder Arnold, pp. 773–9.
3. Lalla RV, Peterson DE (2009). Oral symptoms. In: Walsh TD, Caraceni AT, Fainsinger R, Foley K, et al. (eds.), *Palliative Medicine*. Philadelphia: W. B. Saunders, pp. 937–46.
4. Lovelace TL, Fox NF, Sood AJ, Nguyen SA, Day TA (2014). Management of radiotherapy-induced salivary hypofunction and consequent xerostomia in patients with oral head and

neck cancer: metanalysis and literature review. *Oral Surg Oral Med Oral Pathol Oral Radiol* May;117(5):595–607.

5. Brimhall J, Jhaveri MA, Yepes JF (2013). Eficacy of cevimeline vs. pilocarpine in the secretion of saliva: a pilot study. *Spec Care Dentist* May–Jun;33(3):123–7.

6. Smith HS (2009). Hiccups. In: Walsh TD, Caraceni AT, Fainsinger R, Foley KM, et al. (eds.), *Palliative Medicine*. Philadelphia: W. Bl. Saunders, pp. 894–8.

7. Thomas T, Wade R, Booth S (2006). Other respiratory symptoms (cough, hiccup, and secretions). In: Bruera E, Higginson IJ, Ripamonti C, von Gunten C (eds.), *Textbook of Palliative Medicine*. Oxford: Hodder Arnold, pp. 663–72.

8. Ramierz FC, Graham DY (1992). Treatment of intractable hiccup with baclofen: results of a double-blind randomized, controlled, cross-over study. *Am J Gastroenterol* 87(12):1789–91.

9. Summey BT. Pruritus (2009). In: Walsh TD, Caraceni AT, Fainsinger R, Foley K, et al. (eds.), *Palliative Medicine*. Philadelphia: W. B. Saunders, pp. 910–3.

10. Pittelkow MR, Loprinzi CL (2004). Pruritus and sweating in palliative medicine. In: Doyle D, Hanks G, Cherny N, Calman K (eds.), *Oxford Textbook of Palliative Medicine*. New York: Oxford University Press, pp. 573–87.

11. Fleischer AB, Dalgleish D (2002). Pruritus. In: Berger AM, Portenoy RK, Weissman DE (eds.), *Principles and Practice of Palliative Care and Supportive Oncology*. Philadelphia: Lippincott Williams & Wilkins, pp. 299–306.

12. Misery L, Brenaut E, Le Garrec R, Abasq C, Genestet S, Marcorelles P, Zagnoli F (2014). Neuropathic pruritus. *Nat Rev Neurol* Jul;10(7):408–16.

13. Davidson S, Moser H, Giesler G (2014). Ascending pathways for itch. In: Carstens E, Akiyama T (eds.), *Itch: Mechanisms and Treatment*. Boca Raton, FL: CRC Press.

14. Schulz VN, Kozell KM, Martins LM (2009). Pressure ulcers and wound care. In: Walsh TD, Caraceni AT, Fainsinger R, Foley K, et al. (eds.), *Palliative Medicine*. Philadelphia: W. B. Saunders, pp. 478–84.

15. Froiland KG (2006). Pressure ulcers/wounds. In: Bruera E, Higginson IJ, Ripamonti C, von Gunten C (Eds.), *Textbook of Palliative Medicine*. Oxford: Hodder Arnold, pp. 768–72.

16. Reddy M, Gill SS, Kalkar SR, et al. (2008). Treatment of pressure ulcers: a systematic review. *JAMA* 300(22):2647–62.

17. Gillespie BM, Chaboyer WP, McInnes E, Whitty JA, Thalib L (2014). Repositioning for pressure ulcer prevention in adults. *Cochrane Database Syst Rev* Apr 3;4:CD009958.

18. Towers A (2009). Lymphedema. In: Walsh TD, Caraceni AT, Fainsinger R, Foley K, et al. (eds.), *Palliative Medicine*. Philadelphia: Saunders, pp. 474–8.

19. Clein LJ. Edema (2009). In: Walsh TD, Caraceni AT, Fainsinger R, Foley K, et al. (eds.), *Palliative Medicine*. Philadelphia: W. B. Saunders, pp. 881–6.

20. Guo Y, Konzen B (2006). Lymphedema. In: Bruera E, Higginson IJ, Ripamonti C, von Gunten C (eds.), *Textbook of Palliative Medicine*. Oxford: Hodder Arnold, pp. 787–96.

21. Szolnoky G, Dobozy A, Kemeny L (2014). Towards an effective management of chronic lymphedema. *Clin Dermatol* Sept–Oct;32(5):685–91.

22. Leung EY, Tirlapur SA, Meads C (2014). The management of secondary lower limb lymphedema in cancer patients: a systematic review. *Palliat Med* Aug 18. Pii: 0269216314545803.

23. Groninger H, Muir JC (2009). Seizures and movement disorders. In: Walsh TD, Caraceni AT, Fainsinger R, Foley K, et al. (eds.), *Palliative Medicine*. Philadelphia: W. B. Saunders, pp. 961–5.

24. Lawlor P, Lucey M, Creedon B (2009). Opioid side effects and overdose. In: Walsh TD, Caraceni AT, Fainsinger R, Foley K, et al. (eds.), *Palliative Medicine*. Philadelphia: W. B. Saunders, pp. 1411–6.

25. Burhard PR (2014). Acute and subacute drug-induced movement disorders. *Parkinsonism Relat Disord* Jan;20(Suppl 1):S108–12.

26. Dulin JD, Noreika DM, Coyne PJ (2014). Management of refractory status epilepticus in an actively dying patient. *J Pain Palliat Care Pharmacother* Sep;28(3):243–50.

Management of Cancer Treatment–Related Adverse Effects

David Hui

Introduction

A growing proportion of advanced cancer patients seen by palliative care clinicians are on antineoplastic agents, including chemotherapy, hormonal therapy, and targeted agents. This can be attributed to the increasing availability of therapeutic options, as well as to earlier palliative care referral for symptom control.

While antineoplastic agents may improve patients' symptoms through tumor shrinkage or stabilization, they can also be associated with significant adverse effects. Thus, palliative care specialists caring for patients with advanced cancer should be familiar with the management of common side effects associated with these agents.

This chapter provides a brief review of the clinical management of a number of common adverse effects related to antineoplastic agents, including febrile neutropenia, cytopenia, chemotherapy-induced nausea and vomiting (CINV), oral mucositis, diarrhea, drug rash, and peripheral neuropathy.

Cancer-related fatigue, another side effect frequently experienced by cancer patients on treatment, is discussed in Chapter 5.

A detailed discussion of all adverse effects associated with each antineoplastic agent is beyond the scope of this chapter. Readers are referred to other resources for further information (e.g., NCCN guidelines, Up-To-Date).

Clinical Pearl

- Effective management of adverse effects related to antineoplastic agents requires a sound understanding of the common and serious side effects related to each drug, frequent symptom assessments, patient education, and early initiation of treatment.

Cytopenia and Febrile Neutropenia

In this section, some of the common management strategies for chemotherapy-induced bone marrow toxicities (Table 17.1) and febrile neutropenia are highlighted.

Anemia

Patients with significant anemia (hemoglobin [Hb] < 8.0 g/dL) may benefit from packed red blood cell (RBC) transfusions. For patients with underlying ischemic heart disease or pulmonary disorders, the threshold for transfusion may be lower (e.g., Hb < 9.0 g/dL).

Erythropoiesis-stimulating agents such as epoetin-alfa and darbepoetin are generally not given and should be avoided in patients with advanced cancer who are not on chemotherapy. Erythropoiesis-stimulating agents are associated with not only a risk of thromboembolism but also increased mortality, which is thought to be related to stimulation of tumor growth.[1]

Neutropenia

Neutropenia (absolute neutrophil count [ANC] < 1000/mm³) on its own is not life threatening, but it may predispose patients to febrile neutropenia and overwhelming sepsis.

Granulocyte colony–stimulating factor (GCSF) should generally not be used to treat neutropenia in the absence of fever, although it has a role in primary or secondary prophylaxis for patients at risk of developing febrile neutropenia.

Febrile Neutropenia

Febrile neutropenia is one of the most common oncological emergencies, defined as the presence of fever > 38.3°C (or > 38°C for > 1 hour) and neutrophil count < 500/mm³ (or < 1000/mm ³ and expected to decrease

Table 17.1 National Cancer Institute Common Terminology Criteria for Adverse Events, Version 4.03: Hematological Toxicities[4]

Grade	Hemoglobin	Neutrophil Count	Platelet Count
1	< LLN–10.0 g/dL	< LLN–1500/mm³	< LLN–75,000/mm³
2	< 10.0–8.0 g/dL	< 1500–1000/mm³	< 75,000–50,000/mm³
3	< 8.0 g/dL	< 1000–500/mm³	< 50,000–25,000/mm³
4	Life-threatening consequences; urgent intervention indicated	< 500/mm³	< 25,000/mm³

LLN = lower limit of normal.
National Cancer Institute (2006). National Cancer Institute Common Terminology Criteria for Adverse Events (CTCAE) v4.03. Last accessed May 2013.

further). Any patient who develops fever while on chemotherapy should be assumed to have febrile neutropenia unless proven otherwise—complete blood count (CBC) with differential and cultures should be done urgently.

Once febrile neutropenia is confirmed, broad-spectrum antibiotics should be initiated immediately while waiting for culture results.[2]

Patients at low risk for complications (i.e., no significant signs or symptoms of infection, no comorbidities, ANC > 100/mm^3, and reliable for follow-up) may be treated on an outpatient basis with oral antibiotics, such as amoxicillin-clavulanate 500 mg PO q8h plus ciprofloxacin 500 mg PO bid for 7–10 days.

High-risk patients should be admitted and given intravenous (IV) antibiotics. Common antibiotic regimens include ceftazidime 2 g IV q8h, imipenem 500 mg IV q6h, and piperacillin/tazobactam 4.5 g IV q8h ± gentamicin 2–2.5 mg/kg IV q8h. It is important that clinicians check renal function and local susceptibility pattern before prescribing these drugs. Vancomycin 1 g IV q12h should be added if line infection is suspected. Antifungals should be considered if fever persists for more than 5 days. GCSF should given to patients at high risk of developing complications.[3] Patients with febrile neutropenia should avoid being in direct contact with other infected individuals or fresh flowers, which are laden with bacteria; however, contact isolation is generally unnecessary.

Thrombocytopenia

Platelet transfusions should be considered for patients with a platelet count < 20,000/mm^3 or those with thrombocytopenia and clinically significant active bleeding.

Clinical Pearls

- Any patients who develops a fever while on chemotherapy should be assumed to have febrile neutropenia unless proven otherwise.
- Avoid erythropoietin use, as it is associated with an increased risk of thromboembolism and mortality in advanced-cancer patients.

Chemotherapy-Induced Nausea and Vomiting

Chemotherapy-induced nausea and vomiting (CINV) is one of the most common side effects (20%–50%) experienced by cancer patients and is frequently ranked as the top symptom affecting quality of life during treatment.[5] Clinicians tend to underestimate patients' experience of CINV, particularly the delayed phase.

Prevention is key in the management of CINV. This requires appropriate identification of emetogenic risk and use of anti-emetic prophylaxis. Significant advances in the management of CINV include use of corticosteroids, serotonin receptor antagonists, and, most recently, neurokinin 1 (NK-1) receptor antagonists.

In addition to the prevention and treatment of CINV, it is important to assess hydration status, food intake, and other common treatment-related complications (e.g., mucositis, diarrhea) (see Table 17.2) and to initiate proper therapies, when appropriate.

Patients on chemotherapy may have nausea and vomiting from causes other than CINV, including bowel obstruction, hypercalcemia, brain metastasis, and opioids. Chapter 10 provides further management strategies for nausea and vomiting in palliative care patients not on chemotherapy.

Types of CINV

- *Acute emesis* happens within 24 hours of chemotherapy administration. It usually begins in 1–2 hours and peaks at 4–6 hours.
- *Delayed emesis* happens after 24 hours of chemotherapy administration and can last for 4 days or more. It is most commonly associated with cisplatin but may also occur with carboplatin, cyclophosphamide, and anthracyclines.

Table 17.2 National Cancer Institute Common Terminology Criteria for Adverse Events, Version V4.03: Nausea and Vomiting

Grade	Nausea	Vomiting
1	Loss of appetite without alteration in eating habits	1–2 episodes (separated by 5 minutes) in 24 hours
2	Oral intake decreased without significant weight loss, dehydration, or malnutrition	3–5 episodes (separated by 5 minutes) in 24 hours
3	Inadequate oral caloric or fluid intake; tube feeding, total parenteral nutrition (TPN), or hospitalization indicated	≥ 6 episodes (separated by 5 minutes) in 24 hours; tube feeding, TPN, or hospitalization indicated
4	—	Life-threatening consequences; urgent intervention indicated

- *Anticipatory emesis* is a conditioned response in patients who have experienced severe nausea with previous cycles of chemotherapy. This typically begins 3–4 hours prior to chemotherapy initiation.

Emetogenic Levels of Antineoplastic Agents

- *High risk* (> 90% risk of CINV in the absence of anti-emetic prophylaxis): carmustine, cisplatin, cyclophosphamide (> 1500 mg/m^2), dacarbazine, dactinomycin, mechlorethamine, streptozocin
- *Moderate risk* (31%–90% risk): carboplatin, cyclophosphamide P1500 mg/m^2), cytarabine (> 1000 mg/m^2), daunorubicin, doxorubicin, epirubicin, idarubicin, ifosfamide, irinotecan, oxaliplatin
- *Low risk* (10%–30% risk): bortezomib, cetuximab, cytarabine P1000 mg/m^2), docetaxel, etoposide, fluorouracil, gemcitabine, ixabepilone, lapatinib, methotrexate, mitomycin, mitoxantrone, paclitaxel, pemetrexed, temsirolimus, topotecan, trastuzumab
- *Minimal risk* (< 10% risk): bevacizumab, bleomycin, busulfan, cladribine, fludarabine, vinblastine, vincristine, vinorelbine, rituximab

Clinical Pearl

- Prevention is key in the management of CINV. Identify the emetogenic risk category and prescribe prophylaxis accordingly.

Management of Chemotherapy-Induced Nausea and Vomiting

Selection of anti-emetic agents for prophylaxis should be based on the highest emetogenic level among the intravenously administered antineoplastic agents (see Table 17.3).

Table 17.3 Prevention and Treatment of Acute and Delayed CINV: A Practical Approach

	Any High-Risk Agents or AC Chemotherapy	Any Moderate-Risk Agents	Any Low-Risk Agents	Minimal-Risk Agents
1. 5HT3 antagonist (choose one)				
Dolasetron (Anzemet)	100 mg PO/IV on day 1	100 mg PO/IV on day 1, then 100 mg PO days 2–3	—	—
Granisetron (Kytril)	1 mg IV or 2 mg PO on day 1	1 mg IV or 2 mg PO on day 1, then 1 mg PO bid on days 2–3	—	—
Ondansetron (Zofran)	8–12 mg IV or 16–24 mg PO on day 1	8 mg IV or 8 mg PO bid on day 1, then 8 mg PO bid on days 2–3	—	—
Palonosetron (Aloxi)	0.25 mg IV on day 1	0.25 mg IV on day 1	—	—
Tropisetron (Navoban)	5 mg PO/IV on day 1	5 mg PO/IV on day 1, then 5 mg on days 2–3	—	—
2. Dexamethasone (Decadron)	12 mg PO/IV on day 1, then 8 mg PO days 2–4	12 mg PO/IV on day 1, then 8 mg PO daily or 4 mg PO bid days 2–3	8 mg PO/ IV day 1	—
3. NK1 antagonist (choose one)				
Fosaprepitant (Emend)	150 mg IV on day 1	—	—	—
Aprepitant (Emend)	125 mg PO on day 1, then 80 mg PO days 2–3	—	—	—

(continued)

Table 17.3 (Continued)

	Any High-Risk Agents or AC Chemotherapy	Any Moderate-Risk Agents	Any Low-Risk Agents	Minimal-Risk Agents
4. As needed for breakthrough CINV (choose one or more)				
Metoclopramide (Reglan)		5–10 mg PO/IV q4h PRN		
Prochlorperazine (Compazine)		5–10 mg PO/IV q4h PRN		

Adapted from Kris MG, Hesketh PJ, Somerfield MR, Feyer P, Clark-Snow R, Koeller JM, Morrow GR, Chinnery LW, Chesney MJ, Gralla RJ, Grunberg SM (2006). American Society of Clinical Oncology guideline for antiemetics in oncology: update 2006. *J Clin Oncol* 24(18):2932–2947.[6]

Oral Mucositis

Oral mucositis, defined as inflammation and ulceration of membranous mucosa, can occur throughout the gastrointestinal tract (see Table 17.4). It is very common among cancer patients, with an incidence of 20%–40%.

Risk factors for mucositis include chemotherapy (e.g., 5-fluorouracil, cytarabine, methotrexate, bleomycin, capecitabine, chlorambucil, doxorubicin, etoposide, and vinblastine), radiation to the head and neck region, specific cancer primaries (requiring previously noted treatment modalities), younger age, poor oral hygiene, smoking, and alcohol use.

Severe cases (grades 3–4) can lead to complications such as severe pain, bleeding, and superinfections (bacteremia, febrile neutropenia), and may result in hospitalization.

For patients on chemotherapy, the presence of oral mucositis may indicate that other parts of the alimentary tract are involved. Thus, one should always assess for the presence of diarrhea, abdominal pain, nausea, and vomiting. Patients should be encouraged to ensure good oral intake and oral hygiene.

Management of Oral Mucositis

Prevention is key to the management of mucositis. A number of resources are available on this topic.[7] For patients on 5-fluorouracil, edatrexate, or high-dose melphalan, cryotherapy with ice chips is reasonably tolerable, easily assessable, and cheap. Treatment of established oral mucositis consists of the following.

Hydration and Oral Hygiene

Maintenance of good oral hygiene and adequate hydration is essential.
- Use of a soft tooth brush for at least 90 seconds twice daily
- Daily flossing
- Denture care (where applicable)
- Bland rinses include 0.9% saline, baking soda, or salt and baking soda solution (mix 1 teaspoon of baking soda and one-half teaspoon of salt in 1 L of water). The patient should take a tablespoon every 4 hours, swish for at least 30 seconds, and spit out rinse right afterward.

Table 17.4 National Cancer Institute Common Terminology Criteria for Adverse Events, Version 4.03: Oral Mucositis

Grade	
1	Asymptomatic or mild symptoms; intervention not indicated
2	Moderate pain; not interfering with oral intake; modified diet indicated
3	Severe pain; interfering with oral intake
4	Life-threatening consequences; urgent intervention indicated

National Cancer Institute (2006). National Cancer Institute Common Terminology Criteria for Adverse Events (CTCAE) v4.03. Last accessed May 2013.

Analgesia

Topical analgesia may be useful for short-term pain relief of mucositis.

- Different preparations of Magic (or Miracle) mouthwashes may vary, but they generally consist of lidocaine for pain control. One example is a 100 mL solution of hydrocortisone 25 mg, glycerin 95% 2 mL, normal saline 52 mL, lidocaine 2% 25 mL, and nystatin 2,083,300 IU or 20.833 mL. Use 10 mL swish and spit q4h to q6h.
- Morphine sulfate 2 mg/mL in 15 mL of water, swish and spit, q4h to q6h
- Lidocaine viscous 2% 10 mL, swish and spit, q4h PRN

Pharmacological Treatment

- Systemic opioids remain the mainstay in management of pain associated with mucositis (e.g., morphine 5 mg PO q4h PRN, titrating up as needed). For patients who cannot tolerate the oral route, patient-controlled analgesia (PCA) with parenteral opioids may be considered.
- Current guidelines from the Multinational Association of Supportive Care in Cancer (MASCC) and the European Society for Medical Oncology (ESMO) recommend against the use of chlorhexidine mouthwash in the prevention and treatment of mucositis.

Infections

- For patients with oral candidiasis, treatment with nystatin 500,000 IU swish and swallow qid, clotrimazole troches, or fluconazole should be considered.
- Acyclovir or valacyclovir may be given for suspected herpes simplex virus (HSV) infection after cultures have been taken.

Clinical Pearls

- Patients with painful oral mucositis should be prescribed adequate analgesia (topical agents or systemic opioids), and monitored for dehydration.
- CINV, oral mucositis, and chemotherapy-induced diarrhea often coexist. When one of these is present, inquire about the others.

Chemotherapy-Induced Diarrhea

Chemotherapy-induced diarrhea (CID) (Table 17.5) occurs in 20%–40% of cancer patients on treatment and is commonly associated with fluoropyrimidines (5-fluorouracil and capecitabine) and irinotecan. Other causative agents include cisplatin, docetaxel, paclitaxel, doxorubicin, cyclophosphamide, methotrexate, cytosine arabinoside, and topotecan. Targeted agents such as imatinib, erlotinib, sunitinib, and sorafenib may also cause diarrhea.

The pathophysiology of CID is incompletely understood. CID may be caused by treatment-induced intestinal mucosal damage, leading to reduced transit time and decreased water absorption.

Other factors, such as alteration in intestinal microflora, may also play a role. Irinotecan causes both an early secretory and delayed severe diarrhea in up to 60%–80% of patients. This is partly related to its active metabolite SN30, which causes damage of the intestine.

Management of Chemotherapy-Induced Diarrhea

A clinical practice guideline is available for CID:[8]
- First-line treatment: loperamide 4 mg PO, followed by 2 mg every 2 hours (or 4 mg every 4 hours) until 12 hours has elapsed without any diarrhea.
- Second-line treatment: octreotide 100–150 mcg SC as needed. Octreotide is a somatostatin analog that slows intestinal transit and decreases fluid secretion into the small intestine.
- For irinotecan-induced diarrhea, neomycin, pentoxifylline, kampo medicine, and chrysin represent a number of potential treatment options; however, the evidence supporting their use remains limited.

It is also important to ensure adequate hydration and to assess for other symptoms such as oral mucositis, nausea, and vomiting. Remember to hold all laxatives in patients who have diarrhea.

Table 17.5 National Cancer Institute Common Terminology Criteria for Adverse Events, Version 4.03: Diarrhea

Grade	
1	Increase of < 4 stools per day over baseline; mild increase in ostomy output compared to baseline
2	Increase of 4–6 stools per day over baseline; moderate increase in ostomy output compared to baseline
3	Increase of ≥ 7 stools per day over baseline; incontinence; hospitalization indicated; severe increase in ostomy output compared to baseline; limiting self-care ADL
4	Life-threatening consequences; urgent intervention indicated

Treatment-Related Skin Lesions

Dermatological complications of antineoplastic agents include alopecia, palmar plantar erythrodysesthesia, xerosis, skin rash, hair and nail changes, and phototoxicity. In this section, discussion is focused on palmar plantar erythrodysesthesia and rash related to epidermal growth factor receptor (EGFR) inhibition.

Palmar Plantar Erythrodysesthesia

Palmar plantar erythrodysesthesia,[9] also known as hand-foot syndrome (Table 17.6), is commonly associated with capecitabine, 5-fluorouracil, docetaxel, doxorubicin (including liposomal formulation), and cytarabine. Multi-kinase inhibitors such as sorafenib and sunitinib can also be associated with a hand-foot skin reaction, which tends to be more localized and hyperkeratotic than classic palmar planter erythrodysesthesia.

Early recognition and modification of treatment regimen are key to managing this syndrome. Supportive measures to keep the skin moist and intact include topical Bag Balm and petroleum jelly. Appropriate analgesia should be given if pain becomes an issue. The role of systemic or topical corticosteroids remains undefined.

Table 17.6 National Cancer Institute Common Terminology Criteria for Adverse Events, Version 3.0: Hand-Foot Syndrome

Grade	Criteria
1	Minimal skin changes or dermatitis (e.g., erythema, or hyperkeratosis) without pain
2	Skin changes (e.g., peeling, blisters, bleeding, edema, or hyeprkeratosis) with pain; limiting instrumental ADL
3	Severe skin changes (e.g., peeling, blisters, bleeding, edema, or hyperkeratosis) with pain; limiting self-care ADL
4	—

National Cancer Institute (2006). National Cancer Institute Common Terminology Criteria for Adverse Events (CTCAE) v4.03. Last accessed May 2013.

Skin Lesions Associated with EGFR Inhibition

Targeted agents that inhibit the EGFR pathway, including erlotinib, gefitinib, cetuximab, and panitumumab, are commonly associated with a rash involving the face, chest, and upper back. This reaction typically peaks after 1–2 weeks of therapy.

It is papulopustular or macropapular in nature and frequently is mistaken for an acneiform eruption. Importantly, the presence of skin rash is a predictive marker of treatment response to EGFR inhibitors.

The following proposed classification is based on symptom severity:[10]

- *Mild toxicity*: generally localized papulopustular reaction that is minimally symptomatic, with no sign of superinfection, and no impact on daily activities
- *Moderate toxicity*: generalized papulopustular reaction, accompanied by mild pruritus or tenderness, with minimal impact on daily activities and no signs of superinfection
- *Severe toxicity*: generalized papulopustular reaction, accompanied by severe pruritus or tenderness, that has a significant impact on daily activity and has the potential for superinfection or has become superinfected.

Patients with EGFR inhibitor–associated skin rash should be advised to avoid sun exposure. Specific management is based on rash severity:[10]

- *Mild toxicity*: consider observation alone, topical hydrocortisone 1%–2.5% cream, or clindamycin 1% gel. Continue EGFR inhibitor at the same dose and monitor carefully.
- *Moderate toxicity*: topical hydrocortisone 2.5% cream or clindamycin 1% gel or pimecrolimus 1% cream, plus either doxycycline 100 mg PO bid or minocycline 100 mg PO bid. Continue EGFR inhibitor at the same dose and monitor carefully.
- *Severe toxicity*: topical hydrocortisone 2.5% cream or clindamycin 1% gel or pimecrolimus 1% cream, plus either doxycycline 100 mg PO bid or minocycline 100 mg PO bid. Consider dose reduction of EGFR inhibitor and monitor carefully.

Treatment-Induced Peripheral Neuropathy

Peripheral neuropathy is one of the major adverse effects associated with antineoplastic agents, including taxanes (docetaxel, paclitaxel), platinum agents (oxaliplatin, cisplatin, carboplatin), vinca alkalodis (vincristine, vindesine, vinblastin, vinorelbine), epothilones (ixabepilone, patupilone), thalidomide, lendalidomide, and bortezomib.

Cisplatin and carboplatin are mainly associated with sensory neuropathy, whereas the rest may also have a motor component.[11] Oxaliplatin is associated with both acute neuropathy (cold hypersensitivity and muscle contractions) and chronic sensory peripheral neuropathy that is closely associated with the cumulative dose.

Risk factors for the development of peripheral neuropathy include high treatment dose, prior or concurrent use of neurotoxic agents, and preexisting neuropathy due to comorbidities such as diabetes.

Severe peripheral neuropathy has a negative impact on quality of life (see Table 17.7) and is an important dose-limiting toxicity that frequently results in early termination of cancer treatments.

Management of Peripheral Neuropathy

If patients develop significant peripheral neuropathy (grade 2 or above), dose reduction or delay or discontinuation of treatment may be required. Early diagnosis can minimize development of more neurotoxicity. The neuropathy may not improve (and may sometimes worsen) until several weeks or months after discontinuation of the antineoplastic agent. In some cases, the neurotoxicity may be irreversible.

Table 17.7 National Cancer Institute Common Terminology Criteria for Adverse Events, Version V4.03: Neuropathy

Grade	Peripheral Sensory Neuropathy	Peripheral Motor Neuropathy
1	Asymptomatic; loss of deep tendon reflexes or paresthesia	Asymptomatic; clinical or diagnostic observations only; intervention not indicated
2	Moderate symptoms; limiting instrumental ADL	Moderate symptoms; limiting instrumental ADL
3	Severe symptoms; limiting self-care ADL	Severe symptoms; limiting self-care ADL; assistive device indicated
4	Life-threatening consequences; urgent intervention indicated	Life-threatening consequences; urgent intervention indicated

National Cancer Institute (2006). National Cancer Institute Common Terminology Criteria for Adverse Events (CTCAE) v4.03. Last accessed May 2013.

Specific prophylactic strategies for oxaliplatin-induced peripheral neuropathy include stop-and-go administration schedules and neuromodularlory agents such as Ca/Mg infusions. For neuropathic pain, gabapentin, carbamazepine, and venlafaxine have also been used with variable success.

References

1. Bohlius J, Schmidlin K, Brillant C, Schwarzer G, Trelle S, Seidenfeld J, Zwahlen M, Clarke M, Weingart O, Kluge S, Piper M, Rades D, Steensma DP, Djulbegovic B, Fey MF, Ray-Coquard I, Machtay M, Moebus V, Thomas G, Untch M, Schumacher M, Egger M, Engert A (2009). Recombinant human erythropoiesis-stimulating agents and mortality in patients with cancer: a meta-analysis of randomised trials. *Lancet* 373(9674):1532–42.
2. Hughes WT, Armstrong D, Bodey GP, Brown AE, Edwards JE, Feld R, Pizzo P, Rolston KV, Shenep JL, Young LS (1997). Guidelines for the use of antimicrobial agents in neutropenic patients with unexplained fever. Infectious Diseases Society of America. *Clin Infect Dis* 25(3):551–73.
3. American Society of Clinical Oncology (1994). Recommendations for the use of hematopoietic colony-stimulating factors: evidence-based, clinical practice guidelines. *J Clin Oncol* 12(11): 2471–508.
4. National Cancer Institute (2006). National Cancer Institute Common Terminology Criteria for Adverse Events (CTCAE) v4.03. Last accessed May 2013.
5. Hesketh PJ (2008). Chemotherapy-induced nausea and vomiting. *N Engl J Med* 358(23):2482–94.
6. Kris MG, Hesketh PJ, Somerfield MR, Feyer P, Clark-Snow R, Koeller JM, Morrow GR, Chinnery LW, Chesney MJ, Gralla RJ, Grunberg SM (2006). American Society of Clinical Oncology guideline for antiemetics in oncology: update 2006. *J Clin Oncol* 24(18):2932–47.
7. Keefe DM, Schubert MM, Elting LS, Sonis ST, Epstein JB, Raber-Durlacher JE, Migliorati CA, McGuire DB, Hutchins RD, Peterson DE; Mucositis Study Section of the Multinational Association of Supportive Care in Cancer and the International Society for Oral Oncology (2007). Updated clinical practice guidelines for the prevention and treatment of mucositis. *Cancer* 109(5):820–31.
8. Benson AB, Ajani JA, Catalano RB, Engelking C, Kornblau SM, Martenson JA Jr, McCallum R, Mitchell EP, O'Dorisio TM, Vokes EE, Wadler S (2004). Recommended guidelines for the treatment of cancer treatment–induced diarrhea. *J Clin Oncol* 22(14):2918–26.
9. Nagore E, Insa A, Sanmartín O (2000). Antineoplastic therapy–induced palmar plantar erythrodysesthesia ('hand–foot') syndrome: incidence, recognition and management. *Am J Clin Dermatol* 1(4):225–34.
10. Lynch TJ Jr, Kim ES, Eaby B, Garey J, West DP, Lacouture ME (2007). Epidermal growth factor receptor inhibitor–associated cutaneous toxicities: an evolving paradigm in clinical management. *Oncologist* 12(5):610–21.
11. Behin A, Psimaras D, Hoang-Xuan K, Leger JM (2008). Neuropathies in the context of malignancies. *Curr Opin Neurol* 21(5):534–9.

Radiotherapy and Palliative Care

Elizabeth A. Barnes

Introduction

Radiotherapy (RT) plays an important role in the multidisciplinary management of patients with cancer. Approximately half of all RT treatment is given with palliative and not curative intent. Local RT is used in the palliative setting to relieve symptoms resulting from tumor mass effect.

The goal of palliative RT is to use a short treatment schedule to provide effective and durable symptom relief with minimal treatment-related side effects. Typically, one RT treatment (fraction) is given per day, 5 days a week (Monday through Friday). Small doses per fraction (2 Gy or less) reduce the risk of late toxicity and are used in the curative setting. For symptom palliation, a high total dose is not required and palliative fractionation schedules can therefore be shorter, using a higher dose per fraction, thus minimizing patient visits to the cancer center. Commonly used palliative RT regimes include 8 Gy in a single fraction, 20 Gy in 5 fractions, and 30 Gy in 10 fractions.

Treatment-related side effects are defined as acute (≤ 90 days after treatment start) or late (> 90 days). As RT is a local treatment, side effects depend on the area treated. A description of the common acute side effects from palliative RT and the management is given in Table 18.1.

Late toxicity is usually not a problem in the palliative setting, given the low total dose used and the limited life expectancy of this population. However, care needs to be taken with RT retreatment, and with the use of stereotactic radiosurgery, where very high dose per fraction is utilized.

Table 18.1 Acute Side Effects from Palliative Radiotherapy and Management

Site	Symptom	Management
Head and neck	Mucositis	Soft diet, viscous xylocaine PRN, treat infection
Chest	Dysphagia	Soft diet, viscous xylocaine PRN, treat infection
Abdomen	Nausea and vomiting	Anti-emetics (ondansetron)
Pelvis	Diarrhea	Low-fiber diet, loperamide or diphenoxylate/atropine as required
Skin	Erythema	Skin hygiene (mild soap and water)
	Dry desquamation	Moisturizer (plain, unscented, lanolin-free hydrophilic cream), hydrocortisone for pruritis
	Moist desquamation	Topical antibiotics, moist wound dressings

Palliative RT is usually very effective for relieving pain, bleeding, and other symptoms due to tumor mass effect. Treatment is usually well tolerated with minimal acute side effects. Indications for palliative RT are summarized and details on the most common clinical scenarios are given in Box 18.1.

Box 18.1 Common Indications for Palliative Radiotherapy

Pain
- Bone metastases, lung tumor invading chest wall, tumor mass compressing nerve or soft tissue

Neurological Symptoms
- Spinal cord compression, brain metastases

Bleeding
- From GYN, GI, GU, lung, or skin tumors

Obstruction
- Esophageal, airway, ureteric, or rectal obstruction from tumor mass
- Superior vena cava obstruction

Skin Ulceration and Fungation
- Skin cancer or other tumors (e.g., breast) eroding through the skin

Bone Metastases

Indications

Bone metastases are common in patients with advanced cancer and are the most common cause of cancer pain. RT is a very effective modality for palliating painful bone metastases.[1]

Dose

There has been some controversy over the optimal dose fractionation schedule, with numerous randomized trials published on the subject since the 1980s. Eight Gy is the most commonly given single-fraction (SF) dose,[2] and various multiple-fraction (MF) regimes are used in clinical practice. The latest meta-analysis (2012) reviewed 25 randomized trials of SF versus MF RT for palliation of painful uncomplicated bone metastases.[3] No significant difference was found in pain relief between SF and MF RT. For intent-to-treat patients, the overall response rates for pain were 60% (SF) and 61% (MF), and complete response rates were 23% (SF) and 24% (MF). No statistically significant difference was found between the two arms in the rates of pathological fracture or spinal cord compression. The retreatment rate was 2.6-fold higher after SF RT (20% vs. 8% for MF). The results from this meta-analysis confirm conclusions from previous clinical practice guidelines and consensus documents stating that SF RT should be the standard of care considering patient convenience, cost-effectiveness, and resource implications for the given RT department.

Retreatment can be considered for patients who experience initial pain relief followed by a relapse, have incomplete pain relief, or experience no pain relief after the initial treatment. A randomized trial of SF versus MF for repeat radiation of painful bone metastases found 8 Gy SF to be non-inferior and less toxic than 20 Gy/5 fr. [4]

Large Field Treatment

For diffuse bony metastatic disease, half-body irradiation (HBI) and systemic radionuclides can be used to simultaneously target all bony lesions. HBI encompasses either the upper half (base of skull to iliac crest) or lower half (iliac crest to ankles) of the body in a single large RT field. Systemic radionuclides are deposited at the site of osteoblastic bony metastases, mirroring the uptake seen on bone scan. Radionuclides have been studied mainly in patients with prostate cancer, as bone metastases are osteoblastic (rather than the osteolytic or mixed metastases seen with other primary tumors). The acute gastrointestinal toxicity associated with HBI requires pre-medication and IV hydration, and there are concerns of late toxicity to visceral structures. The use of systemic radionuclides is limited by cost and availability. Both HBI and systemic radionuclides are associated with transient myelosuppression, which delays the use of chemotherapy.

Fracture Risk

Prophylactic surgical fixation should be considered for good-performance status patients with bone lesions at high risk of fracture. Postoperative RT is routinely given, as it is thought to improve functional status, decrease pain, and reduce the risk of refracture. Lesions at high risk of fracture include those with > 50% cortical destruction of a long bone; femoral lesions > 25 mm in the neck; subtrochanteric, intertrochanteric, or supracondylar regions; and diffuse lytic involvement of a weight-bearing bone that is especially painful. An analysis of femoral metastases from the Dutch Bone Metastasis Study found that the risk of fracture was mostly dependent on the amount of axial cortical involvement.[5] These investigators recommend prophylactic fixation for lesions > 30 mm, or in nonsurgical candidates MF RT to decrease fracture occurrence.

Spinal Cord Compression

Spinal cord compression (SCC) if untreated can result in pain, paralysis, sensory loss, and sphincter dysfunction.[6] Management includes corticosteroids, followed by either urgent surgery and/or RT. Treatment recommendations depend on the patient's neurological status, performance status, and life expectancy, extent of spinal disease, and spinal stability. Surgery should be considered for patients with good prognosis who are operable, especially those with spinal instability. Radiation is typically given postoperatively. Radiation should be given to nonsurgical patients. Poor prognosis patients can receive an SF of 8 Gy. For those with good prognosis, 30 Gy/10 fr can be considered, as although functional outcomes and overall survival were found to be similar to short-course RT in one trial, 12-month progression-free survival and local control were significantly improved.

Stereotactic Body Radiotherapy

Stereotactic body radiotherapy (SBRT) is an emerging technology that delivers high doses to metastatic spinal disease with a steep dose gradient while sparing adjacent neural structures.[7] This treatment option may provide superior pain relief and local control benefit (particularly with radio-resistant histologies). Given this is a resource-intensive treatment, as well as demanding for the patient (requiring near-rigid body immobilization), patients should have good performance status and prognosis. Stereotactic body radiotherapy may be used for patients with new or recurrent spinal metastases, and in the postoperative setting. However, efficacy and safety data are mostly retrospective single-institution series.[1] Reported complications include higher rates of vertebral compression fracture and radiation myelopathy compared to conventional RT.[7]

Brain Metastases

Brain metastases occur in approximately 20%–40% of cancer patients. Various treatment options exist, including whole brain RT (WBRT), surgery, stereotactic radiosurgery, and best supportive care.[8] Treatment decisions are based on patient factors (age, performance status) and tumor factors (number and size of brain metastases, histology, extent of extracranial disease).

Patients with limited life expectancy (< 3 months) and multiple brain metastases may be best managed with supportive care. An ongoing Medical Research Council trial (QUARTZ) randomizes patients with inoperable brain metastases from non-small-cell lung cancer to supportive care alone (corticosteroids) versus supportive care plus WBRT. Interim analysis shows no detriment to quality of life, overall survival, or QALYs for patients in the supportive care alone arm.[9]

Thirty to forty percent of patients present with a single brain metastasis. For this population with good performance status and limited extracranial disease, surgical excision followed by WBRT has been shown to improve survival over WBRT alone.[10] The use of postoperative WBRT after surgical excision of a single metastasis has been shown to improve local brain control. Radiosurgery may be considered in lieu of surgery for nonoperable patients (with lesions < 3–4 cm). For good performance status patients, a radiosurgery boost after WBRT has been shown to improve survival for those with a single brain metastasis (< 4 cm), and to improve functional autonomy for those with 2–3 metastases (all < 4 cm).[11]

Patients with multiple brain metastases may be treated with WBRT alone, WBRT with a radiosurgery boost, or radiosurgery alone.[8] There are no trials showing a survival difference between these options. Neurocognition and quality of life may be improved with the omission of WBRT. However, with radiosurgery alone there is an increased risk of brain recurrence; therefore these patients need to be followed with imaging, as symptomatic recurrence may not recover despite salvage treatment.

There is no difference in overall survival or symptom control with the commonly used different WBRT fractionation regimes, including 30 Gy/10 fr or 20 Gy/5 fr.[8]

Lung Cancer

Lung cancer is one of the most common causes of cancer death worldwide. More than two-thirds of patients with non-small-cell lung cancer present with incurable locally advanced or metastatic disease. The overall prognosis is poor, with a median survival of less than 1 year.

Thoracic symptoms can be effectively palliated with local RT, with overall response rates of 80% from hemoptysis, 50% cough, and 64% chest pain.[12] A systematic review of 13 randomized controlled trials found higher-dose palliative regimes (eg 30 Gy/10 fr) provided modest improvements in survival and total symptom score, particularly in patients with good performance status. This was associated with higher rates of esophagitis, therefore lower-dose regimes (eg 20 Gy/5 fr, 17 Gy/2 weekly fr or 10 Gy/1 fr) can be considered for patients with poor performance status or wanting a shorter treatment course.[13]

Pelvic Disease

Locally advanced and recurrent pelvic malignancies arising from gastrointestinal, gynecological, or genitourinary sites can result in many disabling symptoms. These include hemorrhage, necrotic vaginal discharge, pain (due to adenopathy, tumor invasion of bone, lumbosacral plexus, and soft tissue), lower extremity edema, fistula formation, gastrointestinal tract obstruction, and renal failure due to bilateral ureteric obstruction.

Patients presenting with locally advanced bladder cancer are often elderly, smokers, and those with medical comorbidities. Palliative RT can provide effective palliation of urinary symptoms. Several hypofractionated regimes have been reported in the literature. One randomized trial compared 35 Gy/10 fr versus 21 Gy/3 fr on alternate days over 1 week and found no difference between regimes, with a 68% overall improvement in bladder symptoms at 3 months and late bowel toxicity rate of < 1%.[14] Other groups have looked at delivering 5–6 weekly fractions of 6 Gy and also found effective symptom palliation.

Cervix cancer is prevalent in developing countries, with many women presenting with advanced disease. Palliative RT can provide relief of vaginal bleeding and pelvic pain. There is a dearth of information in the literature regarding the optimal palliative RT regime.[15] Recurrent ovarian cancer is typically treated with chemotherapy; however, RT can offer excellent symptom palliation, even in patients with platinum-resistant disease. A review of 53 patients found a symptom response rate of 100%, with a complete response of 68%.[16]

Locally advanced and recurrent rectal cancer can cause pelvic pain, bleeding, and bowel obstruction. A systematic review of palliative RT found the pooled overall symptom response rate was 75%. Reporting of QOL and toxicity was lacking, and no optimal RT regime was found. [17] Concurrent fluorouracil is often given as a radiosensitizer.

Emerging Technologies

The development of SBRT, based on improvements in RT delivery with intensity-modulated and image-guided RT, allows delivery of ablative doses of RT to extracranial sites. [18] The aim of SBRT in this setting is to achieve local control and delay progression. This may be a treatment option for selected patients with 1–3 metastases, small metastases, breast histology, and long disease free interval. Randomized trials are needed to test whether SBRT really does improve progression-free and overall survival.[18]

Conclusion

Palliative RT provides effective and efficient palliation of symptoms due to locally advanced or metastatic disease experienced at the end of life. Side effects are often minimal, and the time to symptom response is rapid; for painful bone metastases or bleeding, response can be seen within a week.

Clinical Pearls

- A single fraction of RT can often palliate distressing symptoms due to local disease.
- Palliative RT may not be suitable for patients with uncontrolled pain, severe orthopnea, or delirium, as they must lie still, supine, and unattended for 10–15 minutes for RT planning and treatment delivery.
- The acute side effects of palliative RT are usually mild and transient.
- Ongoing trials will help determine the optimal role of stereotactic RT in palliation.

References

1. Lutz S, Berk L, Chang E, et al. (2011). Palliative radiotherapy for bone metastases: an ASTRO evidence-based guideline. *Int J Radiat Oncol Biol Phys* 79(4):965–76.
2. Dennis K, Makhani L, Zeng L, Lam H, Chow E (2013). Single fraction conventional external beam radiotherapy for bone metastases: a systematic review of randomized controlled trials. *Radiother Oncol* 106(1):5–14.
3. Chow E, Zeng L, Salvo N, Dennis K, Tsao M, Lutz S (2012). Update in the systematic review of palliative radiotherapy trials for bone metastases. *Clin Oncol* 24(2):112–24.
4. Chow E, van der Linden YM, Roos D, et al. (2014). Single versus multiple fractions of repeat radiation for painful bone metastases: a randomised, controlled, non-inferiority trial. *Lancet Oncol* 15(2):164–71.
5. Van der Linden YM, Kroon HM, Dijkstra SP, et al. (2003). Simple radiographic parameter predicts fracturing in metastatic femoral bone lesions: results from a randomised trial. *Radiother Oncol* 69(1):21–31.
6. Loblaw DA, Mitera G, Ford M, Laperriere NJ (2012). A 2011 updated systematic review and clinical practice guideline for the management of malignant extradural spinal cord compression. *Int J Radiat Oncol Biol Phys* 84(2):312–7.
7. Sahgal A, Bilsky M, Chang EL, et al. (2011). Stereotactic body radiotherapy for spinal metastases: current status, with a focus on its application in the postoperative patient. *J Neurosurg Spine* 14(2):151–66.
8. Tsao MN, Rades D, Wirth A, et al. (2012). Radiotherapeutic and surgical management for newly diagnosed brain metastasis(es): an American Society for Radiation Oncology evidence-based guideline. *Pract Radiat Oncol* 2(3):210–25.
9. Langley RE, Stephens RJ, Nankivell M, et al. (2013). Interim data from the Medical Research Council QUARTZ Trial: does whole brain radiotherapy affect the survival and quality of patients life with brain metastases from non-small cell lung cancer? *Clin Oncol* 25(3):e23–30.
10. Patchell RA, Tibbs PA, Walsh JW, et al. (1990). A randomized trial of surgery in the treatment of single metastases to the brain. *N Engl J Med* 322(8):494–500.
11. Andrews DW, Scott CB, Sperduto PW, et al. (2004). Whole brain radiation therapy with or without stereotactic radiosurgery boost for patients with one to three brain metastases: phase III results of the RTOG 9508 randomised trial. *Lancet* 363(9422):1665–72.
12. Fairchild A, Harris K, Barnes E, et al. (2008). Palliative thoracic radiotherapy for lung cancer: a systematic review. *J Clin Oncol* 26(24):4001–11.
13. Rodrigues G, Videtic GM, Sur R, et al. (2011). Palliative thoracic radiotherapy in lung cancer: an American Society for Radiation Oncology evidence-based clinical practice guideline. *Pract Radiat Oncol* 1(2):60–71.
14. Duchesne GM, Bolger JJ, Griffiths GO, et al. (2000). A randomized trial of hypofractionated schedules of palliative radiotherapy in the management of bladder carcinoma: results of medical research council trial BA09. *Int J Radiat Oncol Biol Phys* 47(2):379–88.
15. van Lonkhuijzen L, Thomas G (2011). Palliative radiotherapy for cervical carcinoma, a systematic review. *Radiother Oncol* 98(3):287–91.
16. Choan E, Quon M, Gallant V, Samant R (2006). Effective palliative radiotherapy for symptomatic recurrent or residual ovarian cancer. *Gynecol Oncol* 102(2):204–9.
17. Cameron MG, Kersten C, Vistad I, Fossa S, Guren MG (2014). Palliative pelvic radiotherapy of symptomatic incurable rectal cancer: a systematic review. *Acta Oncol* 53(2):164–73.
18. Tree AC, Khoo VS, Eeles RA, et al. (2013). Stereotactic body radiotherapy for oligometastatses. *Lancet Oncol* 14(1):e28–37.

Hospice Approach to Palliative Care

Joan K. Harrold and Charles F. von Gunten

Hospice Care in the United States

Hospice care is palliative care at the end of life. Hospices differ as to how early in the course of an illness they provide care, so it is important to know the scope and timing of services provided by your local hospices. Nearly all hospices, however, provide care for patients with life expectancies of 6 months or less.

In the United States, 80% of hospice care is paid for by Medicare, the federal system of healthcare coverage for the elderly and the disabled. The Medicare Hospice Benefit (MHB) pays for comprehensive medical, nursing, counseling, and bereavement services to terminally ill patients and their families[1] (Box 19.1). These services are provided

---

Box 19.1 Medicare Hospice Benefit

Covered Services (100%; No Copay)

- Nursing care: to provide intermittent (usually 1–3 times/week) assessment, support, skilled services, treatments, and case management services
- 24-hour availability for assessment and management of changes, crises, and other acute needs
- Social work: supportive counseling, practical aspects of care (other community services), and planning (healthcare surrogates, advance directives)
- Counseling services: including chaplaincy
- Home health aid and homemaker services
- Speech therapy, nutrition, physical therapy (PT), and occupational therapy (OT) services
- Bereavement support to family after the death
- Medical oversight of plan of care (POC) by hospice medical director
- All medications and supplies for management and palliation of the terminal illness (hospices may collect a small copay for medications)
- Durable medical equipment (e.g., hospital bed, commode, wheelchair, etc.)
- Short-term general inpatient care for medical problems that cannot be managed at home, such as pain, dyspnea, delirium, acute skilled needs
- Short-term respite to permit family caregivers to take a break
- Continuous care at home for short episodes of acute medical need

Services Not Covered by Medicare Hospice Benefit

- Continuous nursing or nurse aid care
- Medications unrelated to the terminal illness
- Physician visits for direct medical care (billed to Medicare separately)
- Residential (non-acute) care in a facility

by an interdisciplinary team that meets at least biweekly to review the plan of care and its effectiveness in advancing the goals expressed by the patient, family, and other caregivers. The services can be provided in the patient's home, a nursing home, an inpatient hospice unit, or a hospital.

Although hospice provides end-of-life care, referral for hospice care does not shorten life expectancy. For certain diagnoses, hospice enrollment is associated with longer survival times.

Referring for Hospice Care

Referral for hospice care is appropriate when the patient has a limited prognosis and the most important goals are comfort and symptom management.

The number one complaint about hospice care from patients and families is that no one told them about it sooner. The second most common complaint is that no one told them about the practical benefits; there was too much talk about the philosophy of care and not enough about who would help and how.

When patients elect coverage using the MHB, the hospice agency becomes responsible for coordinating and paying for all treatments and medications related to the primary hospice diagnosis. Patients can continue to receive care for diseases unrelated to the terminal illness (e.g., dialysis for renal failure if the patient is dying of cancer, cataract removal) using regular Medicare coverage.

Most Medicaid and commercial insurers use the Medicare Hospice Benefit Model for coverage of hospice care.

Medicare Hospice Benefit Eligibility

To pay for hospice care, Medicare requires both the attending physician and hospice physician to certify that the patient has a life expectancy of 6 months or less if the disease or condition runs its normal course. If patients improve or resume disease-directed therapy with the primary goal of extending life expectancy, they can be discharged and can resume services later without penalty.

Individual patients can continue to be eligible if they live longer than 6 months as long as the physician believes that death is more likely than not within 6 months. The patient does not need a do-not-resuscitate (DNR) order to be eligible for hospice care. There is no limit to the number of days a patient can receive hospice care. There is no penalty if the patient outlives the diagnosis.

Prognosis

Physicians overestimate prognosis when compared with actual survival by a factor of 3 or greater. Prognostication may be more accurate for cancer because of the pattern of decline that precedes death (Box 19.2).

Although trajectories of other terminal conditions are less well defined, there are a variety of factors to consider and resources to use when assessing prognosis and considering hospice referral (Box 19.3).

Box 19.2 Cancer: Prognostic Factors

General
- Performance status:
- Karnofsky ≤ 50, ECOG ≤ 3
- Most of the time in bed or lying down

Signs Associated with Prognosis ≤ 6 Months
- Malignant pericardial or pleural effusions
- Malignant ascites
- Multiple brain metastases
- Carcinomatous meningitis
- Malignant bowel obstruction
- Serum albumin < 2.5 mg/dL
- Hypercalcemia (except in newly diagnosed breast cancer or myeloma expected to receive standard treatment)

Cancers Associated with Prognosis ≤ 6 Months
- Metastatic lung cancer
- Unresectable pancreas cancer
- Progressive metastatic breast or prostate cancer with poor or decreasing functional status
- Metastatic solid tumor, acute leukemia, or high-grade lymphoma forgoing chemotherapy

Box 19.3 Non-Cancer Prognostic Factors

Heart Disease

- Functional capacity, comorbidities, recent cardiac hospitalization, systolic blood pressure < 100 mmHg and/or pulse > 100 bpm, cachexia, anemia, hyponatremia, elevated BUN and/or creatinine ≥ 1.4 mg/dL, left ventricular ejection fraction ≤ 45%, ventricular dysrhythmias (treatment resistant); Seattle Heart Failure Model

Lung Disease

Ambulatory Patients

- FEV_1, age, exercise capacity, low body mass index (BMI), low PaO_2, resting pulse > 100 beats per minute, subjective estimates of dyspnea

Hospitalized Patients

- Age, functional status, comorbidities, severity of illness (APACHE II score), need for mechanical ventilation, hypoxia, hypercarbia, low serum albumin, low hemoglobin

Dementia

- Age, significant comorbidities, cardiac dysrhythmias, peripheral edema or laboratory data consistent with hypoalbuminemia, aspiration, bowel incontinence, recent or ongoing weight loss, episodic dehydration, recurrent fevers, multiple and/or non-healing stage 3–4 pressure ulcers, seizures, shortness of breath, dysphagia, low oral intake, not awake for most of the day, low BMI, recent need for continuous oxygen, recent hospitalization for pneumonia or hip fracture

Renal Disease

- Age, functional status, comorbidities, albumin < 3.5 g/dL, refusal or discontinuation of dialysis

Liver Disease

- Age, comorbidities, ascites, encephalopathy, bilirubin, albumin, prolonged prothrombin time, hepatorenal syndrome, hepatocellular carcinoma, rate of clinical decompensation; MELD Score

Some of these factors are deemed decisive by Medicare when determining eligibility. Because the prognostic utility of all of these factors changes according to advances in medical research, they should be used in conjunction with clinical judgment to guide assessment of hospice eligibility and timely planning by patients and families.

Plan of Care (POC)

The hospice program approves, coordinates, and pays for services that are reasonable and necessary for palliation and/or management of the terminal illness. The POC is based on the patient's diagnosis and needs, orders of the attending physician, and, as necessary, collaboration with the hospice medical director.

Physician Role

The attending physician is indicated by the patient at the time of enrollment. Sometimes the patient will select a hospice physician for this role.

The attending physician is responsible for working with the hospice team to determine appropriate care. Direct patient care services by the attending physician are billed to Medicare in the usual fashion.

Places of Care

Home

The majority (95%) of hospice care takes place in the home because that's where patients say they want to be. Hospice team members visit the patient and family on an intermittent basis. Care continues as long as the patient remains eligible and wants the care. Medicare rules do not require a primary caregiver in the home.

Nursing Home or Other Long-Term Care Facility

This is the patient's home, and the patient's "family" frequently includes the staff. Hospice care is specialty care provided in addition to usual nursing home care.

Hospice Inpatient Unit

Dedicated units that are free-standing or within other facilities such as nursing homes or hospitals are sometimes available. Permitted length of stay varies, as some are for residential care and others for short-term acute care.

Hospital

Occasionally, pain and other symptoms or other conditions related to the terminal illness cannot be managed at home and the patient is admitted to an inpatient hospital or other contracted inpatient facility for more intensive management. The inpatient facility must have a contract with the hospice program.

Payment to the Hospice

Medicare pays for covered services using a *per diem* capitated arrangement in one of four categories:

- *Routine home care*: care at home or nursing home
- *Inpatient respite care*: care in an inpatient setting (usually a nursing home or inpatient hospice unit) for up to 5 days to give family caregivers a break
- *General inpatient care*: acute inpatient care for conditions related to the terminal illness (e.g., pain and symptom control, caregiver breakdown, impending death and the patient doesn't want to die at home)
- *Continuous home care*: provides acute care at home with around-the-clock care for a crisis that might otherwise lead to inpatient care.

Payment to Attending and Consulting Physicians

Direct patient care services by the attending physician for care related to the terminal illness are covered by Medicare, but not under the Medicare Hospice Benefit.

If the attending physician is not associated with the hospice program, the physician bills Medicare Part B in the usual fashion. The bill must indicate that the physician is not associated with the hospice program, or the claim may be denied.

If the attending physician is associated with the hospice program or is a consultant, the physician submits the bill to the hospice program, which in turn submits the claim to Medicare under Part A. The physician is reimbursed on the basis of a contract with the hospice program.

Discussing Hospice Care

One of the biggest barriers to timely referral for hospice care is physician discomfort with the discussion.[2-7]

Clinical Pearls

- Discuss hospice care in the context of the larger goals of care, using a step-wise approach.

Establish the Setting

Ensure comfort and privacy; sit down next to the patient. Ask if family members or others should be present. Introduce the subject with a phrase such as "I'd like to talk with you about our overall goals for your care."

What Does the patient Understand?

Ask open-ended questions to elicit patient understanding about his or her current health situation. It is important to get the patient talking; if the doctor is doing all the talking, it is unlikely that the rest of the conversation will go well. Consider starting with phrases such as "What do you understand about your current health situation?" or "What have the doctors told you about your cancer?"

Listen for phrases like "I know I'm going to die of this cancer," or "I know I don't have much time left," or "I know the cancer is getting worse." If the patient does not know or appreciate his or her current status, this is the time to review that information.

What Does the Patient Expect?

Next, ask the patient to consider the future. Examples of ways to start this discussion are "What do you expect in the future?" or "What goals do you have for the time you have left—what is important to you?" This step allows you to listen while the patient describes a real or imagined future. Most patients with advanced cancer use this opening to voice their thoughts about dying—typically mentioning comfort, family, and home as their goals of care. If there is a sharp discontinuity between what you expect and what the patient expects, this is the time to clarify.

Listen carefully to the patient's responses; most patients have thought a lot about dying, they only need permission to talk about what they have been thinking. Setting up the conversation in this way allows the physician to respond with clarifying and confirming comments, such as, "So what you're saying is, you want to be as independent as possible and stay out of the hospital," or "What you've said is, you don't want to be a burden on your family."

Use the opportunity to teach patients about what to expect if they express inaccurate or exaggerated fears—pain can be controlled; they can avoid returning to the emergency department or hospital. Consider asking what other experiences they have had. Some have seen (or read or heard about) "bad" deaths that can be prevented by modern care.

Discuss Hospice Care

Use language that the patient will understand, and give information in small pieces. Never say, "There's nothing more we can do." "Nothing" is abstract and easily misinterpreted. To a patient, "nothing" means abandonment.

Consider summarizing the patient's goals as part of introducing a discussion of hospice care. For example: "You've told me you want to be as independent and comfortable as possible. Hospice care is the best way I know to help you achieve those goals."

Listen carefully to the response. Many patients have distorted views of hospice care. Others have never heard the term. Ask what the term means to them. Patients frequently describe hospice as a place to go to die or what you do when you give up. Respond by asking why they think that. Probe for previous experiences or how they developed their point of view.

Respond by describing hospice as a program that helps the patient and family achieve the goals the patient just described. It's a team of people that help the doctor meet the patient's and family's physical, psychological, social, and spiritual needs.

Offer to ask someone from the hospice to come by to give information. You don't have to be the expert. Tell the patient you can talk again after they have more information.

Offer your recommendation: "From what you've told me, I think it would be best if we got the hospice involved," or "I always recommend the hospice to get involved for my patients at this stage of their illness."

Reassure the patient and family that, if they get better, or if there is a new treatment discovered, they can be discharged (or graduate) from hospice care to receive that care. Nationally, 10% of hospice patients are discharged alive.

Respond to Emotions

Strong emotions are expected when discussing death. Typically, the emotional response is brief. The most profound initial response a physician can make is silence, providing a reassuring touch, and offering tissues. The most frequent mistake is to talk too much.

Establish a Plan

Clarify the plan. For example, "I'll ask the hospice to come by to talk with you, and then you and I can talk again."

Common Questions and Dilemmas

- My patient has end-stage disease and wants CPR. Can I still refer him to hospice?
  - Yes. A DNR order is not required to be eligible for hospice care. Since CPR is unlikely to be successful, however, discuss your patient's goals for such treatment. If he still wants CPR, revisit the plan after hospice care has been established. If he wanted CPR because going to the hospital for care was his only experience, the patient may have different goals once he has experienced care in his home.
- My patient has a prognosis of 4–6 months, but her symptoms are controlled. When should I make the referral to hospice?
  - Now. Your patient and her family can get to know the hospice team, begin to establish trust, and be monitored for new or worsening symptoms before a crisis occurs. They will also receive emotional and spiritual support, coordination of care and resources, and preparation for what to expect with disease progression.

- The hospice does not cover the pain medication that my patient is taking unless other medication has failed him. What do I do?
  - Call the hospice medical director and discuss the treatment plan. Tell him or her if other medications were ineffective prior to hospice care. If not, ask why the hospice prefers certain medications as first-line therapy.
- If I refer my patient to hospice, will I still be her doctor, or will the hospice physicians take over her care?
  - The patient chooses the physician to manage her care. If you are willing to do so, your patient can choose to have you as her attending physician. Some physicians prefer to have the hospice physician manage or co-manage their patients. Let the hospice know if you prefer that model so that your patient can make an informed choice.
- My patient has a prognosis of about 6 months, but she may need chemotherapy or radiation therapy to help manage her symptoms. Will hospice cover the treatments?
  - Hospice coverage may vary according to the goals of care, expected effectiveness, and resources. Many hospices will cover treatments that are expected to significantly reduce symptoms. Some hospices will cover all treatments as long as they are unlikely to increase the patient's life expectancy past 6 months. Most hospices will help assess if the benefits outweigh the burdens relative to the patient's life expectancy. Larger programs with more resources may be able to cover treatments that smaller programs cannot. If radiation therapy or chemotherapy is indicated, call the hospice medical director and discuss the treatment plan.
- I want to prescribe a treatment for my patient, but the hospice does not cover it and recommends that he revoke the MHB. What does that mean?
  - Your patient can revoke the MHB if he wants to use his regular Medicare benefits to cover his care. This is not a decision to be taken lightly, as the patient forfeits all of his hospice services when he revokes the MHB unless he re-elects to use the MHB in the future. He should not revoke just for the treatments and then re-elect the MHB in between, as this is inconsistent with the intent of the MHB. If you believe that the treatment should be included in the hospice coverage, call the hospice medical director and discuss the treatment, goals of care, and reasons that it is not covered.
- The hospice says that my patient has an extended prognosis and no longer qualifies for hospice services. What happens now?
  - If a patient no longer has a life expectancy of 6 months or less given the natural course of the disease process, he or she cannot be certified as eligible for the MHB. The hospice is expected to establish a discharge plan with the patient to ensure that care needs can be met in other ways.
- My patient has improved since she was referred to hospice. Why doesn't the hospice discharge her?
  - Some patients appear to "improve" after admission to hospice because symptoms are managed, support is provided, and care needs are met. These improvements do not change the patient's prognosis

or eligibility for hospice care. Other patients have illnesses marked by fluctuations and exacerbations. If the patient's death appeared imminent but the patient rallied, the longer-term prognosis may still be poor and consistent with eligibility.

- My patient lives in a nursing home. Why would he need hospice, too?
  - Hospice care augments the care to residents living the end of their lives in nursing homes. Hospice provides expertise in pain and symptom management, coverage of medications and other treatments, additional care for complex needs, and support for family members and other caregivers. The nurses, aides, counselors, and volunteers from hospice work with the staff of the nursing home to provide comprehensive end-of-life care, increased presence to comfort patients and families, and support and recognition of the efforts of nursing home staff as they face the death of a resident to whom they may have become attached.

- My patient only has days to live. Isn't it too late for hospice care?
  - Although patients are eligible for hospice care with a life expectancy of 6 months or less, referral at any time has been shown to benefit patients and families.[8,9] In addition to helping during an often difficult time, bereavement support will also be offered to your patient's family.

- My patient is likely to die during this hospital admission. Can hospice still help her?
  - Hospices are sometimes able to provide end-of-life care in hospitals as general inpatient care. Although you may be managing physical symptoms quite well, the additional presence of hospice staff may be especially helpful to patients and families coping with death and dying in the hospital setting. Even if your patient does not enroll in hospice, the hospice may still provide bereavement support to the family based on your referral.

References

1. Centers for Medicare and Medicaid Services (2003). Medicare Hospice Benefits. Publication No. CMS 02154. Revised July 2003.
2. Emanuel LL, von Gunten CF, Ferris FD (eds.) (1999). The EPEC Curriculum. The EPEC Project. Retrieved January 31, 2009, from www.epec.net.
3. End of Life/Palliative Education Resource Center (EPERC). Fast facts and concepts. Retrieved January 31, 2009, from www.eperc.mcw.edu/ff_index.htm.
4. Diem SJ. Lantos JD. Tulsky JA (1996). Cardiopulmonary resuscitation on television: miracles and misinformation. N Engl J Med 334(24):1578–82.
5. Junkerman C, Schiedermayer D (1998). Practical Ethics for Students, Interns and Residents, 2nd ed. Hagerstown, MD: University Publishing Group.
6. Council on Ethical and Judician Affairs, American Medical Association (1999). Council report: medical futility in end-of-life care. JAMA 281:937–41.
7. Buckman R (1992). How to Break Bad News: A Guide for Health Care Professionals. Baltimore, MD: Johns Hopkins University Press.
8. Taylor DH, Ostermann J, Van Houten CH, et al. (2007). What length of hospice use maximizes reduction in medical expenditures near death in the US Medicare program? Soc Sci Med 65(7):1466–78.
9. Connor SR, Pyenson B, Fitch K, et al. (2007). Comparing hospice and nonhospice patient survival among patients who die within a three-year window. J Pain Symptom Manage 33(3):238–46.

Psychosocial and Cultural Considerations in Palliative Care

V. S. Periyakoil

Common Psychological Issues in Palliative Care Patients

There is often a complex interplay of medical and psycho-sociocultural issues in the setting of any chronic and/or serious life-limiting illness. The conventional biomedical model (which works very well for any acute illness) often minimizes and tends to ignore the role of these issues in patient health care and well-being. A stance that focuses narrowly on only the biological and physical aspects and ignores the underlying psycho-sociocultural aspects will lead to poor care outcomes, resulting both in increased patient and family distress as well as clinician frustration. It can also result in consumption of ineffective and burdensome treatments that diminish quality of life while increasing costs of care. This chapter will identify common psychosociocultural issues in palliative care, provide key clinical pearls regarding assessment and management, as well as identify resources for further self-directed learning.

Preparatory Grief

Preparatory grief is the normal grief reaction to perceived losses experienced by persons who are dying. Persons who are dying prepare for their death by mourning the losses implicit in death. The anticipated separation from loved ones is an obvious one. Simple pleasures of living may be grieved. People may reflect on their past and relive great moments and disappointments, and mourn for missed opportunities. Looking to the future, they may grieve the loss of much-anticipated experiences, such as a child's graduation or the birth of a grandchild. Distinguishing[1-3] between grief and depression in patients who are dying can be difficult. Many of the signs and symptoms traditionally used to diagnose depression are also present in patients who are grieving (see Figure 20.1).

Figure 20.1. Overlap of processes in patients with advanced illnesses.

Clinical Pearls
- Many patients with serious life-limiting illness will experience grief.
- Grief is a normal part of the dying process and responds well to support.
- Grief can mimic depression, and the two should be differentiated as the management is different.

Depression

Major depression is defined[4] by persistent low mood, or anhedonia (pervasive loss of interest or pleasure), that lasts for 2 weeks or more and is accompanied by at least four of the following nine symptoms: sleep disruption (especially early morning insomnia), weight loss or change in appetite, psychomotor retardation or agitation, fatigue or loss of energy, feelings of worthlessness or excessive guilt, diminished ability to think or concentrate, and recurrent thoughts of death or suicidal ideation. False positives are very common in a palliative care setting (see Figure 20.2) as the illness per se can cause many of the somatic (appetite, weight, sleep, libido, energy changes, etc.) and affective (sadness, fleeting thoughts of death/suicide crying, limiting social activities, etc) symptoms.

Clinical Pearls
- Depression is *not* a normal part of the terminal illness process.
- Presence of hopelessness, helplessness, worthlessness, pervasive loss of pleasure (anhedonia), and persistent dysphoria are signs of depression in palliative care patients, and their presence should trigger an in-depth screening.
- Anxiety and depression often coexist in a palliative care setting.
- Depression is under diagnosed and under treated. Depression can and should be treated (see Figure 20.2) will improve the quality of life of palliative care patients.
- Medication choice in treating depression in a palliative care setting is determined by patient prognosis, drug–drug interactions, and medication side effects. Selective serotonic reuptake inhibitors (SSRIs) are the drug of choice for depression in a palliative care setting and are usually well tolerated. SSRIs have a latency of onset of a few weeks and thus are not useful in patients with an anticipated life span of hours to days.
- Common SSRIs used include citalopram 20–60 mg/d, escitalopram 10–20 mg/d, fluoxetine 20–60 mg/d, fluvoxamine 50–150 mg bid, paroxetine 20–50 mg/d and sertraline 50–200 mg/d. These medications typically take at least 4–6 weeks for full effect and this late onset of action is particularly problematic in patients with advanced illness and an expected prognosis of days to weeks.
- Common SSRI side effects include nausea, diarrhea, headache, insomnia, anxiety, anorexia, dizziness, tremor, sweating, and sexual dysfunction.
- Depressed patients with anticipated prognosis of days to weeks can be treated with psychostimulants like methylphenidate.

Anxiety

About 18% of American adults have anxiety disorders. Anxiety is a state of apprehension and fear resulting from the perception of a current or

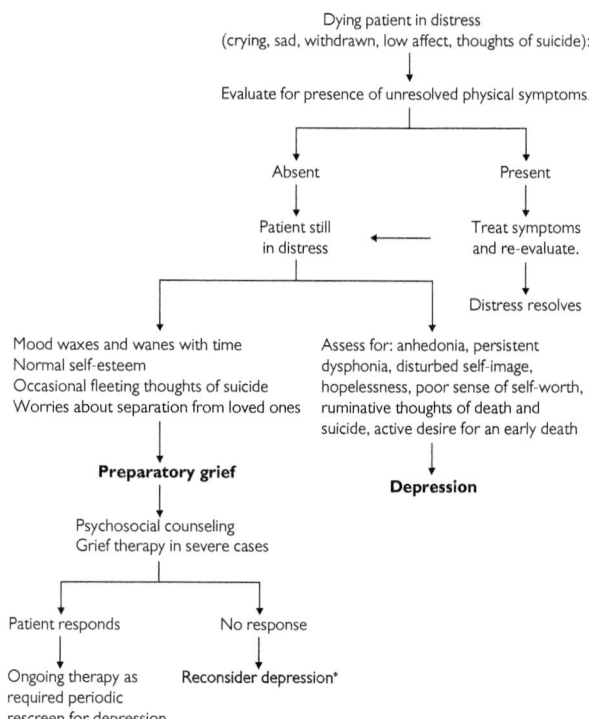

Figure 20.2. Differentiating preparatory grief from depression in patients with terminal illness.

future threat to oneself. At least 25% of cancer patients and 50% of CHF and COPD patients experience significant anxiety. Anxiety[5, 6] is often seen secondary to poorly managed acute or chronic pain, dyspnea, nausea, and other distressing symptoms. Anxiety can also be precipitated by medications like corticosteroids, psychostimulants, and some antidepressants, as well as due to withdrawal of alcohol, opioids, benzodiazepines, nicotine, clonidine, antidepressants, and corticosteroids. In addition, death anxiety and existential and psychosocial concerns about dying, disability, loss, legacy, family, finances, and religion/spirituality can also precipitate anxiety. Anxiety is a predominant symptom of the following psychiatric disorders, which are common in palliative care patients:

1. *Generalized anxiety disorder (GAD)*: Anxiety and fear occur commonly in the dying patient. However, disabling anxiety and/or panic is not a normal aspect of the dying process. Patients with generalized anxiety

disorder can't seem to shake their worries, which are usually also accompanied by physical symptoms, especially fatigue, headaches, muscle tension, muscle aches, difficulty swallowing, trembling, twitching, irritability, sweating, and hot flashes. It is to be further noted that panic disorder (PD) diagnosis in the patient's caregiver can be associated with patient generalized anxiety disorder (GAD), and patient GAD can be associated with caregiver PD.

2. *Panic disorder*: A panic[7,8] attack is defined in the *DSM-IV* as a discrete period of intense fear or discomfort, in which four (or more) of the following symptoms develop abruptly and reach a peak within 10 minutes: palpitations, pounding heart or accelerated heart rate, sweating, trembling or shaking, sensations of shortness of breath or smothering, feeling of choking, chest pain or discomfort, nausea or abdominal distress, feeling dizzy, unsteady, lightheaded or faint, derealization or depersonalization, fear of losing control or going crazy, fear of dying. Derealization is a sensation of feeling estranged or detached from one's environment. Depersonalization is an altered and unreal perception of self, feelings, and/or situation (described by one patient as "feeling like you are on the outside looking in").

Clinical Pearls
- Panic disorder is more common in palliative care patients with chronic dyspnea.
- Medical management is influenced by anticipated life span and severity of panic symptoms.
- SSRI monotherapy or SSRI therapy augmented with low-dose benzodiazepines for a period of 3–4 weeks, followed by SSRI monotherapy (taper off benzodiazepines after 3 weeks), is indicated in patients with an anticipated life span of at least several weeks.
- SSRIs can exacerbate anxiety in some patients during the first few days of therapy. Consider adding benzodiazepines as needed for the first few weeks in such cases.
- Benzodiazepine monotherapy should be considered in patients with anticipated life span of days to weeks.

Post-traumatic stress disorder (PTSD)

An estimated 25% of patients with past history of traumatic life events can develop post-traumatic stress disorder (PTSD). Traumatic events that trigger PTSD[9,10] include exposure to robbery, physical assault, sexual assault, natural disasters, fires/arson, or environmental hazards; tragic death of a close friend or family member by means of accident, suicide, or homicide; cancer diagnosis; motor vehicle crash; war combat. In DSM-5, PTSD has been moved from the class of anxiety disorders into new class of "trauma & stress related disorders" PTSD can develop when a person has experienced, witnessed, or was confronted with an event(s) that involved actual or threatened death or serious injury, or a threat to the physical integrity of self or others. PTSD can manifest as anxiety, agitation, nightmares, and hyperarousal.

Clinical Pearls
- A simple four-item screen helps identify PTSD (see Box 20.1)

- SSRIs are the drug of choice for PTSD. While the FDA has approved both sertraline and paroxetine for PTSD, other SSRIs like citalopram are effective and well tolerated.
- SSRIs help palliate all symptom groups (re-experiencing, avoidance, hyperarousal) of PTSD.
- TCAs are second line for treatment of PTSD and are thought to alleviate intrusive symptoms, anxiety, depression, and insomnia.
- SNRI class of antidepressants, such as venlafaxine and nefadazone, are effective in treating PTSD.

Advance Directives

An advance directive is a form that documents the patient's expressed wishes about what kind of care she or he would like to have if she or he becomes incapable of making medical decisions (when in a coma or due to dementia). The advance directive should guide the physicians and the family when making healthcare decisions on behalf of the patient. Advance directives can take many forms and, more important, the laws about advance directives are different in each state. Physicians must have a good understanding of the local institutional policy as well as the state laws governing care.

Clinical Pearls

- A living will is one type of advance directive that describes the kind of medical treatments or life-sustaining treatments a patient would want if she or he were to become seriously or terminally ill. A living will doesn't let the patient name a surrogate decision-maker.
- A durable power of attorney (DPA) for health care is another kind of advance directive. A DPA documents the person(s) chosen by the patient to make healthcare decisions on his or her behalf in event she or he becomes incapable of making such decisions. A DPA becomes active any time a patient is unable to make medical decisions. A DPA is generally more useful than a living will. But a DPA may not be a good choice if you don't have another person you trust to make these decisions for you.

Box 20.1 Screening for Post-Traumatic Stress Disorder

In your life, have you ever had any experience that was so frightening, horrible, or upsetting that, in the past month, you ...
1. Have had nightmares about it or thought about it when you did not want to?
2. Tried hard not to think about it or went out of your way to avoid situations that reminded you of it?
3. Were constantly on guard, watchful, or easily startled?
4. Felt numb or detached from others, activities, or your surroundings?
Screen is positive if patient answers "yes" to any two of these.

Prins A, Ouimette P, Kimerling R, Cameron RP, Hugelshofer DS, Shaw HJ, Thraikill A, Gussman FD, Sheikh JI (2009). The primary care PTSD screen (PC-PTSD): development and operating characteristics. *Prim Care Psychiatry* 9:9–14.

- Physician Orders for Life-Sustaining Treatment (POLST): A POLST[11] form is a brightly colored, medical order form used to write orders indicating life-sustaining treatment wishes for seriously ill patients. The POLST accomplishes two major purposes: (1) it turns treatment wishes of an individual into actionable medical orders; (2) it is portable from one care setting to another.
- The POLST form remains with a patient if he or she is moved between care settings, regardless of whether the patient is in the hospital, at home, or in a nursing home. The POLST is legally used in some states in the United States; in these states, when a patient has a completed POLST form, the form must be honored by all healthcare providers.
- The Letter Project (http://med.stanford.edu/letter.html) is a simple tool available in multiple languages that provides a framework for sensitive end of life discussions. It was created after extensive research with multi-ethnic patients and families as well as with multi-specialty doctors. The free App is called "Stanford Letter Project" and is available in the Apple Appstore (https://itunes.apple.com/us/app/stanford-letter-project/id1010816774?mt=8) and Google Playstore. (https://play.google.com/store/apps/details?id=com.stanford.letterproject&hl=en)
- Letter to Directive Tool: This tool is designed to help patients easily complete advance directives. Patients are asked to answer some simple questions in English. The tool takes their responses to auto-fill and advance directive that they then edit, print and sign. They can also email it to their doctor and their family members. This tool is available as an online form (http://med.stanford.edu/letter/advancedirective.html). It is also available as a free Stanford App called "Advance Directives" in the Apple Appstore and Google Playstore

Cultural Issues

Culture has a great influence on how people make healthcare decisions, and their preferences for care interventions, including advance care planning as well as heroic life-prolonging measures. It also has a huge influence on rituals related to death and dying and after-death care.

Clinical Pearls

- Cultural differences persist[12–14] in all of health care, including end-of-life care, and ethnicity has been shown to be a marker of common cultural beliefs and values that, in combination, influence decision-making at the end of life.
- Review of ethnic variations in hospice use also indicates that minorities use services disproportionately less than white patients, even after researchers control for specific sociodemographic and clinical characteristics.
- Another recent study[14] showed that compared with white patients, black and Hispanic patients are less likely to consider themselves terminally ill and more likely to want intensive treatment and less likely to have an advance care planning.

Explanatory Model

Sometimes patients and families from diverse cultural backgrounds may have very different ways of understanding their illness, its consequences, and how it needs to be treated, that is, a different "explanatory model of illness," as described by Kleinman.[15] This is especially true for recent immigrants and those who are not acculturated to the mainstream American culture and who are are still unfamiliar with Western biomedicine. Eliciting the patient's understanding of his or her illness process in a culturally competent manner will help the clinician better understand the patient's stance, be better able to tailor healthcare interventions, avoid frustration, and promote adherence to the care plan. See Box 20.2 for the trigger questions that help elicit the explanatory model.

Box 20.2 The Explanatory Model of Illness: A Culturally Sensitive Approach to Asking about a Health Problem

- What do you call your problem?
- What do you think caused your problem?
- Why do you think started when it did?
- What does your sickness do to you? How does it work?
- How severe is it? How long do you think you will have it?
- What do you fear most about your illness?
- What are the chief problems your sickness has caused you?
- What have you done so far to treat your illness?
- What treatments do you think you should receive?
- What important results do you hope to receive from the treatment?
- Who should be involved in making healthcare decisions for you?
- Who else can help you?

Nondisclosure and the Concept of Protective Truthfulness

In some cultures and ethnic minorities, the family may request nondisclosure of terminal illness; that is, they may request that the physician withhold the diagnosis from the patient (e.g., "Doctor, please don't tell my father that he has cancer. If he finds out that he has cancer, he will lose all hope and just give up and die"). Requests for nondisclosure may cause clinicians considerable distress and ethical conflict. Some may feel that it is the patient's right to know his or her diagnosis and that withholding diagnostic and prognostic information is ethically questionable. In addition, physicians may feel that it is not possible to obtain informed consent for interventions like chemotherapy and radiation therapy if the patient does not know her diagnosis. The following points will hopefully guide the clinician in dealing with requests for nondisclosure.

Clinical Pearls

- Request for nondisclosure are usually motivated by the concept of "protective truthfulness" (i.e., truth-telling is thought to be an insincere and potentially harmful act if a patient were to lose hope and confidence in life after learning of his or her disease). Thus it is to be noted that the intent of the family is to protect the patient and not to harm the patient.
- When the family asks you to withhold the truth, use the explanatory model of open-ended questions to elicit their concerns, as follows:
  - Why do you want me to withhold the information?
  - What are you concerned about?
  - What do you think will happen if the patient were to hear the truth?
  - Discuss with the family about how you are going to approach the patient and what you are going to talk about.
  - Approach the patient and explore the sensitive subject gently. For example, "Mr. Patel, I understand from your family that you do not want to know the details about your illness and that you want them to make decisions for you regarding your health care." If the patient requests "not to know" and wants the family to make decisions, this is ethically acceptable as she or he is exercising autonomy by choosing not to know.
  - Reassure the patient that anytime he or she wants to know more information, you are always available to discuss his or her medical situation.
- Autonomy, or the right to exercise free will, can be invoked by the patient in not wanting to know diagnostic and prognostic information related to the illness (i.e., the patient has the right to refuse to learn about the diagnosis and defer all decision-making to the designated decision-maker).

Working with Medical Interpreters

Communicating with patients and families with limited English proficiency is particularly challenging. Lack of adequate communication could result in loss of critical information, resulting in suboptimal care and poor patient and family satisfaction. In communicating with patients with limited English proficiency, physicians must use a *professional medical interpreter*. Such services are and should be available in all healthcare systems (some systems have interpreters on staff, and others use commercial telephone-based interpreter services).

Clinical Pearls

- Family members should not serve as interpreters. The gold standard is to use a professional medical interpreter.
- Interpreters should be from the same culture as the patient. Interpreters not only translate the patients' words but also interpret it within the cultural context (i.e., they should serve as cultural brokers and translate the concept and the meaning from the patient's language to English).
- The professional medical interpreter should similarly interpret the physician's explanations and proposed interventions and explain these to the patient and family.
- Professional medical interpreters are bound by the standard HIPPA regulations and should treat all information learned as confidential.
- The professional medical interpreter should *not* influence the opinion and actions of the patient.
- When communicating through a professional medical interpreter, using short simple sentences (avoiding jargon), asking them to translate a few sentences at a time, frequently checking in with them, and debriefing with them after the interaction will help foster accuracy and collegiality.
- For practical resources and tips for working with medical interpreters please go to https://geriatrics.stanford.edu/medical-interpreters.html

References

1. Periyakoil VS, Hallenbeck JL (2002). Identifying and managing preparatory grief and depression at the end of life. *Am Fam Physician* 65(5):883–90. http://www.aafp.org/afp/20020301/883.html.
2. Periyakoil VS, Kraemer HC, Noda A, Moos R, Hallenbeck J, Webster M, Yesavage JA (2005). The development and initial validation of the Terminally III Grief or Depression Scale (TIGDS). *Int J Methods Psychiatr Res* 14(4):202-12
3. Periyakoil VS (2005). Is it grief or depression? In: Lisa Pelzek-Braun (ed.), *End-of-Life Physician Education Resource Center*. Retrieved November 8, 2008, from <http://www.aahpm.org/cgi-bin/wkcgi/view?status=A%20&search=177&id=226&offset=0&limit=151>.
4. *Diagnostic and Statistical Manual of Mental Disorders*, 4th ed. (*DSM-IV*). (1994). Washington, DC: American Psychiatric Association.
5. Anxiety in palliative care: causes and diagnosis. Retrieved November 8, 2008, from http://www.eperc.mcw.edu/fastFact/ff_186.htm.
6. Retrieved November 8, 2008, from http://www.nimh.nih.gov/health/publications/generalized-anxiety-disorder.shtml.
7. Periyakoil VS, Skultety K, Sheikh J (2005). Panic, anxiety and chronic dyspnea at the end of life. *J Palliat Med* 8(2):453–9.
8. Periyakoil VS (2005). Fast facts and concepts #145: panic disorders at the end of life. In: Lisa Pelzek-Braun (ed.), *End-of-Life Physician Education Resource Center*. Retrieved November 8, 2008, from http://www.aahpm.org/cgi-bin/wkcgi/view?status=A%20&search=177&id=646&offset=0&limit=25.
9. Feldman DB, Periyakoil VS (2006). Posttraumatic stress disorder at the end of life. *J Palliat Med* 9(1):213–8.
10. Prins A, Ouimette P, Kimerling R, Cameron RP, Hugelshofer DS, Shaw HJ, Thraikill A, Gussman FD, Sheikh JI (2003). The primary care PTSD screen (PC-PTSD): development and operating characteristics. *Prim Care Psychiatry* 9:9–14.
11. Physician orders for life-sustaining treatment paradigm. Retrieved November 8, 2008, from http://www.ohsu.edu/ethics/polst/.
12. Johnson KS, Kuchibhatla M, Tulsky JA (2008).What explains racial differences in the use of advance directives and attitudes toward hospice care? *J Am Geriatr Soc.*
13. Cohen LL (2008). Racial/ethnic disparities in hospice care: a systematic review. *J Palliat Med* 11(5):763–8.

14. Smith AK, McCarthy EP, Paulk E, Balboni TA, Maciejewski PK., Block SD, Prigerson HG (2008). Racial and ethnic differences in advance care planning among patients with cancer: impact of terminal illness acknowledgment, religiousness, and treatment preferences. *J Clin Oncol* 26(25):4131–7.
15. Kleinman A (1978). Culture, illness and cure: clinical lessons from anthropologic and cross-cultural research. *Annals Int Med* 88:251–8.

Further Reading

1. Periyakoil VS. *Stanford End of Life Curriculum*. Retrieved November 8, 2015, from http://palliative.stanford.edu.
2. Letter Project: A multi-lingual resource for advance care planning discussions Retrieved November 8, 2015, from http://med.stanford.edu/letter.html
3. Ethnogeriatrics portal: A virtual textbook with ethnic-specific care information on 13 common ethnic groups in the US. Retrieved November 8, 2015, from http://geriatrics.stanford.edu

Spiritual Issues
in Palliative Care

**Christina M. Puchalski, Betty R. Ferrell,
and Edward O'Donnell**

Introduction

Since the inception of hospice and the development of palliative care, spirituality has been recognized as an essential element of palliative care. Saunders described the concept of "total pain" as encompassing spiritual distress as well as psychosocial and physical distress.[1] Her model was eventually described as the biopsychosocial-spiritual model, which is the framework for palliative care.[2] The model emphasizes the totality of a patient's experience in the context of his or her illness and/or dying.

While the primary diagnosis may be cancer, for example, the span of the clinician's assessment of that patient includes the physical signs and symptoms of the cancer, the patient's emotional response to the illness, the social ramifications of the cancer on the patient and his or her family and friends, and, finally, the spiritual issues that may present as a result of the illness. Integrating all dimensions of a patient's experience with illness is key to patient-centered care.

Spirituality as part of patient-centered care, particularly in palliative care, is supported by ethical as well as empirical literature.[3-6] Studies have demonstrated that spiritual care affects healthcare outcomes including quality of life,[7-9] will to live,[9,10] survival,[11,12] and coping.[13]

Surveys demonstrate that patients want their spiritual issues formally addressed in the clinical setting[14,15] and want their spiritual needs attended to by healthcare professionals.[16,17] In hospital settings, the degree to which spiritual needs of patients are attended to is the strongest predictor of patient satisfaction with care and with patient perception of quality of care.[18] Studies have also indicated that spiritual or religious beliefs can impact end-of-life decision-making.[19] The Picker Institute has noted that respecting patients' beliefs and values may improve patients' healthcare outcomes and is critical to the practice of patient-centered care.[20]

The National Consensus Project for Quality Palliative Care (NCP), a coalition of leading palliative care organizations in the United States, represents the nation's 4700 hospices, 9000 hospice and palliative care nurses, 1400 hospital-based palliative care programs, and 4000 members of American Academy of Hospice and Palliative Medicine. In 2004, the NCP developed guidelines to strengthen new and existing palliative care services.[21] The guidelines were updated in 2009.[22] Spiritual care is one of the eight distinct domains within the NCP guidelines, and spiritual and existential concerns are mentioned throughout as aspects of pain, psychological concern, and grief.

The National Quality Forum (NQF), one of the leading forces in health care, accepted the NCP domains and created preferred practices to operationalize the NCP guidelines.[22,23] These preferred practices are all relevant to clinical practice (see www.nationalconsensusproject.org).

The NQF framework presents 38 best practices across the eight domains of the NCP framework. These practices are evidence based or endorsed through expert opinion, and apply to both hospice and palliative care provided across settings.[23] The NCP guidelines are a significant contribution in acknowledging the importance of spiritual care in palliative medicine and provide a foundation for the broader integration of spirituality into medical care.

Despite these guidelines, the implementation of spiritual care is not uniform in palliative or other care settings. Reasons for this include confusion over the definition of spirituality, lack of resources and tools, inadequate professional education, and lack of practical implementation tools. The variability in approaches to spirituality in palliative care underscores the need to articulate a definition of spirituality and to set common guidelines for spiritual care as a dimension of palliative care.

In 2009, Puchalski and Ferrell co-led a national Consensus Conference to develop recommendations for implementing the spiritual care domain of the NCP guidelines for palliative care. The project was a collaboration between the George Washington Institute for Spirituality and Health and the City of Hope National Medical Center. Forty leaders in palliative care and spiritual care who were from various disciplines were invited to develop specific and practical recommendations for the implementation of interdisciplinary spiritual care in palliative care, which was defined as starting from initial diagnosis of a serious or chronic illness.

Specific recommendations, as well as models for spiritual care implementation and interdisciplinary spiritual care education, were developed. The resultant recommendations were then reviewed nationally; they were approved through a consensus process and were published for widespread dissemination as a consensus document, titled "Improving the Quality of Spiritual Care as a Dimension of Palliative Care."[24] More detailed information was published in a handbook of spiritual care in palliative care.[25]

As part of this initiative, resources for spiritual care are available on a national repository for spirituality and health, called SOERCE, on the website of the George Washington Institute for Spirituality and Health (www.gwish.org). The goal of this seminal work is to provide resources and tools for the increased integration of spiritual care into palliative care and into medical care in general.

Implementing Spirituality in Clinical Settings

The key to implementing spirituality in clinical settings is to have a practical model for implementation that allows all clinicians to recognize and integrate patients' spiritual issues into the treatment or care plan. A key outcome of the Consensus Conference was the development of a spiritual care implementation model (Figure 21.1).

This model, which is based on a generalist–specialist model in which board-certified chaplains are recognized as the spiritual care experts, includes the following features:

- All patients receive a spiritual screening, history, and assessment by the appropriate healthcare professional.
- Spiritual screenings are admissions questions to screen for spiritual distress. Screening is limited to two questions: Is spirituality or religion important for you? Are your spiritual or religious beliefs helping you right now? A "yes/no" combination to these questions triggers a referral to a board-certified chaplain.
- Spiritual histories are more detailed and are done by clinicians who determine treatment or care plans. The spiritual history can be taken by means of a tool, such as the FICA (Faith, Importance, Community, Action),[26] HOPE (sources of Hope, Organized religion, Personal spirituality and Practices, Effects on medical care and End-of-life issues),[27] or SPIRIT (Spiritual belief system, Personal spirituality, Integration with a spiritual community, Ritualized practices and restrictions, Implications for medical care, and Terminal events planning) instruments.[28] All of these tools were developed for clinicians.
- Spiritual diagnoses are made by clinicians, ideally in an interdisciplinary team setting with the input of board-certified chaplains, who will also integrate spirituality into the treatment and care plan.
- There is an ongoing follow-up and modification of the plan, as needed.
- Clinicians receive professional training in practicing spiritual care.

Once the clinician obtains the information from the history, he or she integrates it into the treatment plan. This includes making a diagnosis of spiritual distress or pain, or identification of spiritual issues or spiritual goals, if appropriate, and determining and implementing the appropriate spiritual interventions.

There are two possible pathways once a diagnosis is made: the simple and the complex. For simple issues, such as a patient wanting to learn about yoga or meditation, the clinician can make the appropriate referral or course of action.

For more complex spiritual and religious issues, such as the need for forgiveness and/or reconciliation of self or others, severe existential distress, or lack of connection or love of others or God, referral to a chaplain and other spiritual care professionals is critical. Each of these elements is discussed in depth in the title report of the Consensus Conference, which includes decision-tree algorithms (Figure 21.2).

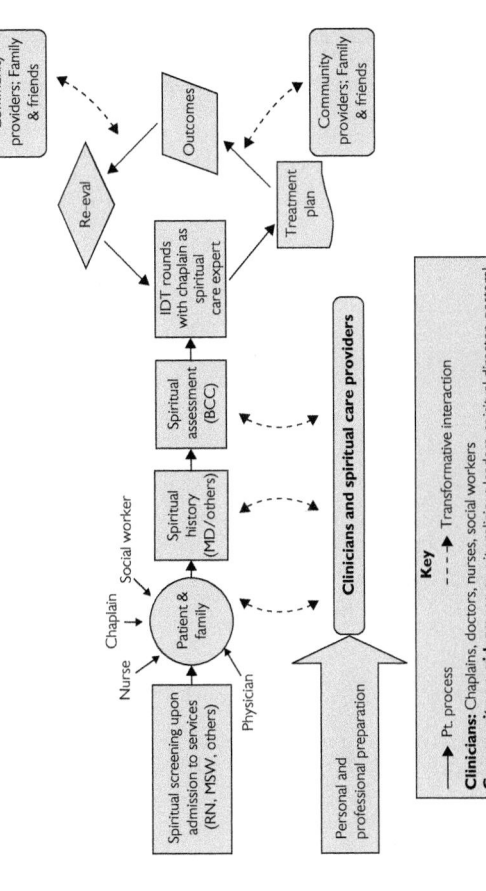

Figure 21.1. Spiritual care implementation model.

Reprinted with permission from Puchalski CM, Ferrell B, Virani R, et al. (2009). Improving the quality of spiritual care as a dimension of palliative care: the report of the Consensus Conference. *J Palliat Med* 12(10):885–904. The publisher for copyrighted material is Mary Ann Liebert, Inc., publishers.

In the final analysis, the spiritual care model is a relational model in which the patient and clinicians work together in a process of discovery, collaborative dialogue, treatment, and ongoing evaluation and follow-up.

Thus, an integral part of this model is ongoing professional development of the clinician in his or her ability to provide compassionate, patient-centered care. This would include attention to the spiritual needs of the healthcare professional as related to his or her call to serve others in an altruistic, compassion-based model of professional practice.

Clinicians should also attend to their biopsychcosocial-spiritual issues, with the goal of having balance in their lives and healthy approaches to stress management and to the issues that arise in caring for seriously ill patients (Figure 21.2).

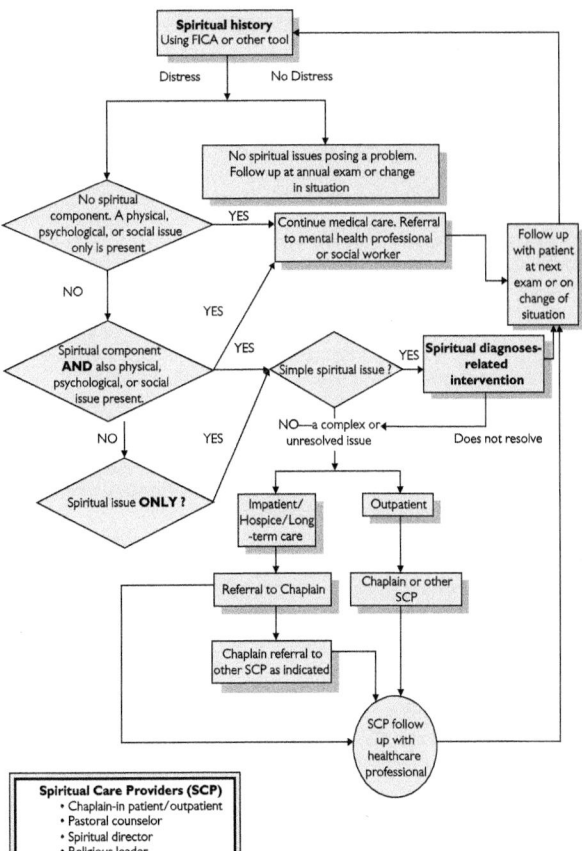

Figure 21.2. Spiritual care algorithm.

Reprinted with permission from Puchalski CM, Ferrell B, Virani R, et al. (2009). Improving the quality of spiritual care as a dimension of palliative care: the report of the Consensus Conference. *J Palliat Med* 12(10):885–904. The publisher for copyrighted material is Mary Ann Liebert, Inc., publishers.

Spiritual Issues and Diagnosis

Spirituality may be defined as that part of the person that seeks meaning in life and finds coherence in the midst of disorder and purpose in his or her life. Spirituality has been described as the essence of the human being, the search for meaning and purpose,[29] the expression of connection to others, God, or the transcendent or sacred,[24] and the basis for the healing relationships that clinicians form with patients.[30] The definition agreed upon for palliative care in the Consensus Conference is as follows: "Spirituality is the aspect of humanity that refers to the way individuals seek and express meaning and purpose, and the way they experience their connectedness to the moment, to self, to others, to nature, and to the significant or sacred."[24]

There is some concern in the field about labeling spiritual issues as "diagnosis." Spiritual or religious concerns are thought to be so integral to a person's being that caution has been raised about labeling spirituality as pathology, as this is an aspect of a human being, not a disorder.[31]

Yet spirituality and religion in the context of illness may also present as distress. Religion may have negative effects on health,[13] and spirituality in general may result in distress, pain, or suffering.[32] In this context, we would argue that spiritual or existential issues may in some circumstances be classified as diagnosis, in those cases where patients are experiencing distress or where beliefs may be impacting health adversely.

Spiritual issues include the following:

- Despair and hopelessness
- Lack of meaning and purpose
- Grief and loss
- Guilt and shame
- Anger
- Abandonment by God or others
- Isolation
- Reconciliation
- Concerns about relationship with deity
- Conflicted or challenged beliefs.

Each of these spiritual issues may present as part of a person's life without causing distress or even affecting the illness with which the patient presents. For example, patients may be experiencing demoralization, finding no meaning or purpose in their lives. This may be experienced as part of a transition in life, such as during a divorce, illness, or as a mid-life crisis. A patient may simply be questioning meaning in life as a reflective process. This would be identified as a spiritual issue that may or may not be affecting the presenting medical or health problem.

On the other hand, a patient may experience deep suffering and distress from a lack of meaning in life. We would suggest that in times when meaninglessness produces pain, suffering, or distress, it should be identified as a diagnosis and treated as a symptom equal to physical pain.

Forgiveness or reconciliation might be understood as a spiritual or religious practice, but in certain contexts the inability to forgive might impact the illness or the person in such as a way as to cause severe distress or suffering or may even be a contributing cause of clinical depression.

It is important that clinicians be able to differentiate the full spectrum of how spirituality presents in patients' lives in the context of their illness and how it presents in the clinical environment. Integral to this process of differentiation is working with board-certified chaplains who are trained in distinguishing spiritual pathology from normal spiritual developmental issues.

Spiritual Development Issues

Spiritual growth and development is a lifelong journey. Spiritual development often parallels emotional development.[33] In childhood, the main psychosocial tasks include development of trust, autonomy, and initiative. Spiritually, children start making meaning of a world that is new to them, a world that is gradually becoming part of their life.

Religion often plays a role at this time if the family is religious. This is a time of extrinsic religiosity, a time when children are exposed to the rituals and religious customs of the family. Clinically, this might be manifested as a clear, concrete vision of what life after death may mean, as, for example, a picture of heaven with a grandfather-like God.

In adolescence, the primary psychosocial task is to form identity. Spiritually, the adolescent begins to accept conventional ways of finding meaning in life but also begins to question what has been offered to him or her by parents and teachers. It is a time of movement from extrinsic to intrinsic faith. Clinically, a dying adolescent might struggle with what she believes but might revert back to what the conventional beliefs are if she has not determined what her own beliefs are.

Early adulthood is a time of establishing a career and intimate relationships. Spiritually, the young adult develops a personal faith or way of making meaning in life by reflecting on what has been passed on to him and determining what elements of this faith or meaning-making he will integrate as his own. This is often called a time of *intrinsic faith*.

A young adult who has established his or her own faith will use that as a foundation for dealing with illness. But many people sacrifice attention to spiritual development in favor of intellectual and career development. So in times of crisis they may revert back to childhood faith, sometimes called "foxhole faith."

In adulthood, generativity is the key psychosocial task, one of establishing oneself securely in one's professional and family or relational life. At this time, spirituality is expressed in the integration into oneself of much that was suppressed or unrecognized in the interest of a career or family. Some refer to this stage as *holistic spirituality*. It may be a deep time of searching for what is meaningful beyond the external.

Spirituality may be expressed in religious terms but also in nature, beauty, pets, people, or other beliefs. Clinically, illness may actually push an adult onto a spiritual path, especially if the illness prevents the person from working or from doing the things that once were meaningful.

As people grow older, they often become satisfied with the achievement of career goals and find a deep sense of meaning for life in themselves and the world. This is also a time of acknowledging loss and disappointments, of navigating the joys as well as the sorrows of life. Many arrive at a place of peace and understanding regarding the universal value and goodness of life and of all that constitutes one's world. The adult who goes through this part of spiritual growth, called gerotranscendence, comes to an acceptance of the paradoxes of life.

Clinically, this journey may be intensified in illness, particularly in end-of-life care, and some patients may not arrive at this peace. In this situation, one goal of care would be to provide the support and environment for the patient to explore these deep issues of existence and find some peace or acceptance of his or her life.

Spiritual development often does not move along in a linear fashion.[34] Also, spiritual growth many times does not parallel professional or personal development. Illness or dying may be the triggers for deeper questioning.

But if people have not had the opportunity to focus on spiritual developmental issues, they may experience spiritual distress in the context of illness and may need to revert to their childhood spirituality for support. The beliefs and practices they valued as children may not support them or help them in their time of illness and stress.

Awe is the primary spiritual attitude that children experience. But when a religious dimension is added to the child's life, it can either foster or diminish that spiritual awakening. Religion fosters this awakening if ritual and dogma support a growing awareness of the transcendent, so that the growth of awe in the life of the child is nourished and encouraged. Religion can diminish or retard spiritual development in the childhood stage if it is rule centered or emphasizes a punishment-and-reward approach to dealing with the transcendent.[34]

Neglect or abuse can also dampen or destroy a child's enthusiasm for the transcendent. This can be evident in the way people handle illness, stress, or dying.

If people's sense of the transcendent has been nurtured, they are likely to have positive religious coping. If they have had a rule-centered approach, it is more likely that they will experience negative religious coping. Pargament et al.[13] have demonstrated this pattern in their work on religious coping.

People who have a partnership relationship with God or find support in their religious communities have better psychological coping than those who see the illness as a punishment from God.

Spiritual Diagnosis

While there has been some attempt to develop diagnosis codes for spiritual issues that impact health (e.g., National Comprehensive Cancer Network), this is still an area that needs further work. In the Consensus report we set up a potential model for framing these issues within clinical care. In general, a spiritual issue becomes a diagnosis if the following criteria are met:

- A spiritual issue leads to distress or suffering. Examples include lack of meaning, conflicted religious beliefs, and inability to forgive.
- A spiritual issue is the cause of psychological or physical diagnosis such as depression, anxiety, or acute or chronic pain. Examples include severe meaninglessness that leads to depression or suicidal ideation, or guilt that leads to chronic physical pain.
- A spiritual issue is a secondary cause or affects the presenting psychological or physical diagnosis—for example, hypertension that is difficult to control because the patient refuses to take medications because of religious beliefs.

Treatment or Care Plans

Palliative care is based in the biopsychosocial-spiritual model of care.[2] Thus, spiritual treatment or care plans should be developed by an interdisciplinary team, with the board-certified chaplain as the expert in spiritual care, and should be documented in the framework of the whole patient.

For example, if a patient expresses a lack of meaning and purpose in his or her life, the spiritual issue or diagnosis would be meaninglessness or demoralization. The primary care clinician would make that diagnosis and then would discuss the management of that with the interdisciplinary team, specifically the chaplain. If there is no team or no chaplain, as in outpatient settings, the clinician would determine the appropriate treatment modality.

In Table 21.1, possible treatment options are listed. These include continued presence and support from the clinician, referral to an outpatient spiritual care professional such as a chaplain or pastoral counselor, meaning-centered group therapy, reflection and journaling, or other spiritual support group.

In diagnosing and documenting spiritual issues, it is important to also recognize that the spiritual issue may be affecting the physical, emotional, or social domains. So a patient who finds no meaning in life may experience greater physical pain, may feel unengaged from treatment and be noncompliant, may have depressive symptoms, or may be isolated from his or her community of support.

Table 21.1 Examples of Spiritual Health Interventions

Therapeutic communication techniques	Compassionate presence
	Reflective listening, query about important life events
	Support patient's sources of spiritual strength
	Open-ended questions to illicit feelings
	Inquiry about spiritual beliefs, values, and practices
	Life review, listening to the patient's story
	Continued presence and follow-up
Therapy	Guided visualization for "meaningless pain"
	Progressive relaxation
	Breathing practice or contemplation
	Meaning-oriented therapy
	Referral to spiritual care provider as indicated
	Use of storytelling
	Dignity-conserving therapy
Self-care	Massage
	Reconciliation with self or others
	Support groups
	Meditation
	Sacred or spiritual readings or rituals
	Yoga, tai chi
	Exercise
	Art therapy (music, art, dance), journaling

In documentation, therefore, the assessment and plan should include the diagnosis and plans for all four domains, as illustrated in Table 21.1.

Case Example: Assessment and Plan

Mrs. M. is a 78-year-old female who has had a recent stroke, which has left her with mild cognitive impairment, as well as some loss of motor function. Her source of meaning was being a political activist and making a difference in people's lives. She feels useless now and without meaning and purpose. Her support group consists of other activists for the homeless.

Physical	s/p CVA, rehab, speech therapy, Plavix, resume enalapril and monitor blood pressure
Emotional	Referral to counselor for support; however, patient declined.
Social	Explore possible other work with activist group; encourage patient to explore options with her group. Social worker to record patient's life story and help her explore themes.
Spiritual	Referral to chaplain; patient willing to explore meaning issues; continued supportive care and listening, explore what gave meaning in past and how that can occur with present physical limitations, referral to social work for narrative medicine as above.

Demonstration Projects: INSPIR

Integrating Spirituality in Hospital Settings

This successful study involved training interdisciplinary teams of healthcare professionals in five hospitals. Each site had 1 year to develop and pilot spiritual care interventions specifically focused on training providers to do a spiritual history. Part of the training included how to provide spiritual care.

Program evaluation included quantitative patient and provider outcome measurements at 3, 6, and 12 months. The pilot studies demonstrated that healthcare professionals find greater meaning at work and have a greater ability to provide compassionate care if they address patients' spiritual issues and focus on whole-person care, and also have the opportunity to focus on their own spirituality and call to service within the professional context.

Results of the study included culture changes in test units, improved patient satisfaction with care, increased staff satisfaction, lower burnout, and lower turnover.

These pilot studies also provide examples of practical tools used for spiritual care and enhance the knowledge of best practices in clinical environments.[17] Some examples of these tools are listed in Box 21.1.

> **Box 21.1 Tools for Integrating Spirituality into Clinical Settings**
>
> - Education for staff: brown bag lunches, workshops, grand rounds (didactic, experiential), in-service talks
> - Team activities: huddle, group activities centered around spirituality and compassionate care
> - Artwork, posters, inspirational quotes on hospital walls and in staff lounges
> - Rituals in clinical practice (e.g., moment of silence when a patient dies, journal at bedside of patient where staff can write comments, thoughts, blessings), rituals to honor transitions (birth, death of patients, or transitions for staff)
> - Recognition of excellence in spiritual care (beads, certificates)
> - Institutionalized spiritual assessment, interdisciplinary spiritual histories, spiritual screening
> - Reminders of calling to profession (chimes, rituals, reinforcement from administration)
> - Accountability measures for spiritual care

Conclusion

Patients with chronic and serious illness have spiritual needs that can impact their care and affect health outcomes. While there are national guidelines requiring that spiritual care be provided for seriously ill patients, surveys demonstrate that most patients do not have their spiritual issues addressed in their care.

Based on a national consensus process, a model has been developed for the implementation of spiritual care within a medical model that can be implemented in palliative care settings and in settings where seriously ill patients are treated. This model includes the identification or diagnosis of spiritual issues, as well as integration of patients' spirituality into the treatment or care plan in conjunction with board-certified chaplains who function as the spiritual care experts.

Integral to this model is the recognition that clinicians should also attend to their own spiritual needs as related to their professional work of service. Examples of practical tools in hospital settings can be used to create more holistic hospital and clinical settings for both the patient and clinician.

References

1. Smith WJ (2009). Dame Cecily Saunders: the mother of modern hospice care passes on. *The Weekly Standard*, March 27.
2. Sulmasy, DP (2002). A biopsychosocial-spiritual model for the care of patients at the end of life [see comment]. *Gerontologist* 42(Spec No. 3):24–33.
3. Sulmasy DP (1999). Is medicine a spiritual practice? *Acad Med* 74(9):1002–5.
4. Astrow AB, Puchalski CM, Sulmasy DP (2001). Religion, spirituality, and health care: social, ethical, and practical considerations. *Am J Med* 110(4):283–7.
5. Ferrell BR, Coyle N (2008). The nature of suffering and the goals of nursing. *Oncol Nurs Forum* 35(2):241–7.

6. Puchalski CM, Lunsford B, Harris MH, Miller RT (2006). Interdisciplinary spiritual care for seriously ill and dying patients: a collaborative model. *Cancer J* 12(5):398–416.

7. Cohen SR, Mount BM, Tomas JJ, Mount LF (1996). Existential well-being is an important determinant of quality of life: evidence from the McGill quality of life questionnaire. *Cancer* 77(3):576–86.

8. Roberts JA, Brown D, Elkins T, Larson DB (1997). Factors influencing views of patients with gynecologic cancer about end-of-life decisions. *Am J Obstet Gynecol* 176(1 Pt 1):166–72.

9. Tsevat J, Sherman SN, McElwee JA, Mandell KL, Simbartl LA, Sonnenberg FA, et al. (1999). The will to live among HIV-infected patients. *Ann Intern Med* 131(3):194–8.

10. Yi MS, Mrus JM, Wade TJ, Ho ML, Hornung RW, Cotton S, et al. (2006). Religion, spirituality, and depressive symptoms in patients with HIV/AIDS. *J Gen Intern Med* 21(Suppl. 5):S21–7.

11. Kimmel PL, Emont SL, Newmann JM, Danko H, Moss AH (2003). ESRD patient quality of life: symptoms, spiritual beliefs, psychosocial factors, and ethnicity. *Am J Kidney Dis* 42(4):713–21.

12. Koenig HG, McCullough ME, Larson DB (2001). *Handbook of Religion and Health.* New York: Oxford University Press.

13. Pargament KI, Smith BW, Koenig HG, Perez L (1998). Patterns of positive and negative religious coping with major life stressors. *J Sci Study Relig* 37(4):710–24.

14. McCord G, Gilchrist VJ, Grossman SD, King BD, McCormick KE, Oprandi AM, et al. (2004). Discussing spirituality with patients: a rational and ethical approach. *Ann Family Med* 2(4):356–61.

15. Ehman JW, Ott BB, Short TH, Ciampa RC, Hansen-Flaschen J (1999). Do patients want physicians to inquire about their spiritual or religious beliefs if they become gravely ill? *Arch Intern Med* 159(15):1803–6.

16. Balboni TA, Vanderwerker LC, Block SD, Paulk ME, Lathan CS, Peteet JR, et al. (2007). Religiousness and spiritual support among advanced cancer patients and associations with end-of-life treatment preferences and quality of life. *J Clin Oncol* 25(5):555–60.

17. Puchalski CM, McSkimming S (2006). Creating healing environments. *Health Prog* 87(3):30–5.

18. Astrow AB, Wexler A, Texeira K, Kai He M, Sulmasy DP (2007). Is failure to meet spiritual needs associated with cancer patients' perceptions of quality of care and their satisfaction with care? *J Clin Oncol* 25(36):5753–7.

19. Phelps AC, Maciejewski PK, Nilsson M, Balboni TA, Wright AA, Paulk ME, et al. (2009). Religious coping and use of intensive life-prolonging care near death in patients with advanced cancer. *JAMA* 301(11):1140–7.

20. Institute for Alternative Futures (2004). *Patient-Centered Care 2015: Scenarios, Vision, Goals & Next Steps.* Alexandria, VA: The Picker Institute. Retrieved from http://www.altfutures.com/pubs/Picker%20Final%20Report%20May%2014%202004.pdf.

21. National Consensus Project for Quality Palliative Care (2004). Clinical practice guidelines for quality palliative care, executive summary. *J Palliat Med* 7(5):611–27. Retrieved from http://search.ebscohost.com/login.aspx?direct=true&db=aph&AN=14963387&site=ehost-live.

22. National Consensus Project for Quality Palliative Care (2009). *Clinical Practice Guidelines for Quality Palliative Care,* 2nd ed. Retrieved from http://www.nationalconsensusproject.org.

23. National Quality Forum (2006). *A National Framework and Preferred Practices for Palliative and Hospice Care Quality.* Washington, DC: National Quality Forum. Retrieved from http://qualityforum.org/publications/reports/palliative.asp.

24. Puchalski C, Ferrell B, Virani R, Otis-Green S, Baird P, Bull J (2009). Improving the quality of spiritual care as a dimension of palliative care: the report of the Consensus Conference. *J Palliat Med* 12(10):885–904.

25. Puchalski C, Ferrell B (eds.) (2010). *Making Health Care Whole: Integrating Spirituality into Healthcare.* West Conshohocken, PA: Templeton Press.

26. Puchalski C, Romer AL (2000). Taking a spiritual history allows clinicians to understand patients more fully. *J Palliat Med* 3(1):129–37.

27. Anandarajah G, Hight E (2001). Spirituality and medical practice: using the HOPE questions as a practical tool for spiritual assessment [see comment]. *Am Fam Physician* 63(1):81–9.

28. Maugans TA (1996). The SPIRITual history. *Arch Fam Med* 5(1):11–6.

29. Frankl VE (1963). *Man's Search for Meaning.* New York: Washington Square Press, Simon & Schuster.

30. Association of American Medical Colleges (1999). Report III. Contemporary issues in medicine. Medical School Objectives Project (MSOP III). Washington, DC: AAMC. Retrieved from https://services.aamc.org/Publications/showfile.cfm?file=version89.pdf&prd_id=200&prv_id=241&pdf_id=89.

31. Griffith JL, Griffith ME (2002). *Encountering the Sacred in Psychotherapy: How to Talk with People about Their Spiritual Lives.* New York: Guilford Press.

32. Doka KJ, Morgan JD (1993). *Death and Spirituality*. Amityville, NY: Baywood.
33. Kelcourse FB (2004). *Human Development and Faith*. A multi-authored textbook for use in human development courses. St. Louis: Chalice Press.
34. Fowler J (1995). *Stages of Faith: The Psychology of Human Development and the Quest for Meaning*. San Francisco: HarperSanFrancisco.

Chapter 22

The Palliative Care Team

Eduardo Bruera

Introduction

From its origins in the United Kingdom in the 1960s and the further development of the field in Canada in the 1970s and the United States in the 1980s, palliative care has evolved and developed a series of principles and practices.

Modern palliative care programs have three major principles:

1. *Multidimensional assessment and management.* This includes the presence of structures, processes, and outcomes needed to address multiple physical symptoms, psychosocial and spiritual distress, and functional, financial, and family concerns.

2. *Interdisciplinary care.* Modern palliative care is recognized as a team effort, including not only physicians and nurses but also social workers, pastoral care, occupational therapy, physiotherapy, pharmacy, counselors, dieticians, and volunteers who work in an integrated fashion for the delivery of assessment and management of patients and families.

3. *Emphasis on caring for patients and their families.* Palliative care teams recognize that the overwhelming majority of the physical and emotional care is delivered by the family and that delivering care at the end of

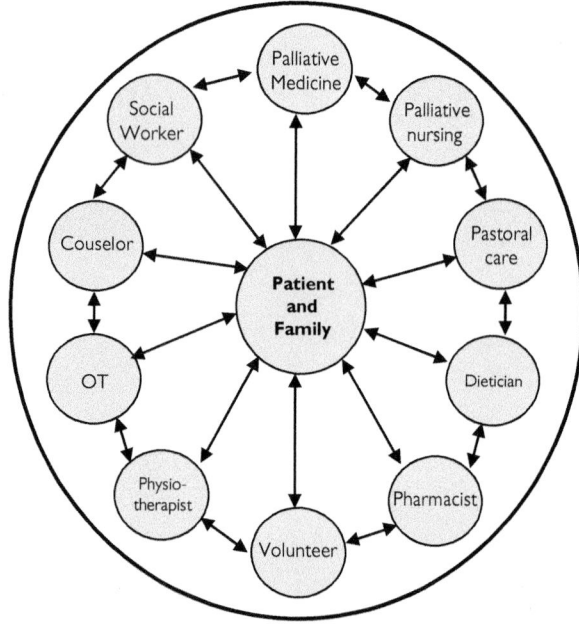

Figure 22.1. The palliative care team.
OT = occupational therapy.

life to a loved one puts an enormous physical, emotional, financial, and existential burden on family members. Palliative care programs consider families the unit of care.

Figure 22.1 summarizes the interdisciplinary nature of care delivered by the palliative care team.

The Palliative Medicine Specialist

In 2008, the United States established hospice and palliative medicine as a formal medical subspecialty after lengthy but ultimately highly successful negotiations led by the American Board of Hospice and Palliative Medicine and the American Academy of Hospice and Palliative Medicine. Palliative medicine was established as a medical specialty in the United Kingdom in 1987 and since then this specialty and/or subspecialty status has been formally established in Canada, Australia, a significant number of European countries, and even several developing countries.

The body of knowledge of palliative medicine is by nature multidimensional. Figure 22.2 summarizes the contribution of different medical and nonmedical fields to palliative medicine.

Pioneers in the field of palliative medicine had to search for information from all of these disparate fields to acquire the necessary knowledge for effectively practicing as clinical and/or academic specialists.

Fortunately, in recent years, the field has developed peer-reviewed journals; national, regional, and international congresses; and a number of excellent textbooks that successfully summarize aspects of the body of knowledge, consisting of different medical and nonmedical disciplines, that is required of the palliative medicine specialist.

Figure 22.2. Contributions to the body of knowledge of a palliative medicine specialist.

The Palliative Care Team

While all the disciplines described in Figure 22.1 are required for the appropriate care of palliative care patients and their families, not all of these disciplines have the body of knowledge and expertise to specialize in the delivery of palliative care.

Palliative nursing has made considerable progress in recent years, including some specific board certification in many countries, the publication of books on palliative nursing, and scientific meetings. Unfortunately, there has been limited success in other areas.

Therefore, the establishment and maintenance of a palliative care team requires much more emphasis on initial orientation and support of members than in other, more established areas of health care.

Acute Care Hospitals

All of the disciplines are readily available in these hospitals. Therefore, ideally outpatient and inpatient programs should be placed geographically within acute care facilities in such a way as to enable allocation of a proportion of healthcare professionals' time to the delivery of interdisciplinary palliative care.

Acute Palliative Care Units

These are the most sophisticated and effective settings for the delivery of palliative care to highly distressed patients and families. In this setting, it is mandatory that the vast majority of patients and families receive assessment and management by all the major disciplines and that all the disciplines meet at least once per week for the purpose of discussing particularly complex problems and continuing education and support.

Consult Teams

These teams see patients in settings where there is no palliative care unit. They are particularly at risk for professional burnout and for achieving less successful outcomes. This situation is aggravated when physicians and nurses working on these teams have no access to an interdisciplinary palliative care team but instead have to interact with ad hoc professionals from areas in the hospital (e.g., for a patient on a surgical ward, the social worker, chaplain, case manager, physiotherapist, and pharmacist will be those assigned to surgery).

These well-intentioned professionals usually have no undergraduate or postgraduate palliative care training. This lack of training complicates communication and planning of care for complex situations such as somatization of physical symptoms, chemical coping, emotional distress, preexisting psychiatric or social problems for the patient or family, advance directives, and conflict among different healthcare teams.

Ideally, consult teams in acute care hospitals that have no palliative care units should develop Internet-based "virtual palliative care units" through which members of an interdisciplinary palliative care team can visit all patients and participate in the necessary assessment, management, family conferences, and discharge planning.

The two main limitations of such virtual units, compared to a palliative care unit, are the absence of a trained, full-time palliative care bedside nurse and the absence of administrative leadership, such as a unit manager capable of allocating resources and inpatient policies and procedures.

Outpatient Palliative/Supportive Care

This can be challenging when patients in severe physical and psychosocial distress and their primary caregivers are asked to make multiple appointments to see members of an interdisciplinary team. Outpatient palliative care clinics should be capable of delivering an assessment by many different disciplines in one single physical setting where patients have access to a full-size bed, proximity to a bathroom, and enough space in the consult room for some relatives to participate in the visit.

Outpatient facilities for palliative care patients should also have extra rooms where split visits can take place. This allows patients and relatives to meet separately with different members of the palliative care team, thereby optimizing the visit time for both patients and families and healthcare professionals.

Home Palliative Care

This is particularly challenging for interdisciplinary teams. Newly developed techniques, including lower-cost videoconferencing, interactive voice response systems, and active telephone visiting, are increasing access to members of the team, such as social workers, counselors, pastoral care, and case management. Unfortunately, the vast majority of patients at home will have very limited access to members of an interdisciplinary team.

One of the challenges for the visiting nurses and physicians is to determine when a patient and family are not coping well at home and when much more intense interdisciplinary care is required. At that point, admission to an acute care hospital, acute palliative care unit, or inpatient hospice facility may be required, depending on the severity of the patient's and family's distress, to provide rapid and interdisciplinary resolution of the distress. Home or inpatient community-based care may be required, depending on the level of patient needs and community-based support.

In addition to formal periodic communication (such as team meetings), daily informal interaction among the different team members is important to coordinate efforts and, most important, to unify goals of care and interactions with patients, families, and primary referring healthcare professionals.

Palliative care teams are only effective when regular and consistent communication and dialogue take place. This is what differentiates a successful interdisciplinary team from the multidisciplinary approach to patient care currently available in most acute care institutions and hospices.

Formal symptom assessment tools, joint charting of findings and recommendations by different members, and a strong commitment from all members of the team to communicate with other members of the team at any time when they make an important observational finding are key to successful outcomes.

The interdisciplinary team should regularly participate in educational activities, ideally based on clinical cases of difficult problems with patients, families, or referring healthcare teams. These joint regular educational sessions are crucial to generating common understanding of the principles and practice of palliative care.

While continued review of all principles and practice is an important intellectual activity for all team members, it is equally important that the team maintain a very consistent message in the communication with every individual patient and/or family. This is the key to dramatically reducing distress and conveying to the patient and family that the team is well integrated and can effectively lead them through very difficult times.

Perhaps the most important member of an interdisciplinary palliative care team in an acute care facility is the bedside nurse. All clinical findings relating to the patient and family, as well as all pharmacological and nonpharmacological interventions or investigations, should be discussed at length with the bedside nurse, and his or her impressions about patient and family distress and coping should be assessed on a daily basis.

Interdisciplinary teams spend a limited amount of time with each admitted patient. The bedside nurse is in charge of the patient 24 hours a day, including off hours when no members of the interdisciplinary team are present. It is therefore crucial that the bedside nurse be made a pivotal member of the interdisciplinary care team for each admitted patient.

Family Conference

Role in Palliative Care

Margaret Isaac and J. Randall Curtis

Introduction

Family conferences can be critical events in the course of an illness, defining goals of care for the patient and shaping the experience of the family and surrogate decision-makers involved in a patient's care. Whether in the ICU, medical ward, clinic, or home setting, family conferences conducted by palliative care providers and other clinicians have an important role in patient care and family support at the end of life.

Role of Palliative Care Specialists in Communication at the End of Life

The presence of palliative care specialists in the hospital and other settings is becoming increasingly common, and the involvement of interdisciplinary palliative care teams has been associated with improved patient satisfaction in both the home[1] and hospital[2] setting.

Role of Families and Surrogate Decision-Makers

Many patients at the end of life are unable to participate in their own medical decision-making, and clinicians often rely on surrogate decision-makers to assist in establishing a plan of care.

Not only is it an ethical obligation for physicians to share medical and prognostic information with surrogates, this information is important for surrogate decision-makers to be able to apply the principle of substituted judgment in making decisions. In addition, even if patients have decisional capacity, many may want to involve their families in decision-making about end-of-life care. Surrogate decision-making is a difficult task, with surrogates needing to balance their duty to represent the wishes of their loved one with their struggle around personal feelings of responsibility or grief related to the anticipated death of their family member, their wishes to pursue any treatment that might bring about clinical recovery, and their responsibility to promote family harmony and well-being.[3] In particular, surrogates without prior experience and those who have not previously discussed end-of-life preferences with their loved one may struggle most in this role and can especially benefit from skilled communication and support from clinicians.[4]

Shared Decision-Making Model

Shared decision-making has several defining characteristics: (1) involvement and participation of both a clinician and patient (and/or surrogate decision-maker); (2) information shared by the clinician, specifically prognosis as well as treatment options and their relative risks and benefits; (3) information shared by the patient and/or surrogate decision-maker about patient's values and goals of care; and (4) consensus between clinician and patient and/or surrogate on treatment decisions.[5]

Shared decision-making is only one of several models, others being parentalism, in which decisions are made unilaterally by clinicians, and autonomy with informed consent, in which information regarding treatment options is given to the patient or surrogate, and decision-making is left entirely in their hands. Shared decision-making has been advocated by many as an optimal way to engage patients and families in medical decisions in the critical care setting. That said, patients and family members vary widely in their desired level of decisional control. Assessing the degree to which patients' families and decision-makers want to be involved in medical decision-making is critical in providing effective, appropriate, and patient- and family-centered end-of-life care.

Approach to Communication during Family Conferences

Evidence-Based Approach to Family Conferences

Communication from clinicians during family conferences can have a significant impact on medical decision-making as well as on patient and family satisfaction. Specifically, statements that include affirmations of nonabandonment, assurances that the patient will not suffer, and support of families' decisions have been associated with higher family satisfaction.[6]

Additionally, increased proportion of family speech has been associated with higher degrees of family satisfaction.[7] Box 23.1 details recommended components of effective family conferences, which were initially developed for the ICU, but are also useful in the acute care hospital, long-term care, clinic, and home settings.

The VALUE mnemonic has been proposed as an effective method in communicating with families in the ICU setting and has been shown to reduce family member symptoms of anxiety and depression after death of a loved one in an ICU.[8] This approach is summarized in Figure 23.1.

Discussing Prognosis

Clinicians have a responsibility to share prognostic information with patients and families, as this information can have an important impact on medical decision-making.[9] Recommendations include using quantitative estimates, framed as information about groups of patients, along with a description of the uncertainty involved in these estimates. It is also important to address the risk of long-term functional impairment and its impact on future quality of life, in addition to death, when discussing prognosis. Patients and family members often care more about prognosis for quality of life and functional status than survival.

Box 23.1 Components of a Family Conference about End-of-Life Care

Before the Conference

- Plan the specifics of location and setting: a quiet, private place.
- Conduct a "pre-conference" with all interdisciplinary team members to review the conference, ensuring that team members share a similar understanding of medical details, the prognosis, the treatment options, and the goals of the discussion.

During the Conference

- Introduce names and roles of the team members and the family.
- Ask the family for their understanding of the current situation to gauge their level of understanding.
- Discuss prognosis frankly in a way that is meaningful to the family.
- Acknowledge uncertainty in the prognosis.
- Review the principle of substituted judgment: "What would the patient want?"
- Make a recommendation about treatment.
- Support the family's decision.
- Make it clear that withholding life-sustaining treatment is not withholding caring.
- If life-sustaining treatments will be withheld or withdrawn, discuss what the patient's death might be like.
- Acknowledge strong emotions and use reflection to encourage patients or families to talk about these emotions.
- Tolerate silence.

Summarizing the Conference

- Summarize the discussion and plans.
- Ask what questions the family might have.
- Ensure a basic follow-up plan and make sure the family knows how to reach you for questions.
- Document the discussion in the medical record.

Adapted from Curtis JR, Patrick DL, Shannon SE, et al. (2001). The family conference as a focus to improve communication about end-of-life care in the intensive care unit: opportunities for improvement. *Crit Care Med* 29:26–33.

V	Value family statements
A	Acknowledge family emotions
L	Listen to the family
U	Understand the patient as a person
E	Elicit family questions

Figure 23.1. VALUE: 5-step approach to improving communication in the ICU.

Adapted from Lautrette A, Darmon M, Megarbane B, et al. (2007). A communication strategy and brochure for relatives of patients dying in the ICU. *N Engl J Med* 356:469–478.

Spirituality and Religion

Spiritual and religious concerns are often prominent at the end of life, although many clinicians can feel uncomfortable discussing these topics. Because of the distinctively personal relationship between a clinician and patient or family, clinicians often have a unique opportunity to explore these issues with patients and families.

Making appropriate referrals to spiritual care providers can improve satisfaction on the part of patients and families. The FICA[10] mnemonic can assist clinicians in better understanding a patient's religious or spiritual values during family conferences and how those values may influence health care (adapted from Puchalski):

F: Faith and Belief"Is Mr. X a spiritual or religious person?"

I: Importance"What importance does faith or belief have in Mr. X's life?"

C: Community"Is Mr. X a member of a spiritual or religious community?"

A: Address in Care"How would Mr. X like us to address these issues in his health care?"

Cross-Cultural Communication

Cultural Competence in Communication about Palliative Care

Discussing end-of-life care can be additionally complex with patients or families from diverse cultural backgrounds. Addressing cultural differences directly, using medical interpreters and cultural mediators, involving the family in decision-making, and reconciling issues of a patient's informed refusal to participate in decision-making can all be helpful.[11] Approaches to cultural competence can include obtaining prior knowledge about common values, attitudes, and perspectives within a given culture, but it is important not to use this information to stereotype individuals who may not subscribe to these cultural norms. A more useful approach is simply to ask open-ended questions about what is important to patients and families and to be open to perspectives different from one's own.

Use of Interpreters and Cultural Liaisons

Use of medical interpreters is critical in facilitating communication with patients and families who speak different primary languages than that of the clinicians. More than simply translating, interpreters can function as "cultural mediators," promoting understanding on both sides, provided that their role in the patient–clinician interaction is clear to all involved.

However, it is important to understand the limitations of working with medical interpreters and to follow basic best practices such as speaking slowly, confirming the patient's or family's understanding, meeting with the interpreter before the clinical encounter to brief the interpreter on topics to be discussed, and debriefing the interpreter after difficult discussions.[12]

Summary

Family conferences are a critical element in medical decision-making for seriously ill patients. By assessing the desired level of involvement in medical decision-making, and using a shared decision-making model as a default, clinicians can provide effective guidance and support to patients and surrogate decision-makers.

Clinical Pearls

- Families often play an important role in family conferences, even if patients have decisional capacity.
- Assess patients' and family members' desired level of involvement in medical decision-making.
- Effective communication in family conferences requires clinicians to adapt to family needs and respond accordingly.
- Using affirming and supportive statements and allowing patients and families to speak more in family conferences increase their satisfaction.
- Spirituality, religion, and culture should be addressed directly with open-ended questions.
- Medical interpreters, when properly trained, can also act as cultural mediators in family conferences.

References

1. Brumley R, Enguidanos S, Jamison P, et al. (2007). Increased satisfaction with care and lower costs: results of a randomized trial of in-home palliative care. *J Am Geriatr Soc* 55:993–1000.
2. Gade G, Venohr I, Conner D, et al. (2008). Impact of an inpatient palliative care team: a randomized controlled trial. *J Palliat Med* 11:180–90.
3. Schenker Y, Crowley-Matoka M, Dohan D, Tiver GA, Arnold RA, White DB (2012). "I don't want to be the one saying 'we should just let him die': intrapersonal tensions experienced by surrogate decision makers in the ICU." *J Gen Intern Med* 27(12): 1657–65.
4. Majesko A, Hong SY, Weissfeld L, White DB (2012). Identifying family members who may struggle in the role of surrogate decision maker. *Crit Care Med* 40(8): 2281–6.
5. Charles C, Gafni A, Whelan T (1997). Shared decision making in the medical encounter: what does it mean? (or it takes at least two to tango). *Soc Sci Med* 44(5): 681–92.
6. Stapleton RD, Engelberg RA, Wenrich MD, et al. (2006). Clinician statements and family satisfaction with family conferences in the intensive care unit. *Crit Care Med* 34:1679–85.
7. McDonagh JR, Elliott TB, Engelberg RA, et al. (2004). Family satisfaction with family conferences about end-of-life care in the intensive care unit: increased proportion of family speech is associated with increased satisfaction. *Crit Care Med* 32:1484–8.
8. Lautrette A, Darmon M, Megarbane B, et al. (2007). A communication strategy and brochure for relatives of patients dying in the ICU. *N Engl J Med* 356(5): 469–78.
9. Murphy DJ, Burrows D, Santilli S, et al. (1994). The influence of the probability of survival on patients' preferences regarding cardiopulmonary resuscitation. *N Engl J Med* 330:545–9.
10. Puchalski CM (2002). Spirituality and end-of-life care: a time for listening and caring. *J Palliat Med* 5:289–94.
11. Kagawa-Singer M, Blackhall LF (2001). Negotiating cross-cultural issues at the end-of-life: "You got to go where he lives." *JAMA* 286:2993–3001.
12. Norris WM, Wenrich MD, Nielsen EL, et al. (2005). Communication about end-of-life care between language-discordant patients and clinicians: insights from medical interpreters. *J Palliat Med* 8:1016–24.

Ethical Aspects of Palliative Medicine

James D. Duffy

Introduction

The clinical practice of palliative medicine is inherently fraught with very significant ethical issues. Patients suffering from incurable and/or chronic physical ailments inevitably face decisions about the goals for their medical care that are colored by the quality of their lives and the values that shape their decisions.

Every patient and family infuses their disease with meaning and constructs their own particular reality of their illness. As clinicians, we often play the role of journeymen as we accompany our patients along their unique path through suffering, not imposing our own agenda but providing a safe space in which our patients can construct their own meaning. Rather than constructing rigid rules, bioethics attempts to provide patients and their clinicians with a framework that outlines the parameters of their decision-making.

The modern palliative care clinician is working at the sharp edge between modern medicine's scientific breakthroughs and the practical concerns of patients to optimize the quality and quantity of their lives. A thorough understanding of bioethical principles is crucial as our field continues to advocate for the interests of our patients while optimizing the benefits of modern medical science.

Bioethical approaches can be broadly defined within four categories.

Principle-Based Bioethical Approach

This (deontological) approach is sometimes described as "duty"- or "obligation"-based ethics and is founded on the principle that clearly defined ethical rules should bind our behaviors. This rule-based approach has significant utility in our complex medical environment because it allows clinicians to clearly assess and communicate the ethical justification for their actions.

The clinical utility of the four principles of deontological ethics (autonomy, justice, beneficence, and nonmaleficence) are discussed in greater detail in the section "Four Major Principles of Bioethics."

Virtue-Based Bioethical Approach

The modern term *ethics* is derived from the Greek word *ethikos*. Aristotle posited that positive moral virtue or intent is the most important determinant in deciding ethical behavior. According to Aristotle, virtue represents the balanced center between two extreme behaviors, for example, pride represents the mean between vanity and humility. In this vein, modern palliative care clinicians strive to enhance their compassion as a motivation for their work.

Although a virtue-based ethical approach might have face validity within the context of the private patient–physician relationship, it is not robust enough to define behaviors within our complex modern medicolegal system.

Utilitarianism (Consequentialism)

This approach asserts that any action should be assessed in the overall context of whether it does more harm than good for all affected by the action. While this approach may have utility in the context of broad public health decisions, it is less useful in bedside clinical decision-making.

Casuistry

Rather than relying on rules, rules, and theories, the casuist approach emphasizes the intimate understanding of a particular clinical situation and uses this information to shape decisions.

Four Major Principles of Bioethics

Respect for Autonomy

In the context of health care, *autonomy* describes the patient's right to act intentionally without any controlling influences that might mitigate against his or her free will. Respect for autonomy does not simply represent an attitude but requires actively acknowledging and supporting the patient's right to choices and actions based on his or her personal values and beliefs.

The respect for autonomy provides the basis for the concept of informed consent. In the context of palliative care, if the patient has decisional capacity, the clinician should actively attempt to both understand and support the patient's preferences—even when these might be contrary to the recommendations and/or wishes of healthcare professionals and family.

The Principle of Nonmaleficence

The ethical principle of nonmaleficence requires that the clinician not *intentionally* harm or injure a patient, through acts of either commission or omission. This principle requires the clinician to be medically competent and able to meet clinical standards of care.

The legal term *negligence* describes harm caused by exposing the patient to unreasonable risk and/or careless behavior on the part of the clinician. In palliative medicine, the clinician often participates in the withholding or withdrawing of treatments.

However, if such actions are undertaken with the primary intention of reducing the patient's suffering and are consistent with the patient's stated preferences, then the action is not considered to be maleficent but rather beneficent.

In some situations, the palliative medicine clinician prescribes a treatment that has both a wanted and an unwanted effect—for example, opiate analgesics produce pain relief but may also suppress respiratory drive and hasten the patient's demise. The ethical construct being invoked in such cases is the *principle of double effect*. The four characteristics of the principle of double effect are as follows:

1. The action must inherently be a neutral or beneficial act (e.g., prescribing an analgesic).
2. The primary intention for the action should be the beneficial effect, not the bad effect (e.g., the relief of pain).
3. The harmful means must not be the means of the good effect (shooting and killing a person is not an acceptable means of treating pain).
4. The beneficial effect of the action must outweigh the negative effect (the relief of the patient's overwhelming suffering is more beneficial than increasing their risk of pneumonia).

The Principle of Beneficence

The duty of the clinician is to be of a benefit to the patient. This principle applies to the patient, his or her family, and society as a whole. Palliative medicine clinicians often encounter situations in which there may be some uncertainty around what action or goal is of most benefit to the particular patient.

The clinician often has an important role in shaping and even directing the patient's decision about the relative benefit (and risk) of various medical decisions. It is imperative that the clinician strive to actively respect the patient's autonomy; however, patients and their families often look to the clinician to provide insights into these risks and benefits.

While the principle of autonomy would appear to prohibit "paternalism" on the part of the clinician, it is also clear that a clinician's honest and informed perspective can be of great benefit and can minimize a patient's ruminative and disabling ambivalence around ambiguous medical decision-making.

In clinical situations where the patient lacks decisional capacity and in the absence of a medical surrogate decision-maker, the clinician is justified in assuming a paternalistic role directed by a beneficent intention for the patient's well-being. Unfortunately, palliative medicine clinicians frequently encounter such situations and must always remain mindful of their responsibility to act with beneficent intention.

The Principle of Justice

Justice describes the "fair" distribution of goods in society and requires a "fair" method for allocating scarce resources. What constitutes a "fair" distribution is ambiguous and is largely determined by the social morality of a particular group. The principle of distributive justice is therefore shaped by many sociopolitical and religious influences, which may include each individual's need, effort, contribution, merit, and influence.

Since most chronically ill and dying patients lack the ability to advocate for themselves, palliative medicine clinicians must frequently act as advocates for their patients' needs. Issues relating to the right to avoid unnecessary suffering raise human rights as they pertain to end-of-life care and often necessitate that the palliative medicine clinician assume an advocacy role that extends far beyond the bedside and sometimes into the political arena.

Decisional Capacity and Informed Consent

The assessment of a patient's decisional capacity is crucial to the provision of effective and appropriate palliative care. Patients have the legal and ethical right to direct what happens to their bodies, and their physician has an ethical and legal responsibility to provide them with the information necessary to make an informed decision.

Informed consent is the process whereby a fully informed patient can actively and voluntarily participate in decisions regarding his or her health care. However, given their often significant cognitive deficits, patients receiving palliative care frequently lack the decisional capacity to make such an informed decision. It is the duty of the physician to fully ascertain whether the patient has the ability to become fully informed.

Although psychiatrists are frequently called upon to provide a clinical opinion regarding a patient's decisional capacity, every time clinicians make a clinical decision, they have de facto made the determination of their patient's decisional capacity. Unfortunately, in practice, this means that a patient's decisional capacity is only questioned when he or she counters the recommendation of the clinician.

A patient is deemed to possess decisional capacity when he or she is considered capable of providing fully informed consent for a specific intervention (i.e., decisional capacity is always task specific and is not a global construct).

The elements of a clinical determination of decisional capacity are the evaluation of the patient's ability to

- Understand what decision is being made
- Understand the alternatives to the proposed intervention
- Understand the relevant risks, benefits, and uncertainties related to each alternative. The degree of understanding required will turn on the importance of the decision to be made. Since palliative medicine often involves life-and-death decisions, the clinician should expect the patient (or surrogate) to exhibit a high degree of understanding of the risks and benefits.
- Maintain consistent reasoning based on the patient's values and goals
- Clearly communicate his or her decision.

How Much Medical Information Is Sufficient?

Clinicians possess far more medical information than is necessary for their patients to be able to make an informed decision. One question that arises is just how much information a patient needs in order to be considered informed. Most states have legislation that determines the required standard for informed consent. This standard may be subsumed under one or more of three approaches:

- *The reasonable physician standard*: that is, what would a competent physician tell the patient about the proposed medical intervention? This standard is predicated on the physician's perspective and may not therefore address the interests of the patient.
- *The reasonable patient standard*: that is, what would the average patient need to know in order to be an informed participant in the decision? This standard is predicated on the "standard" patient and does not address the idiosyncratic needs and perspectives of the patient who is making the informed decision.
- *The specific patient standard*: that is, what would this particular patient need to know and understand in order to make an informed decision? This standard is somewhat ambiguous and may sometimes be difficult to accomplish. However, it is likely to be the most effective strategy to ensuring that a patient is informed.

If the patient is determined to be incapacitated and lacking the decisional capacity to make a particular medical decision, a surrogate decision-maker must speak for the patient.

Different states have their own laws that define the hierarchy of appropriate surrogate decision-makers (e.g., the patient's spouse is typically the first person who assumes the surrogate role). In the event of a medical emergency, if no appropriate surrogate decision-maker can be contacted, the physician is expected to act in the best interest of the patient.

Telling the Truth and Withholding Information

Research indicates that the great majority of patients want their physicians to tell them the truth about their diagnosis, prognosis, and all therapeutic options. Any discussion of treatment planning and goals of care should always include a discussion with the patient about how much information he or she wishes to receive.

Only fully informed patients are able to act as autonomous agents in their decision-making and make value-based decisions about their goals of care. These discussions should, however, always be sensitive to the particular sociocultural and religious beliefs of the patient.

In situations where the physician is unfamiliar with the social or religious perspectives of a patient, it is advisable to obtain consultation from a professional (e.g., chaplain or religious adviser) who can provide insight and guidance on these issues.

It is difficult to justify the deception of a patient under any circumstance unless this is in the context of a larger social context and belief system (e.g., some communities consider it damaging to tell the person information about the negative side effects of an intervention).

Advance Directives and Living Wills

An *advance directive* (AD) is a document or recording in which a legally competent individual specifies his or her healthcare preferences in the event that he or she is unable to participate in medical decision-making. Advance directives full under two broad categories: *instructive* (e.g., living wills, DNR directive) and *proxy* (e.g., designation of a durable power of attorney for health care).

The principle of advance directives is recognized in all 50 states. If the AD is constructed in accordance with the requirements of that particular state, it is considered legally binding. Advance directives should only be invoked when the patient lacks decisional capacity.

Unfortunately, since the AD is frequently written in ambiguous terms, the healthcare team and family must frequently attempt to interpret the patient's stated preferences. In situations where the patient's family and decisional surrogates disagree with the patient's AD, the clinician should attempt whenever possible to assist the family in understanding the ethical and legal weight of the AD.

Only in situations where medical circumstances arise that were unpredictable to the patient (e.g., discovery of a new medical option) should the patient's surrogate be allowed to override the AD. In situations where the patient's family refuses to accept the patient's clearly stated AD, a hospital ethics committee should be requested.

Withholding and Withdrawing Life-Sustaining Treatments

A patient with decisional capacity has the legal and ethical right to accept and/or refuse any and all potentially life-sustaining treatments. Patients may have clearly communicated their preferences regarding withdrawing or forgoing treatment in their advance directive (e.g., living will, DNR).

Physicians are not required to, and should not, prolong a patient's stated wishes. It is important to recognize that the patient's decision to withdraw or forgo life-sustaining treatments does not release the physician of the obligation to offer the patient effective palliative interventions.

There is no ethical distinction between withholding and withdrawing an intervention. Withdrawing unwanted treatment is entirely consistent with the four ethical principles of beneficence, nonmaleficence, autonomy, and justice.

It is important to remember that medical treatments in themselves are ethically neutral, and their relative benefit can only be ascertained from the specific patient's particular diagnosis, prognosis, quality of life, goals of care, and beliefs and values.

In palliative care, issues relating to quality of life (rather than cure) are likely to frame the patient's decision. When the patient who has undergone treatment eventually dies from the underlying disease process, the physician is not morally responsible for that patient's death.

Concerns that an intervention will later be withdrawn should not preclude time-limited trials of a palliative treatment, for example, treating a patient's metabolic abnormality to determine if it will enhance the patient's cognitive status and enhance his or her quality of life.

Decisions about the withdrawal of treatment are often framed by the patient's religious or spiritual belief system. In this regard, it is important to recognize that certain religions indicate that life be prolonged no matter what the quality. It is therefore important that the clinician clarify the patient's belief system as part of any conversation around the withdrawal of medical interventions.

Discussions with patients or their decisional surrogate on withdrawing and withholding treatments should include a review of the following:
- The patient's medical status and prognosis
- A review of any previous advance directives
- The benefits and burdens of specific interventions
- The patient's beliefs and values and how they are impinged upon by the various treatment options
- The proposed treatment plan and clarification that ineffective and/or unwanted interventions can be withdrawn at any time.

It is crucial that all decisions regarding the withdrawal and withholding of treatment be clearly documented in the chart (including DNR forms) and that ALL members of the treatment team are clearly informed about the patient's preferences. Each facility or treatment team should establish effective and unambiguous methods for communicating such information (e.g., computer alerts, chart flags).

Clinical sites where the withdrawal of mechanical life support is implemented should establish effective and clearly defined guidelines for the procedures that minimize the patient's distress and are consistent with the doctrine of double effect (see discussion earlier in this chapter).

AAHPM Statement on Withdrawal and Withholding of Nonbeneficial Medical Interventions

AAHPM endorses the ethically and legally accepted view that withholding and withdrawing nonbeneficial medical interventions are morally indistinguishable, and are appropriate when consistent with the patient's goals of care.[1] Withdrawing or withholding nonbeneficial medical interventions is acceptable throughout the course of progressive, life-limiting illness, although patients with whom these discussions are held are often close to death.

When considering withholding or withdrawing a nonbeneficial medical intervention, clinicians should systematically

- Assess the decision-making capacity of the patient. For patients lacking capacity, review all appropriate advance care planning documents and discuss decisions about withholding and withdrawing interventions with the designated surrogate decision-maker, who should use substituted judgment. It is the responsibility of the physician and all members of the care team to keep the focus of decision-making on the patient's preferences and best interests, rather than on the surrogate's beliefs.
- Identify the overall goals of treatment and care for the patient, considering the current disease status and the social, familial, psychological, and spiritual dimensions of the patient's situation.
- Identify the intended goals of the intervention under consideration, including the potential burdens and benefits of that therapy.
- Assess the burdens and benefits of starting (or withholding) or continuing (or withdrawing) an intervention. The assessment should include objective medical data, and assessment of the likely outcome for the patient with the proposed intervention, as well as alternative interventions. When the outcome of a proposed intervention is uncertain, clinicians should consider a time-limited trial of the specific intervention.
- Make a recommendation concerning continuing/starting or withdrawing/withholding a nonbeneficial intervention that is based on the patient's values, goals, and expected likelihood of success.
- Explain what treatments will be continued and what additional treatments will be added if a specific medical intervention is to be withheld or withdrawn and emphasize the types of support that can be provided to either the patient or family. Engage an ethics committee or other institutional committee in cases of disagreement.

Withdrawing Artificial Nutrition and Hydration

Artificial nutrition-hydration (ANH) is an invasive medical procedure that requires the placement of a tube into the gastrointestinal tract (e.g., PEG tube, nasogastric tube), into the vascular system, or below the skin. ANH does not include simple noninvasive assisted nutrition such as assistance with oral feeding.

The withdrawal or withholding of ANH remains a contentious issue. Patients' families and clinicians frequently equate nutrition with nurturance and caring. With the exception of total parenteral nutrition in cancer patients, there is very little empirical evidence to support the efficacy of ANH in improving the quality or quantity of a patient's life.

The absence of any clear risk associated with ANH compounds the ambiguity around its utility. The issue is even more complex in patients experiencing a persistent vegetative state; ANH may prolong the survival of patients who are unable to communicate their quality of life and preferences.

In response to increasing public debate and controversy over the issue of ANH, in 2013 the American Academy of Hospice and Palliative Medicine updated its position statement.[2]

Background

Artificial nutrition and hydration were originally developed to provide short-term support for patients who were acutely ill. When used in patients near the end of life, the available data suggest that these measures are seldom effective in preventing suffering or prolonging life.

Patients with advanced, life-limiting illness often lose the capacity to eat and drink and/or the interest in food and fluids. Ethical issues may arise when patients, families, or caregivers request ANH even if there is no prospect of recovery from the underlying illness.

AAHPM Statement on Artificial Nutrition and Hydration Near the End of Life

> … AAHPM endorses the ethically and legally accepted view that ANH, whether delivered parenterally or through the gastrointestinal tract via a tube (including nasogastric tubes), is a medical intervention. Like other medical interventions, it should be evaluated by weighing its benefits and burdens in light of the patient's clinical circumstances and goals of care. ANH may offer benefits when administered in the setting of acute, reversible illness, or as a component of chronic disease management, when the patient can appreciate the benefits of the treatment and significant burdens are not disproportionate. Near the end of life, some widely assumed benefits of ANH, such as alleviation of thirst, may be achieved by less invasive measures including good mouth care or providing ice chips. The potential burdens of ANH depend on the route used and include sepsis (with

total parenteral nutrition) aspiration and diarrhea (with tube feeding), pressure sores and skin breakdown, and complications due to fluid overload. In addition, agitated or confused patients receiving ANH may need to be physically restrained to prevent them from removing a gastrostomy tube, nasogastric tube, or central intravenous line.[2]

AAHPM advocates respectful and informed discussions of the effects of ANH near the end of life among physicians, other health care professionals, patients, and families, preferably before the patient is close to death. It is incumbent on physicians, and other healthcare providers to describe the options that exist when considering the implementation, continuation, or discontinuation of ANH, and establish goals of care with the patient and/or surrogate decision maker. Before the patient or family specify their preferences, the physician or other palliative care provider should ensure that they have adequate information to make a decision. The patient and family should also understand that appropriate medical interventions would continue, even if ANH is not implemented. Ideally, the patient will make his or her own decision about the use of ANH based on a careful assessment of potential benefits and burdens, consistent with legal and ethical norms that permit patients to accept or forgo specific medical interventions. Such choices are best made in concert with family, and should routinely be communicated to the patient's health care proxy. For patients who are unable to make or communicate decisions, the evaluation of benefits and burdens should be carried out by the patient's designated surrogate or next of kin, using substituted judgment whenever possible, in accordance with local laws.

AAHPM recognizes that in some faith traditions ANH is considered basic sustenance, and for some patients and families, ANH is of symbolic importance, apart from any measurable benefits for the patient's physical well-being. Such views should be explored, understood, and respected, in keeping with patient and family values, beliefs, and culture. Good communication is necessary to allow caregivers to learn about patient and family fears about "starvation" and other frequently expressed concerns. At the same time, communication is essential to explain the patient's clinical condition and that the inability to eat and drink can be a natural part of dying that is generally not associated with suffering. Judicious hand feeding and, in some situations, particularly if there is uncertainty about whether a patient will benefit from ANH, a time-limited trial of ANH may be useful. When a time-limited trial of ANH is pursued, clear, measurable end points should be determined at the beginning of the trial. The caregiving team should explain that, as with other medical therapies, ANH can be withdrawn if it is not achieving its desired purpose.

Key Elements

- Recognize that ANH is a form of medical therapy that, like other medical interventions, should be evaluated by weighing its benefits and burdens in light of the patient's goals of care and clinical circumstances.
- Acknowledge that ANH, like other medical interventions, can ethically be withheld or withdrawn, consistent with the patient's wishes and the clinical situation.
- Establish open communication between patients/families and caregivers, to assure that their concerns are heard and that the natural history of advanced disease is clarified.
- Respect patient's preferences for treatment, once the prognosis and anticipated trajectory with and without ANH have been explained.

Sedation at the End of Life

Unfortunately, a significant percentage of patients experience severe or unbearable symptoms at the end of their lives. *Therapeutic sedation* (the term *terminal sedation* is discouraged) refers to the last-resort use of high-dose sedatives specifically to relieve the patient's extreme suffering.

Therapeutic sedation is limited to patients with a terminal prognosis (i.e., usually days to weeks) for whom other therapeutic interventions have proved ineffective in relieving their severe symptoms. Whenever the clinician is considering therapeutic sedation, it is important to include the family and surrogate decision-makers and to obtain a second opinion from another palliative medicine physician and relevant specialist.

It is also important to obtain the input from clinical staff involved in the immediate care of the patient and to obtain consent for their participation in this form of care.

In 2006, the American Academy of Hospice and Palliative Medicine published their statement on palliative sedation.[3]

Background

Palliative care seeks to relieve suffering associated with disease. Unfortunately, not all symptoms associated with advanced illness can be controlled with pharmacological or other interventions. Patients need and deserve assurance that suffering will be effectively addressed, as both the fear of severe suffering and the suffering itself add to the burden of terminal illness.

AAHPM Statement on Palliative Sedation

The AAHPM believes that distinctions must be made among the following uses of sedatives in medical practice.[3]

Healthcare providers serving patients near the end of life have a responsibility to offer sedatives in appropriate circumstances, usually targeted at specific symptoms ("ordinary sedation"). Palliative sedation (PS) is occasionally necessary to relieve otherwise intractable suffering, with the degree of sedation proportionate to the severity of the target symptom.

PS to unconsciousness should only be considered in the rare circumstance that thorough interdisciplinary assessment and treatment of a patient's suffering has not resulted in sufficient relief (or is associated with unacceptable side effects), and when sedation to unconsciousness is needed to meet the patient's goal of relief from suffering.

As with all treatment, the use of PS requires informed consent. Treatment of pain and other symptoms should be continued with PS, as sedation may decrease the patient's ability to communicate symptoms.

Ethical principles and legal rulings support the use of palliative sedation even to the level of unconsciousness to relieve otherwise refractory suffering. With regard to PS, the AAHPM position statement states that PS is ethically defensible when used:[3]

- After careful interdisciplinary evaluation and treatment of the patient.
- When palliative treatments that are not intended to affect consciousness have failed or, in the judgment of the clinician, are very likely to fail.
- Where its use is not expected to shorten the patient's time to death.

• Only for the actual or expected duration of symptoms.

In clinical practice, PS usually does not alter the timing or mechanism of a patient's death, as refractory symptoms are most often associated with very advanced terminal illness. The possibility that PS might hasten death as an unintended consequence should be assessed by the healthcare team in its consideration of PS, and then addressed directly in the process of obtaining informed consent.

Institutional bioethics committees may be consulted in cases where there is disagreement regarding the provision of PS.

Medical Futility

Although the term is frequently invoked in medical discussions about goals of care, there is currently no universally accepted definition of the term *medical futility*. The ethical authority to render a medical intervention as medically futile rests with the medical profession as a whole and not with individual patients and/or clinicians.

Any discussion around medical futility must therefore be cognizant of generally accepted standards of medical care. Although the ethical principle of autonomy states that a patient has the right to choose from the available medical interventions, it does not entitle the patient (or his or her surrogate) to receive medical interventions that are considered by acceptable standards of medical care to be futile. It is important to remember that medical futility is not equivalent to rationing.

When considering the definition of medical futility, two approaches are employed:

- *Quantitative futility* applies to an intervention that has a very low likelihood of being effective (usually defined as less than 1%).
- *Qualitative futility* is where the intervention will not result in any improvement in the quality of a patient's life (e.g., improving the patient's physiological parameters without addressing the larger aspects of the patient's suffering).

When a patient and/or family members request a medical intervention that the physician considers to be futile, that physician should make every attempt to clearly communicate the treatment options available and their utility.

Language such as "giving up" and "a waste of time" should be avoided, and attempts to define the goals of care in terms of quality rather than quantity should be stressed. In situations where agreement cannot be reached, the physician should obtain a second opinion from an appropriate medical specialist and request a consultation from the ethics committee.

Physician-Assisted Suicide

The issue of physician-assisted suicide is controversial and complex, with opponents and proponents for the concept both presenting valid justifications for their position.

A meaningful review of these issues is beyond the scope of this brief text; however, the recent position statement by the American Academy of Hospice and Palliative Medicine includes the key principles.[4]

Background

Suffering near the end of life arises from many sources, including relentless pain, depression, loss of sense of self, loss of control and dignity, fear of the future, and/or fear of being a burden on others. A primary goal of the American Academy of Hospice and Palliative Medicine is to promote the development, use, and availability of palliative care to relieve patient suffering and to enhance quality of life while upholding respect for patients' and families' values and goals.

Excellent medical care, including state-of-the-art palliative care, can control most symptoms and augment patients' psychosocial and spiritual resources to relieve most suffering near the end of life. On occasion, however, severe suffering persists; in such a circumstance, a patient may ask his physician for assistance in ending his life by providing physician-assisted death (PAD).

PAD is defined as a physician providing, at the patient's request, a lethal medication that the patient can take by his or her own hand to end otherwise intolerable suffering. The term *PAD* is used in this document with the belief that it captures the essence of the process in a more accurately descriptive fashion than the more emotionally charged designation *physician-assisted suicide*.

Subject to safeguards, PAD has been legal and carefully studied in Oregon since 1997. Washington, Vermont and California have also very recently recently passed legislation legalizing PAD.

Situations in which PAD is requested are particularly challenging for physicians and other healthcare practitioners because they raise significant clinical, ethical, and legal issues.

AAHPM Statement on Physician-Assisted Death

> ... When a request for assistance in hastening death is made by a patient, the AAHPM strongly recommends that medical practitioners carefully scrutinize the sources of fear and suffering leading to the request with the goal of addressing these sources without hastening death.
>
> A systematic approach is essential.
>
> Evaluation of requests includes the following elements.

Determine the Nature of the Request

> Is the patient seeking assistance right now? Is he or she seriously exploring the clinician's openness to the possibility of a hastened death in the future? Is he or she simply airing vague thoughts about ending life?

Clarify the Cause(s) of Intractable Suffering

Is there severe pain or another unrelieved physical symptom? Is the distress mainly emotional or spiritual? Does the patient feel he or she is a burden? Has the patient grown tired of a prolonged dying?

Evaluate the Patient's Decision-Making Capacity

Does the patient have cognitive impairment that would affect their judgment? Does the patient's request seem rational and proportionate to the clinical situation? Is their request consistent with the patient's past values?

Explore Emotional Factors

Do feelings of depression, worthlessness, excessive guilt, or fear substantially interfere with the patient's judgment?

Initial responses to requests for hastened death include the following:

- Respond empathically to the patient's emotions.
- Intensify treatment of pain and other physical symptoms.
- Identify and treat depression, anxiety, and/or spiritual suffering when present.
- Consult with specialists in palliative care and/or hospice.
- Consult with experts in spiritual or psychological suffering, or other specialty areas depending on the patient's circumstances.
- Use a caring and understanding approach to encourage dialogue and trust and to ensure the best chance of relieving distress.
- Commit to the patient to work toward a mutually acceptable solution for his suffering.

When unacceptable suffering persists, despite thorough evaluation, exploration, and provision of standard palliative care interventions as outlined above, a search for common ground is essential. In these situations, the benefits and burdens of the following alternatives should be considered:

- Discontinuation of potentially life-prolonging treatments, including corticosteroids, insulin, dialysis, oxygen, or artificial hydration or nutrition
- Voluntary cessation of eating and drinking as an acceptable strategy for the patient, family, and treating practitioners
- Palliative sedation, even potentially to unconsciousness, if suffering is intractable and of sufficient severity (AAHPM Statement on Palliative Sedation)

Despite all potential alternatives, some patients may persist in their request specifically for PAD. The AAHPM recognizes that deep disagreement persists regarding the morality of PAD.

Sincere, compassionate, morally conscientious individuals stand on either side of this debate. The AAHPM takes a position of "studied neutrality" on the subject of whether PAD should be legally regulated or prohibited, believing its members should instead continue to strive to find the proper response to those patients whose suffering becomes intolerable despite the best possible palliative care. Whether or not legalization occurs, AAHPM supports intense efforts to alleviate suffering and to reduce any perceived need for PAD.

For physicians practicing in regions where PAD is legal, the AAHPM advises great caution before instituting PAD, including assurance that

- The patient has received the best possible palliative care. The permissibility of PAD is dependent upon access to excellent palliative care. No patient should be indirectly coerced to hasten their death because he or she lacks the best possible medical and palliative care.
- Requests for PAD emanate from a patient with full decision-making capacity.
- All reasonable alternatives to PAD have been considered and implemented if acceptable to the patient
- The request is voluntary. Safeguards should focus in particular on protection of vulnerable groups, including the elderly, frail, poor, or physically and/or mentally handicapped. Coercive influences from family or financial pressure from payers cannot be allowed to play any role.
- The practitioner is willing to participate in PAD, never being pressured to act against his or her own conscience if asked to assist a patient in dying.

Whenever PAD is being considered by a patient with his or her physician, patients should continue to receive the best possible palliative care. Although many hospice and palliative care practitioners find it morally unacceptable to participate in PAD even where legal, neither a person requesting PAD nor the family should be deprived of any other measure of ongoing palliative care during the dying process and period of bereavement.

The most essential response to the request for PAD in the practice of palliative care is to attempt to clearly understand the request, to intensify palliative care treatments with the intent to relieve suffering, and to search with the patient for mutually acceptable approaches without violating any party's fundamental values.

Ethics Committees and Ethics Consultations

Most hospitals in the United States have an ethics committee that should provide an invaluable resource to clinicians who are dealing with challenging ethical situations. The ethics committee should include a diverse group of healthcare professionals and community representatives whose goal is to support patients and staff in understanding and applying ethical principles to health care.

The ethics committee performs clinical consultations at the request of clinicians and/or patients. These consultations may be performed by one individual (typically an ethics consultant with professional credentials in clinical ethics) or a team consisting of members of the committee.

Ethics consultations should be considered when there is a perceived ethical problem in the care of a patient that cannot be resolved by the parties concerned. Most so-called ethical problems are usually a breakdown in communication and/or can be resolved through facilitated meetings involving the consultation team.

Clinicians and patients should be encouraged to request ethics consultations without any fear of negative repercussions.

Clinical Pearls

- The four principles of bioethics are autonomy, nonmaleficence, beneficence, and justice.
- Withdrawing unwanted treatment is consistent with the principles of bioethics.
- Every time we enter into a treatment contract with a patient, we are making a de facto determination of his or her decisional capacity.
- The physician's intent is the key to the doctrine of double effect.
- Most "ethical problems" can be resolved through better communication among the parties involved.

References

1. AAHPM. (2011). Statement on Withdrawing and Witholding Non Beneficial Medical Interventions. November 2011.
2. AAHPM. (2013). Statement on Artificial Nutrition and Hydration Near the End of Life. September 2013.
3. AAHPM. (2014). Statement on Palliative Sedation. Approved by the Board of Directors, December 5, 2014.
4. AAHPM. (2007). Statement on Physician-Assisted Death. Approved by the Board of Directors, February 14, 2007.

Further Reading

Beauchamp TL, Childress JF (1979). *Principles of Biomedical Ethics*. New York: Oxford University Press.

Bruera E, Hui D, Dalal S, et al. (2013). Parenteral hydration in patients with advanced cancer: a multicenter, double-blind, placebo-controlled randomized trial. *J Clin Oncol* 31:111–8.

Claessens P, Menten J, Schotsmans P, Broeckaert B (2008). Palliative sedation: a review of the research literature. *J Pain Symptom Manage* 36(3):310–33.

Gavrin JR (2007). Ethical considerations at the end of life in the intensive care unit. *Crit Care Med* 35(2 Suppl):S85–94.

Hasselaar JG, Verhagen SC, Vissers KC (2009). When cancer symptoms cannot be controlled: the role of palliative sedation. *Curr Opin Support Palliat Care* 3(1):14–23.

Kon AA, Ablin AR. (2010). Palliative treatment: redefining interventions to treat suffering near the end of life. *J Palliat Med* 13:643–6.

Lemiengre J, de Casterlé BD, Van Craen K, Schotsmans P, Gastmans C (2007). Institutional ethics policies on medical end-of-life decisions: a literature review. *Health Policy* 83(2–3):131–43.

National Ethics Committee, Veterans Health Administration (2006–2007). The ethics of palliative sedation as a therapy of last resort. *Am J Hosp Palliat Care* 23(6):483–91.

Szalados JE (2007). Discontinuation of mechanical ventilation at end-of-life: the ethical and legal boundaries of physician conduct in termination of life support. *Crit Care Clin* 23(2):317–37.

Tillyard AR (2007). Ethics review: "living wills" and intensive care—an overview of the American experience. *Crit Care* 11(4):219.

Prognostication in Palliative Care

David Hui

Introduction

Prognostication, an underused clinical skill, is an essential component of patient management, along with diagnosis and therapeutics. Patients' predicted survival has a significant impact on many medical decisions, including the initiation of specific medications, avoidance of aggressive therapies, and palliative care and hospice referral. As patients progress over the course of their disease, knowing what to expect can provide them with a sense of control and can facilitate the process of advance care planning.

Prognostication consists of two parts: foreseeing (estimating prognosis) and foretelling (discussing prognosis). *Foreseeing* requires knowledge of the natural history of disease (Figure 25.1), an understanding of how treatment could modify survival, and an appreciation of individual patient-related factors such as comorbidities. *Foretelling* entails the delivery of prognostic information in a clear, sensitive, and compassionate manner and represents a longitudinal process of communication rather than a single discussion.

In this chapter, we discuss the science and art of prognostication, specifically related to patients with advanced cancer, congestive heart failure (CHF), chronic obstructive pulmonary disease (COPD), and dementia.

Clinical Pearl

- Clinicians generally tend to overestimate prognosis. Use of prognostic tools such as the Palliative Prognostic Score for cancer patients can help improve accuracy (Figure 25.1).

Figure 25.1. Trajectories of advanced disease. (A) The trajectory for cancer patients tends to be predictable, with a rapid decline in function close to the end of life. (B) This is in contrast to COPD and CHF, with multiple acute exacerbations and a higher chance of sudden death. (C) Patients with dementia generally experience a slow and steady decline over time.

Prognostication in General Palliative Care and Advanced-Cancer Patients

Much of the literature regarding prognostication is derived from patients with advanced cancer.[1] However, many of the key principles of survival predictions can be applied to other palliative care populations.

Clinician predicted survival (CPS) is formulated solely on the basis of the clinician's knowledge and experience. While this intuitive estimation correlates with survival to a certain extent, clinicians tend to be overly optimistic in their estimations and even more generous when communicating prognosis.

Clinicians who are more experienced and who have not yet established a strong relationship with the patient are more likely to be accurate with their predictions.

Prognostic Factors

A number of signs and symptoms have been found to confer a poor prognosis in advanced-cancer patients:

- Performance status—ECOG performance status, Karnofsky Performance Status (KPS), Palliative Performance Scale (PPS) (Table 25.1)
- Delirium
- Dyspnea
- Cachexia–anorexia–dysphagia.

The following laboratory variables are also associated with a shorter survival:

- Leukocytosis
- Lymphocytopenia
- Hypoalbuminemia
- Elevated lactate dehydrogenase (LDH)
- Elevated C-reactive protein (CRP).

Prognostic Models

A number of prognostic models are available for predicting survival in general palliative care and advanced-cancer patients, with the Palliative Prognostic Score (PaP Score)[2] being the most validated (Table 25.2).

A web-based prognostic model is also available at http://web.his. uvic.ca/research/NET/tools/PrognosticTools/. It provides an estimated survival based on patient's age, gender, cancer diagnosis, and Palliative Performance Scale.

Table 25.1 Palliative Performance Scale (PPS)

PPS Level	Ambulation	Activity and Evidence of Disease	Self-Care	Intake	Conscious Level
100%	Full	Normal activity and work; no evidence of disease	Full	Normal	Full
90%	Full	Normal activity and work; some evidence of disease	Full	Normal	Full
80%	Full	Normal activity with effort; some evidence of disease	Full	Normal or reduced	Full
70%	Reduced	Unable to do normal job/work; significant disease	Full	Normal or reduced	Full
60%	Reduced	Unable to do hobby/housework; significant disease	Occasional assistance necessary	Normal or reduced	Full or confusion
50%	Mainly sit/lie	Unable to do any work; extensive disease	Considerable assistance required	Normal or reduced	Full or confusion
40%	Mainly in bed	Unable to do most activity; extensive disease	Mainly assistance	Normal or reduced	Full or drowsy ± confusion
30%	Totally bed bound	Unable to do any activity; extensive disease	Total care	Normal or reduced	Full or drowsy ± confusion
20%	Totally bed bound	Unable to do any activity; extensive disease	Total care	Minimal to sips	Full or drowsy ± confusion
10%	Totally bed bound	Unable to do any activity; extensive disease	Total care	Mouth care only	Drowsy or coma ± confusion
0%	Death	–	–	–	–

Median survival periods for PPS of 60%–70%, 30%–50%, and 10%–20% are 108 days, 41 days, and 6 days, respectively.
Reprinted with permission © Victoria Hospice Society, BC, Canada (2001) www.victoriahospice.org.

Table 25.2 Palliative Prognostic Score (PaP)

Scoring	
Clinician prediction of survival (weeks)	
> 12	0
11–12	2
7–10	2.5
5–6	4.5
3–4	6
1–2	8.5
Dyspnea	1
Anorexia	1.5
Karnofsky performance status 10–40	2.5
Total WBC count	
8501–11000 cells/mm^3	0.5
> 11000 cells/mm^3	1.5
Lymphocyte percentage	
12%–19.9%	1
0%–11.9%	2.5

Interpretation of PaP Score*

Total Score	Advanced-Cancer Patients (Out/Inpatients)	Advanced-Cancer Patients (Inpatients Only)	Cancer and Noncancer Patients (Consult Service)
0–5.5	87% 76 days	97% 17 weeks	66% 60 days
5.6–11	52% 32 days	59% 7 weeks	55% 34 days
11.1–17.5	17% 14 days	25% ≤ 1 week	5% 8 days

* The percentage on the top row represents 30-day survival, while the number below it represents median survival.

Prognostication in Patients with Heart Failure

Predicting survival in patients with CHF is more challenging than for cancer patients because of the relatively unpredictable disease trajectory, with a 25%–50% chance of sudden death.[3]

Prognostic Factors

Functional capacity indicated by New York Heart Association (NYHA) Class is the most important indicator of prognosis:

- Class II (dyspnea with normal activity): 1-year survival: 90%–95%
- Class III (dyspnea with mild activity): 1-year survival: 85%–90%
- Class IV (dyspnea at rest): 1-year survival: 30%–40%.

Other clinical prognostic factors include the following:

- Decreased left ventricular ejection fraction
- Ventricular arrhythmia
- Hospitalization for cardiac reasons
- Cachexia
- Comorbidities such as diabetes, COPD, cirrhosis, cerebrovascular disease, cancer, and HIV.

Laboratory variables associated with poor prognosis are as follows:

- Anemia
- Hyponatremia
- High creatinine (> 1.4 mg/dL) or urea (above upper normal limit).

Prognostic Models

For hospitalized patients with acutely decompensated heart failure, a three-risk factor model based on admission characteristics provides the probability of in-hospital mortality (Table 25.3).

For longer-term prognostication, the Seattle Heart Failure Model (http://www.SeattleHeartFailureModel.org) includes 24 variables related to demographics, medications, laboratory data, and devices and provides an estimate of 1-, 2-, and 3-year survival with or without interventions.

Table 25.3 Prognostic Model for Inpatient Mortality in Heart Failure

Urea (+43 mg/dL)	Systolic Blood Pressure (< 115 mmHg)	Creatinine (+2.75 mg/dL)	In-Hospital Mortality Predictions
(−)	(−)		2.1%
(−)	(+)		5.5%
(+)	(−)		6.4%
(+)	(+)	(−)	12.4%
(+)	(+)	(+)	21.9%

Prognostication in Patients with COPD

The disease course of COPD is similar to that for CHF, with a gradual deterioration of organ function and increasing frequency of exacerbations over time.[4]

Clinical Prognostic Factors

Forced expiratory volume in 1 second (FEV_1) is the most important indicator of prognosis. Specifically, $FEV_1 < 35\%$ is associated with a 2-year survival of 75% and 4-year survival of 45%. Other factors associated with decreased survival include old age, weight loss, and poor functional status.

Clinical prognostic factors for in-hospital mortality are as follows:

- $PaCO_2$ level > 50 mmH 2 O
- Prolonged (> 72 hours) or recurrent mechanical ventilation
- Comorbidities
- Hypoalbuminemia
- Anemia.

Prognostic Models

The BODE Index is a prognostic model developed and validated for COPD patients (Table 25.4).

For critically ill COPD patients requiring admission to the intensive care unit, the APACHE IV score is a reliable tool for prediction of in-hospital mortality (www.icumedicus.com/icu_scores/apacheIV.php).

Table 25.4 BODE Index

Scoring			
Body mass index (BMI)			
0 = > 21	0		
1 = ≤ 21	1		
Obstruction (post-bronchodilator FEV$_1$)			
≥ 65% predicted	0		
50%–64%	1		
36%–49%	2		
≤ 35%	3		
Distance walked in 6 minutes			
≥ 350 m	0		
250–349 m	1		
150–249 m	2		
≤ 149 m	3		
Exercise MMRC dyspnea			
1	0		
2	1		
3	2		
4	3		

Interpretation of BODE Score*

Total Score	1-Year Mortality	2-Year Mortality	52-Mo. Mortality
0–2	2%	6%	19%
3–4	2%	8%	32%
5–6	2%	14%	40%
7–10	5%	31%	80%

* Hazard ratio for death from any cause per one-point increase in BODE score is 1.34.

Prognostication in Patients with Dementia

Dementia is a neurocognitive syndrome with persistent intellectual and functional decline.[5] The different stages of dementia are shown in Table 25.5.

Prognostic Factors

A number of signs and symptoms are associated with poor prognosis in patients with dementia[6]:

- Older age
- Male sex
- CNS: altered level of consciousness
- Respiratory: dyspnea, supplemental oxygen
- GI: dysphagia, aspiration, anorexia, weight loss, bowel incontinence
- Comorbidities: diabetes, CHF, COPD, cancer
- Recent hospitalization.

Prognostic Models

The Mortality Risk Index (MRI) is a 12-factor prognostic model developed in nursing home residents with advanced dementia and has been validated for this purpose (Table 25.6).

Table 25.5 Functional Assessment Staging

Stages	Functional level
1	No difficulty either subjectively or objectively
2	Complains of forgetting location of objects. Subjective work difficulties
3*	Decreased job functioning evident to coworkers. Difficulty in traveling to new locations. Decreased organizational capacity
4*	Decreased ability to perform complex tasks, e.g., planning dinner for guests, handling personal finances (such as forgetting to pay bills), difficulty marketing, etc.
5*	Requires assistance in choosing proper clothing to wear for the day, season, or occasion, e.g., patient may wear the same clothing repeatedly unless supervised
6*	(A) Improperly putting on clothes without assistance or cueing (e.g., may put street clothes on over night clothes, or put shoes on wrong feet, or have difficulty buttoning clothing) occasionally or more frequently over the past weeks (B) Unable to bathe properly (e.g., difficulty adjusting the bath-water temperature) occasionally or more frequently in the past weeks (C) Inability to handle mechanics of toileting (e.g., forgets to flush the toilet, does not wipe properly or properly dispose of toilet tissue) occasionally or more frequently over the past weeks (D) Urinary incontinence (occasionally or more frequently over the past weeks) (E) Fecal incontinence (occasionally or more frequently over the past weeks)
7	(A) Ability to speak limited to approximately a half a dozen intelligible words or fewer, in the course of an average day or in the course of an intensive interview (B) Speech ability is limited to the use of a single intelligible word in an average day or in the course of an intensive interview (the person may repeat the word over and over) (C) Ambulatory ability is lost (cannot walk without personal assistance) (D) Cannot sit up without assistance (e.g., the individual will fall over if there are not lateral rests [arms] on the chair) (E) Loss of ability to smile (F) Loss of ability to hold head up independently

*Scored primarily on the basis of information obtained from knowledgeable informant.
Reisberg B (1998). Functional assessment staging (FAST). *Psychopharmacol Bull* 24(4):653–9.

Table 25.6 Mortality Risk Index (MRI)

Score Sheet to Estimate 6-Month Prognosis in Nursing Home Residents with Advanced Dementia

Risk Factor from Minimum Date Set	Points	Score
Activites of Daily Living Scale = 28*	1.9	—
Male Sex	1.9	—
Cancer	1.7	—
Congestive Heart Failure	1.6	—
Oxygen Therapy Needed in Prior 14 Days	1.6	—
Shortness of Breath	1.5	—
< 25% of Food Eaten at Most Meals	1.5	—
Unstable Medical Condition	1.5	—
Bowel Incontinence	1.5	—
Bedfast	1.5	—
Age > 83 y	1.4	—
Not Awake Most of the Day	1.4	—

Total Risk Score, Rounded to Nearest Integer
Possible Range, 0–19

* The Activities of Daily Living Scale is obtained by summing the resident's self-performance ratings on the Minimum Date Set for the following 7 functional activities: bed mobility, dressing, toileting, transfer, eating, grooming, and locomotion. In the Minimum Date Set, functional ability is rated on 5-point scale for each activity (0, independent; 1, supervision; 2, limited assistance; 3, extensive assistance; and 4, total dependence). A total score of 28 represents complete functional dependence.

If Total Risk Score is ...	Risk Estimate of Death Within 6 Months, %
0	8.9
1 or 2	10.8
1 or 2	23.2
3, 4, or 5	40.4
6, 7, or 8	57.0
9, 10, or 11	70.0
≥ 12	

Table 25.7 General Strategies for Discussing Prognosis

Key Element	Comments
Context	Ensure a quiet, comfortable, and safe environment. Sit down and speak to the patient at eye level. Ask the patient if he or she wants to be accompanied by family or friends during the discussion.
How much does the patient know?	Explore the patient's understanding of his or her illness and expectations.
How would learning about prognosis help the patient?	A clear understanding of the patient's reasons to explore prognosis can help clinicians to shape their discussion to address the patient's goals and to provide a personalized management plan.
Deliver information	Emphasize the uncertainties in prognostication. Discuss prognosis in terms of days, weeks, and months, rather than providing specific numbers or median survivals. Information should be related such that it is measured to the perceptions of the patient's intellectual comprehension and emotional resilience.
Empathic response	Simple remarks such as "This is a difficult time for you" can be helpful. Be prepared to acknowledge and grieve losses.
Empowering	Take this opportunity to help patients define achievable goals and remain hopeful. Initiate discussions about important advance care planning issues such as philosophy of care, living will, and code status.
Provide follow-up and support resources	Reassure patients regarding non-abandonment and symptom control. Introduce other members of the interprofessional team, such as the chaplain and social worker, who will be able to provide further counseling.

Back AL, Anderson WG, Bunch L, Marr LA, Wallace JA, Yang HB, Arnold RM (2008). Communication about cancer near the end of life. *Cancer* 113(7 Suppl):1897–910.

Communicating Prognosis

Even with the most sophisticated prognostic model, it is important to recognize that there will always be uncertainty in survival predictions given the inherent nature of death, mediated by acute complications such as infections and thromboembolism. Thus, it is imperative for clinicians to not only polish the science of prognostication but also further the art of communication, gently guiding patients and families through times of uncertainty.

Instead of avoiding bad news, most patients prefer to receive honest, realistic, and accurate information regarding their prognosis. At the same time, they want to have control over what, when, and how much information is given.

Physicians tend to underestimate patients' need for information yet at the same time overestimate patients' appreciation of their prognosis.[7] Thus, it is important for clinicians to find out about patients' preferences in communication prior to prognostic disclosure, to frequently assess patients' understanding, and to provide ample opportunities for questions.

With disease progression, patients tend to want more discussions around their psychosocial needs rather than biomedical issues. In fact, patients generally want less information as they get closer to the end of life, whereas caregivers tend to need more. Thus, separate discussions with patients and caregivers may be useful for some situations.

Discussing prognosis can be a challenging task, trying to strike a balance between honesty, hope, and empathy. Rather than destroying hope, prognostic information should be framed in such a way to sustain existing goals and/or to create new ones.

While each patient–physician interaction should be individualized, Table 25.7 lists a number of communication strategies that may be helpful for clinicians when sharing prognosis.

Clinical Pearl

- Patients generally want to know how long they have to live. The art of prognostication is in delivering the appropriate amount of information at the right time, in the proper setting, and in a manner tailored to the patient's level of comprehension and emotional state.

References

1. Glare PA, Sinclair CT (2008). Palliative medicine review: prognostication. *J Palliat Med* 11(1):84–103.
2. Maltoni M, Nanni O, Pirovano M, Scarpi E, Indelli M, Martini C, Monti M, Arnoldi E, Piva L, Ravaioli A, Cruciani G, Labianca R, Amadori D (1999). Successful validation of the palliative prognostic score in terminally ill cancer patients. Italian Multicenter Study Group on Palliative Care. *J Pain Symptom Manage* 17(4):240–7.
3. Reisfield GM, Wilson GR (2007). Prognostication in heart failure. *J Palliat Med* 10(1):245–6.
4. Childers JW, Arnold RM, Curtis JR (2007). Prognosis in end-stage chronic obstructive pulmonary disease. *J Palliat Med* 10(3):806–7.
5. Tsai S, Arnold RM (2007). Prognostication in dementia. *J Palliat Med* 10(3):807–8.
6. Reisberg B (1998). Functional assessment staging (FAST). *Psychopharmacol Bull* 24(4):653–9.
7. Parker SM, Clayton JM, Hancock K, Walder S, Butow PN, Carrick S, Currow D, Ghersi D, Glare P, Hagerty R, Tattersall MH (2007). A systematic review of prognostic/end-of-life communication with adults in the advanced stages of a life-limiting illness: patient/caregiver preferences for the content, style, and timing of information. *J Pain Symptom Manage* 34(1):81–93.
8. Back AL, Anderson WG, Bunch L, Marr LA, Wallace JA, Yang HB, Arnold RM (2008). Communication about cancer near the end of life. *Cancer* 113(7 Suppl):1897–1910.

Frequent Pharmacological Interactions in Palliative Care

**Mary Lynn McPherson
and Kashelle Lockman**

Medications are indispensable in managing symptoms associated with advanced illness. According to the Kaiser Foundation, the average US resident acquired 12.1 prescription medications for acute or chronic conditions in 2011.[1] The risk for experiencing an adverse drug-related outcome is increased by patient fragility, comorbid conditions, and increased age. These patients also take more medications. On average, US residents 65 years or older were prescribed 28 medications per person in 2011.[1] Patients entering hospice also have a high medication burden, with one report showing an average of 18 medication orders at admission.[2] Palliative care practitioners frequently add medications to the patient's regimen to control symptoms as a disease progresses, but we should also take away medications as a patient declines and therapeutic goals change. It is imperative that palliative care practitioners understand the clinical effects of both adding and taking away medications from a patient's medication regimen.

A drug interaction is defined as "a measurable modification (in magnitude or duration) of the action of one drug by prior or concomitant administration of another substance (including prescription and nonprescription drugs, food, or alcohol)."[3] This includes drug–drug (prescription or nonprescription), drug–food, drug–herbal, drug–lab, drug–disease, and drug–chemical interactions. In this chapter we will focus on interactions between drugs (known as drug–drug interactions). Drug–drug interactions primarily fall into two categories: pharmacodynamic and pharmacokinetic.

Pharmacodynamic Drug Interactions

Pharmacodynamics describes the study of the action and effects of medications on physiologic function. Therefore, drug interactions that are said to be pharmacodynamic in nature result in either an additive, synergistic, or antagonistic pharmacologic effect. Pharmacodynamic drug interactions can affect either the intended pharmacologic effect of a medication, or the adverse effect. An example of an antagonistic pharmacodynamic drug interaction would be using dexamethasone and glyburide in the same drug regimen. Dexamethasone increases blood glucose, while glyburide is used to decrease blood glucose. Frequently we use this type of "interaction" to our advantage; one example is using a stimulant laxative to increase peristalsis to combat opioid-induced slowed peristalsis.

Additive pharmacodynamic drug interactions can also have a beneficial effect, such as using a combination of medications with different mechanisms of action to achieve better blood-pressure lowering effects, or to achieve better analgesia. Conversely, there are several examples of common adverse additive or synergistic pharmacodynamic drug interactions seen in palliative care practice. Some examples include the following:

- Central nervous system (CNS) depression: patients receiving one or more CNS depressant medication(s) may experience sedation, agitation, and/or confusion, and may progress to respiratory depression. Examples include opioids, benzodiazepines, nonbenzodiazepine sedative-hypnotic agents, barbiturates, alcohol, antipsychotic agents, antidepressants, antihistamines (especially the first-generation agents such as diphenhydramine), antiemetics, anticonvulsants, and illicit drugs. Less obvious CNS depressants include medications such as cimetidine, anticholinergic agents, and drugs that reduce glomerular filtration, such as nonsteroidal anti-inflammatory drugs and angiotension converting-enzyme inhibitors).

- Anticholinergic (or, more correctly, antimuscarinic) adverse effects commonly include constipation, urinary retention, blurred vision, dry mouth, and cognitive impairment. Medications that may cause anticholinergic effects include tricyclic antidepressants, antipsychotics, antihistamines, paroxetine, atropine, scopolamine, and hyoscyamine, among others. The Anticholinergic Risk Scale can be used to calculate anticholinergic burden for patients on multiple medications with anticholinergic side effects.[4] Elderly patients are particulary adversely affected by this drug–drug interaction.

- Constipation may be related to anticholinergic drug use as well as a variety of other medications such as opioids, iron and calcium supplements, and many medications for chronic disease states (e.g., antihypertensives and diuretics).

- QTc prolongation: palliative care practitioners think of methadone as one medication associated with long QT syndrome and the associated life-threatening arrhythmia, torsades de pointes. This is just one medication that may cause this effect. Common examples include anti-arrhythmic agents (such as quinidine, procainamide, dofetilide, sotalol, and amiodarone), antihistamines, antibiotics, anti-emetics, gastrointestinal prokinetic agents, antidepressants, and antipsychotic agents. For a more complete listing of medications that can prolong the QTc, refer to the website www.crediblemeds.org. In this database, medications are identified as having known risk versus possible or conditional risk.[5]

- Serotonin syndrome is a potentially life-threatening condition caused by excess serotonergic stimulation of the central nervous system. Clinical findings range from mild symptoms to life-threatening toxicity and include akathisia, tremor, altered mental status, clonus, muscular hypertonicity, and hyperthermia. Drugs known to cause serotonin syndrome include antidepressants, valproic acid, analgesics (meperidine, fentanyl, tramadol, pentazocine, methadone), anti-emetics (ondansetron, granisetron, metoclopramide), sumatriptan, zolmitriptan sibutramine, linezolid, ritonavir, dextromethorphan, some drugs of abuse, some dietary supplements (e.g., tryptophan, St. John's wort, ginseng), and lithium.[6]

- Some medications can lower the seizure threshold, including meperidine, tramadol, phenothiazines (such as chlorpromazine and haloperidol), tricyclic antidepressants, venlafaxine, propofol, and bupropion. Abrupt discontinuation of antiepileptic agents and benzodiazepines can also increase the risk for seizures.

Pharmacokinetic Drug Interactions

Pharmacokinetics describes the process of what the body does to a drug after administration: absorption, distribution, metabolism, and excretion. While there is little consistent information available regarding pharmacokinetic changes associated with terminal illness, some predictable changes have been shown with aging. Examples of these changes and their impact on drug therapy are as follows:[7]

- Absorption
  - Decrease gastrointestinal acidity (decreased absorption of some drugs)
  - Decreased surface area of small bowel (may reduce absorption of some sustained-release drug products)
- Distribution
  - Increase in adipose tissue (may increase half-life of lipid-soluble drugs)
  - Decrease in lean body mass (may increase serum concentration of water-soluble drugs)
  - Reduced serum albumin (increased free fraction of highly albumin-bound drugs)
- Metabolism
  - Reduced phase I metabolism (prolonged half-life of drugs metabolized by this route)
  - Phase II metabolism largely unchanged
- Elimination
  - Reduced glomerular filtration ratio (prolonged half-life of drugs that are renally excreted)
  - Reduced renal plasma flow.

In addition to age-related changes affecting the pharmacokinetics of drug therapy, pharmacogenetic variability may influence drug metabolism, and drug interactions may affect all four phases of pharmacokinetics (absorption, distribution, metabolism, and excretion). A discussion and example of the impact on each phase follows, with an emphasis on the role of drug-metabolizing enzymes in the liver and other organ sites.

Absorption

After administration, most medications must be absorbed into the systemic circulation to be effective (obviously some medications are intended for a local or topical effect at the site of application). Drugs given by the intravenous route of administration are not subject to most variables that may adversely affect absorption because the drug is placed into the systemic circulation. Similarly, medications given by the intramuscular and subcutaneous routes generally have a high degree of absorption. Oral medication administration is subject to variability in gastric emptying, absorption via passive diffusion or an uptake transporter, and presystemic elimination, including transporter-mediated efflux.[8] Examples of drug interactions subject to these variables are as follows:

- Antacids, anticholinergic drugs, and opioids may slow gastric emptying; this may slow the onset of action of co-administered medications.
- Some medications may be inactivated in the acidic environment of the stomach, such as penicillin G and levodopa. Delayed gastric emptying may decrease bioavailability of these agents.
- Metoclopramide enhances gastric emptying and may cause earlier and higher peak concentration of some drugs.
- Some medications require an acidic environment for absorption (such as griseofulvin, itraconazole, ketoconazole, posaconazole, gabapentin, erlotinib, dasatinib, nilotinib, and bosutinib); enhanced gastric emptying may reduce absorption of these medications. Acid suppression by proton pump inhibitors, histamine-2-receptor antagonists, or antacids may also reduce the absorption of these medications.
- Sucralfate, aluminum- and magnesium-containing antacids, calcium, iron, or zinc may reduce the absorption of quinolone antibiotics (e.g., levofloxacin and ciprofloxacin), tetracycline, minocycline, azithromycin, and dolutegravir.
- Cyclosporine, ritonavir, clarithromycin, and verapamil are inhbitors of the efflux transporter P-glycoprotein (P-gp). They may increase the absorption and bioavailability of atorvastatin, dabigatran, digoxin, apixaban, and rivaroxaban, which are P-gp substrates.[8,9]

Distribution

Medications such as phenytoin, diazepam, warfarin, and others are highly bound to serum protein such as albumin or alpha-1-acid glycoprotein (AAG). When combined, some drugs can "bump" other drugs off proteins in the plasma, increasing the free fraction of drug (which is the portion of the drug that causes the pharmacologic and potentially toxic effect). These drug interactions are rarely clinically significant because this effect is transient and results in a compensatory increase in drug elimination.

Metabolism

Variables that can affect the metabolism of medications include rates of metabolism, diet, age, race, genetics, disease states, and drug dosage. Most pharmacokinetic drug interactions are due to altered drug metabolism via the cytochrome P450 (CYP450) enzyme system. Drug metabolism occurs primarily in the liver, but also in the intestinal mucosa and other parts of the body. Generally speaking, drug metabolism converts an active, nonpolar drug to one or more polar metabolites (that may or may not be pharmacologically active). These polar metabolites are generally cleared by the kidneys. Sometimes, drug metabolism converts an inactive "prodrug" into an active metabolite. Prodrugs require drug metabolism to occur in order to exert a therapeutic effect. Clopidogrel is an example of a prodrug.

The CYP system consists of more than 20 families of isoenzymes; the enzymes most important in drug metabolism are CYP1A2, 2B6, 2C9, 2C19, 2D6, and 3A4. The CYP3A4 group accounts for about 40%–60% of all hepatic CYP isoenzymes and is most frequently implicated in drug–drug interactions. Many medications commonly used in palliative care are metabolized by the 3A4 enzyme, such as dexamethasone, prednisone, midazolam, triazolam, alprazolam, methadone, fentanyl, and haloperidol.[10] In addition to being affected by drug–drug interactions, some patient populations may be deficient in CYP2D6 enzyme activity, which is responsible for the metabolism of codeine to morphine. This variation in activity is largely due to polymorphisms in the CYP2D6 allele. CYP2B6 and CYP2C19 are also highly polymorphic metabolizing enzymes.[11] In addition to CYP3A4, methadone is also metabolized by the polymorphic enzymes CYP2B6, CYP2C19, and CYP2D6.[12]

When we consider drug interactions resulting from drug metabolism, the drug or substance being acted upon is known as a "substrate." Some medications act as "enzyme inhibitors," inhibiting the activity of one or more specific enzymes. Enzyme-inhibiting drugs reduce the metabolism of the substrate drug, resulting in an increased serum concentration. For example, when fluconazole, a potent 3A4 inhibitor, is added to an established methadone regimen (methadone is the substrate in this case), the metabolism of methadone is inhibited, increasing the serum methadone concentration and potentially resulting in sedation or respiratory depression.

Conversely, some medications act as "enzyme inducers," increasing the levels, and subsequently the activity, of one or more enzymes. When an enzyme inducer is introduced, metabolism of the substrate drug is enhanced, resulting in a lower serum concentration, possibly causing a loss of effectiveness. Using methadone as an example again, if phenytoin is added to an established methadone regimen, methadone will be metabolized to a greater extent, with a likely loss of analgesia.

Common symptoms experienced by patients with advanced illness include pain, constipation, diarrhea, anorexia, cachexia, nausea, vomiting, dyspnea, confusion, anxiety, depression, insomnia, and fatigue. The International Association for Hospice and Palliative Care (IAHPC) collaborated with other organizations to develop a list of "essential" palliative care drugs.[13] Table 26.1 is a listing of selected moderately severe and severe drug interactions associated with the medications on this list 13, 14. Practitioners are encouraged to consult a more comprehensive description of these drug interactions as needed for patient care activities.[14]

Table 26.1 Selected Moderate and Major Pharmacokinetic Drug Interactions Affecting Metabolism of Sample IAHPC Essential Palliative Care Drugs

	Interacting Medication	Interaction Effect	Probable Mechanism	Severity*	Clinical Management
Antidepressants					
Amitriptyline	Carbamazepine	Decreased amitriptyline effectiveness	Increased amitriptyline metabolism	Mod	Monitor for clinical efficacy of amitriptyline and for signs of carbamazepine toxicity
	Duloxetine	Increased amitriptyline serum concentration	Duloxetine-induced inhibition of CYP2D6 metabolism of amitriptyline	Mod	Use caution with combination; monitor amitriptyline serum concentration.
	Fluconazole	Increased risk of amitriptyline toxicity	Inhibition of amitriptyline metabolism by CYP enzymes	Maj	Use caution with combination
	Fluoxetine	Increased amitriptyline toxicity	Decreased amitriptyline metabolism	Maj	Concurrent use is not recommended
	Phenytoin	Increased risk of phenytoin toxicity	Inhibition of phenytoin metabolism	Mod	Monitor serum levels of both drugs
	Sertraline	Increased amitriptyline serum level	Inhibition of amitriptyline metabolism	Maj	Use caution with concurrent administration
	St. John's wort	Decreased effect of amitriptyline	Induction of metabolizing enzymes	Mod	Avoid concurrent use

	Valproic acid	Increased serum concentrations of amitriptyline	Decreased amitriptyline plasma clearance	Mod	Monitor serum level of amitriptyline
	Warfarin	Increased risk of bleeding	Reduced warfarin metabolism and increased absorption	Mod	Monitor INR closely
Citalopram	Bupropion	Increased plasma level of citalopram	Inhibition of CYP2D6-mediated citalopram metabolism by bupropion	Mod	Use combination with caution and monitor for excessive citalopram adverse effects
	Desipramine	Increased desipramine serum concentration	Inhibition of desipramine metabolism	Mod	Use combination with caution and monitor patient response
	Fluconazole	Increased risk of serotonin syndrome and QT prolongation	Inhibition of CYP2C19-mediated citalopram metabolism by fluconazole	Maj	Use combination with caution and monitor patient for signs and symptoms of serotonin syndrome or other adverse effects from citalopram
	Imipramine	Increase in bioavailability and half-life of desipramine, major metabolite of imipramine	Inhibition of desipramine metabolism, the major metabolite of imipramine	Mod	Use combination with caution and adjust dosing as clinically indicated

(continued)

Table 26.1 (Continued)

	Interacting Medication	Interaction Effect	Probable Mechanism	Severity*	Clinical Management
	Omeprazole	Increased plasma level of citalopram and risk of QT prolongation	Inhibition of CYP2C19-mediated citalopram metabolism by omeprazole	Maj	Use maximum of 20 mg citalopram daily
Gastrointestinal Agents					
Loperamide	Gemfibrozil		Inhibition of CYP2C8-mediated loperamide metabolism	Mod	Use with caution, especially with high loperamide doses. Monitor for loperamide AE including nausea, vomiting, dry mouth, dizziness, or drowsiness.
	St. John's wort	Delirium with symptoms of confusion, agitation, and disorientation	Unknown	Mod	Use with caution, monitor for signs of altered mental status
	Valerian	Delrium with symptoms of confusion, agitation, and disorientation	Unknown	Mod	
Mineral oil enema	Docusate	Inflammation of intestinal mucosa, liver, spleen, and lymph nodes	Enhanced mineral oil absorption (shown with mineral oil liquid paraffin)	Mod	Avoid concurrent oral administration of docusate salts and mineral oil

Senna	Digoxin	Increased risk of digoxin toxicity	Mod	Avoid concurrent use, or monitor potassium serum concentration
	Droperidol	Increased risk of cardiotoxicity (QT prolongation, torsades de pointes, cardiac arrest)	Maj	Droperidol should be used with extreme caution with laxatives
Anticonvulsants				
Gabapentin	Aluminum, and magnesium salts	Reduces gabapentin bioavailability by 20%	Mod	Avoid antacid use within 2 hours of taking gabapentin
Opioids				
Fentanyl	Carbamazepine	Decreased plasma fentanyl concentrations	Mod	Monitor response to fentanyl and increase dose as appropriate
	Clarithromycin Erythromycin	Increased fentanyl toxicity (CNS and respiratory depression)	Maj	Monitor patient and reduce fentanyl dose
	Diltiazem	Severe hypotension and increased risk of fentanyl toxicity (respiratory depression)	Maj	Monitor blood pressure and reduce/adjust fentanyl dose as appropriate

Senna may cause potassium loss with excessive or prolonged use

Senna may cause potassium and magnesium loss with excessive or prolonged use; may precipitate QT prolongation

Decreased gabapentin bioavailability

Induction of CYP enzymes, increasing clearance of fentanyl

Inhibition of CYP3A4-mediated fentanyl metabolism

Inhibition of CYP3A4-mediated fentanyl metabolism

(continued)

Table 26.1 (Continued)

	Interacting Medication	Interaction Effect	Probable Mechanism	Severity*	Clinical Management
	Fluconazole Ketoconazole Posaconazole Voriconazole	Increased fentanyl toxicity	Inhibition of CYP3A4-mediated fentanyl metabolism	Maj	Monitor patient and reduce fentanyl dose
	Phenytoin	Decreased fentanyl serum concentrations	Induction of fentanyl metabolism by phenytoin	Mod	Adjust fentanyl dose as appropriate
Methadone	Clarithromycin Erythromycin	Increased serum methadone concentrations	Inhibition of CYP3A4-mediated methadone metabolism	Mod	Use caution with combination; consider lowering methadone dose
	Fluconazole Ketoconazole Posaconazole Voriconazole	Increased plasma methadone levels	Inhibition of CYP3A4-mediated methadone metabolism	Mod	Monitor therapy closely; consider lowering methadone dose empirically
	Phenobarbital	Decreased methadone effectiveness	Induction of CYP3A4-mediated methadone metabolism	Mod	Combination may result in lower methadone serum concentration; Monitor closely and increase dose as required
	Ritonavir	Decreased methadone levels and effectiveness	Mechanism unknown; possibly through induction of CYP2B6-mediated methadone metabolism	Mod	Combination may result in lower methadone serum concentration; Monitor closely and increase dose as required

Morphine	Cimetidine	Increased morphine toxicity	Unclear, possibly decreased metabolism	Maj	Use caution with combination, start with lower dose of morphine and titrate as appropriate
Tramadol	Amitriptyline	Increased tramadol levels and decreased levels of the active metabolite (M1) of tramadol, increasing risk of seizure while diminishing analgesic effect (M1 is more potent than the parent drug at the mu opioid receptor); increased risk of serotonin syndrome	Inhibition of CYP2D6-mediated tramadol metabolism	Maj	Use caution with combination; monitor patient for signs and symptoms of tramadol overdose and uncontrolled pain
	Bupropion	Increased tramadol levels and decreased levels of the active metabolite (M1) of tramadol, increasing seizure risk	Inhibition of CYP2D6-mediated tramadol metabolism	Maj	Use caution with combination; monitor patient for signs and symptoms of tramadol overdose and uncontrolled pain
	Carbamazepine	Decreased tramadol efficacy	Induction of CYP3A4 metabolism of tramadol by carbamazepine	Maj	Concurrent administration is not recommended
	Erythromycin	Increased tramadol serum level	Inhibition of CYP3A4 metabolism of tramadol by erythromycin	Mod	Monitor patient for signs and symptoms of tramadol overdose

(continued)

Table 26.1 (Continued)

Interacting Medication	Interaction Effect	Probable Mechanism	Severity*	Clinical Management
Fluconazole Ketoconazole Posaconazole Voriconazole	Increased tramadol serum level	Inhibition of CYP3A4 metabolism of tramadol	Mod	Monitor patient for signs and symptoms of tramadol overdose
Methadone	Increased tramadol levels and decreased levels of the active metabolite (M1) of tramadol; decreased tramadol effectiveness and increased risk of seizures; increased risk of serotonin syndrome	Inhibition of CYP2D6-mediated tramadol metabolism	Maj	Use caution with combination; monitor patient for signs and symptoms of tramadol overdose and uncontrolled pain
Paroxetine	Increased tramadol levels and decreased levels of the active metabolite (M1) of tramadol, increasing risk of seizure while diminishing analgesic effect (M1 is more potent than the parent drug at the mu opioid receptor); increased risk of serotonin syndrome	Inhibition of CYP2D6-mediated tramadol metabolism	Maj	Use caution with combination; monitor patient for signs and symptoms of tramadol overdose and uncontrolled pain
St. John's wort	Decreased tramadol serum level	Induction of CYP3A4 metabolism of tramadol by St. John's wort	Mod	Monitor for tramadol efficacy

Non-Opioid Analgesics				
Acetaminophen	Carbamazepine	Increased risk of acetaminophen toxicity	Carbamazepine may induce metabolism of acetaminophen, resulting in an increased level of hepatotoxic metabolites	Mod	At usual therapeutic oral doses of acetaminophen and carbamazepine, no special monitoring is required
	Phenytoin	Decreased acetaminophen effectiveness and increased risk of hepatotoxicity	Phenytoin increases metabolism of acetaminophen by more than 40% and decreases acetaminophen half-life by about 25%. Increases production of toxic acetaminophen metabolites.	Mod	Avoid large or chronic doses of acetaminophen. Monitor patient for signs or symptoms of hepatotoxicity.
	Warfarin	Increased risk of bleeding due to increased hypoprothrombinemic effect of warfarin. Two to 4 grams/day of acetaminophen increase INR within 1–2 weeks.	Acetaminophen may inhibit metabolism of warfarin or interfere with formation of clotting factors	Mod	Limit intake of acetaminophen. Monitor INR for several weeks when acetaminophen added or discontinued in patients taking warfarin.
	Imatinib	Increased risk of acetaminophen toxicity	Imatinib likely inhibits glucoronidation of acetaminophen	Maj	No pharmacokinetic impact of single 1000 mg acetaminophen dose with 400 mg daily imatinib. Avoid chronic acetaminophen use.

(continued)

Table 26.1 (Continued)

	Interacting Medication	Interaction Effect	Probable Mechanism	Severity*	Clinical Management
Ibuprofen	Desipramine	Increased risk of desipramine toxicity	Inhibition of desipramine metabolism by ibuprofen	Mod	Monitor desipramine concentration and monitor for adverse effects
	Lithium	Increased risk of lithium toxicity	Decreased lithium clearance	Mod	Monitor for signs of lithium toxicity; lithium dosage reduction may be necessary
	Phenytoin	Increased risk of phenytoin toxicity	Increased free phenytoin serum concentration and/or altered metabolism of either phenytoin or ibuprofen	Mod	Monitor patients receiving this combination for signs of phenytoin toxicity and monitor serum levels (free and total phenytoin)
Corticosteroids					
Dexamethasone	Carbamazepine	Decreased dexamethasone effectiveness	Increased dexamethasone metabolism	Mod	Monitor response to dexamethasone and increase dose as clinically indicated
	Phenobarbital	Decreased dexamethasone effectiveness	Increased dexamethasone metabolism	Mod	Monitor response to dexamethasone and increase dose as clinically indicated

Phenytoin	Decreased dexamethasone effectiveness	Increased dexamethasone metabolism	Mod	Monitor therapeutic response to dexamethasone and increase dose as clinically indicated
Benzodiazepines				
Diazepam				
Erythromycin, Clarithromycin	Increased benzodiazepine toxicity	Decreased hepatic metabolism	Mod	Monitor patient for excessive benzodiazepine effects and adjust therapy as appropriate
St. John's wort	Reduced diazepam effectiveness	Induction of CYP3A4-mediated metabolism of diazepam	Mod	Monitor for altered therapeutic and adverse effects of diazepam
Lorazepam				
Valproic acid	Increased lorazepam concentration	Decreased rate of lorazepam metabolism (glucuronidation)	Mod	Reduce lorazepam dose by 50% and monitor for increased adverse effects
Midazolam				
Carbamazepine	Decreased efficacy of midazolam	Induction of CYP3A enzymes by carbamazepines	Mod	Larger doses of midazolam may be required to achieve desired response
Clarithromycin	Increased midazolam toxicity	Inhibition of CYP3A4-mediated midazolam metabolism	Mod	Monitor patient and reduce midazolam dose empirically

(continued)

Table 26.1 (Continued)

Interacting Medication	Interaction Effect	Probable Mechanism	Severity*	Clinical Management
Erythromycin	Increased midazolam sedation	Inhibition of CYP3A4-mediated midazolam metabolism	Mod	Monitor patient and reduce midazolam dose empirically
Fluconazole	Increased midazolam serum concentration and toxicity	Inhibition of CYP3A4-mediated midazolam metabolism	Mod	Monitor patient and reduce dose of midazolam
Ketoconazole	Increased midazolam serum concentration and toxicity	Inhibition of CYP3A4-mediated metabolism of midazolam	Maj	Combination not recommended
Phenytoin	Decreased efficacy of midazolam	Induction of CYP3A4-mediated metabolism of midazolam	Mod	Larger doses of midazolam may be required
St. John's wort	Reduced midazolam effectiveness	Induction of CYP3A4-mediated metabolism of midazolam	Mod	Monitor response and increase midazolam dose as required

Non-benzodiazepine Sedatives/Hypnotics

Interacting Medication	Interaction Effect	Probable Mechanism	Severity*	Clinical Management
Trazodone	Amiodarone	Amiodarone and trazodone are both metabolized by CYP3A4, and amiodarone inhibits this enzyme. Combination increases risk of QT interval prolongation and torsade de pointes.	Unknown	Maj	Use caution if these drugs are used in combination and monitor cardiac function.

Carbamazepine	Decreased trazodone plasma concentration.	Induction of CYP3A4 metabolism	Maj	Monitor trazodone serum concentration and response; adjust therapy as needed.
Clarithromycin	An increase in trazodone plasma levels	Inhibition of CYP3A4 metabolism	Mod	Use a lower dose of trazodone in patients receiving clarithromycin and monitor for adverse effects
Digoxin	Increased serum digoxin concentration and possible toxicity	Unknown	Mod	Monitor serum digoxin concentration with combination
Fluoxetine	Increased trazodone toxicity and/or serotonin syndrome and/or QT interval prolongation	Decreased trazodone metabolism by CYP2D6	Maj	Monitor for trazodone toxicity and adjust dose as necessary
Itraconazole, Ketoconazole	Increased trazodone serum concentrations. Combination increases risk of QT interval prolongation and torsades de pointes.	Inhibition of CYP3A4-mediated trazodone metabolism	Mod	Use a lower dose of trazodone and monitor adverse effects
Phenytoin	Increased phenytoin serum concentrations and increased risk of toxicity	Unknown, possibly due to competitive inhibition of phenytoin metabolism, protein binding or excretion	Mod	Monitor serum phenytoin concentration

(continued)

Table 26.1 (Continued)

	Interacting Medication	Interaction Effect	Probable Mechanism	Severity*	Clinical Management
	Ritonavir	Increased trazodone plasma level and increased risk of adverse effects	Inhibition of CYP3A-mediated trazodone metabolism by ritonavir	Mod	Monitor patient for increased sedative effects and hypotension. May require trazodone dosage reduction.
Zolpidem	Ketoconazole	Increased zolpidem plasma level and increased risk of adverse effects	Impaired metabolism of zolpidem	Mod	If used together, monitor for decreased concentration and increased somnolence
Dopamine Antagonists					
Haloperidol	Bupropion	Increased plasma levels of haloperidol	Inhibition of CPY2D6-mediated haloperidol metabolism	Mod	Use combination with caution, and start with lower dose of haloperidol
	Carbamazepine	Decreased haloperidol effectiveness	Increased CYP 2D6 and 3A4-mediated haloperidol metabolism	Mod	Monitor effectiveness of haloperidol and increase dosage as appropriate

Antihistamines/Anticholinergics

Diphenhydramine	Metoprolol	Increased metoprolol plasma concentrations with prolonged negative chronotropic and inotropic effects of metoprolol, especially in poor CYP2D6 metabolizers	Diphenhydramine inhibits CYP2D6 enzyme, which reduces metoprolol metabolism	Mod	Use combination with caution; monitor for increased metoprolol adverse effects

*Severity: Mod = moderate; Maj = major; CI = contraindicated

Elimination

There are few pharmacokinetic interactions caused by alterations in drug elimination because most drugs have multiple mechanisms of elimination (e.g., biliary, renal). Probenecid has been shown to affect drug secretion in the kidney, prolonging the elimination of methotrexate and penicillin and other β-lactam antibiotics. Drug–disease interaction is more likely to cause drug toxicity, specifically renal and/or hepatic impairment.

Conclusion

Medications are commonly used to palliate symptoms associated with advanced illness. Practitioners must be vigilant in monitoring this frail patient population for drug-induced illnesses, including those caused by drug–drug interactions.

References

1. Prescription drugs. The Henry J. Kaiser Family Foundation. Retrieved August 1, 2014, from http://kff.org/state-category/health-costs-budgets/prescription-drugs.
2. Kemp L, Narula P, McPherson M, Zuckerman I (2009). Medication reconciliation in hospice: a pilot study. *Am J Hosp Palliat Med* 26(3):193–9.
3. Wright J (1992). Drug interactions. In: Melmon K, Morrelli H, Hoffman B, Nierenberg D (eds.), *Melmon and Morrelli's Clinical Pharmacology: Basic Principles in Therapeutics.* New York: McGraw-Hill, p. 1012.
4. Rudolph J, Salow M, Angelini M, McGlinchey R (2008). The anticholinergic risk scale and anticholinergic adverse effects in older persons. *Arch Intern Med* 168(5):508–13.
5. QT drug lists by risk group. Arizona Cert: Center for Education and Research on Therapeutics. Retrieved August 1, 2014, from www.crediblemeds.org.
6. Boyer E, Shannon M (2005). The serotonin syndrome. *New Engl J Med* 352:1112–20.
7. Mihelic R (2005). Pharmacology of palliative medicine. *Semin Oncol Nursing* 21:29–35.
8. König J, Müller F, Fromm M (2013). Transporters and drug-drug interactions: Important determinants of drug disposition and effects. *Pharmacol Rev* 65(3):944–66.
9. Gong I, Kim R (2013). Importance of pharmacokinetic profile and variability as determinants of dose and response to dabigatran, rivaroxaban, and apixaban. *Can J Cardiol* 29(7 Suppl):S24–33.
10. Haddad A, Davis M, Lagman R (2007). The pharmacological importance of cytochrome CYP3A4 in the palliation of symptoms: review and recommendations for avoiding adverse drug interactions. *Support Care Cancer* 15:251–7.
11. Zhou SF, Liu JP, Chowbay B (2009). Polymorphism of human cytochrome P450 enzymes and its clinical impact. *Drug Metab Rev* 41(2):89–295.
12. Gerber JG, Rhodes RJ, Gal J (2004). Stereoselective metabolism of methadone N-demethylation by cytochrome CYP4502B6 and 2C19. *Chirality* 16(1):34–47.
13. De Lima L (2012). Key concepts in palliative care: the IAHPC list of essential medicines in palliative care. *Eur J Hosp Pharm* 19:34–7.
14. Micromedex 2.0 [Internet database]. Truven Health Analytics (2014). Retrieved August 9, 2014, from http://www.micromedex.com/.

Pediatric Palliative Care

Donna S. Zhukovsky and Rhonda Robert

What Is Pediatric Palliative Care and Whom Does It Involve?

Definition of Pediatric Palliative Care

Pediatric palliative care (PPC) is a family-centered approach to care for children living with life-threatening illness and their families. The goal of PPC is to manage pain and other physical symptoms while addressing the psychological, social, and spiritual problems of the child and the child's family.

As defined by the World Health Organization,[1] effective palliative care for children

- Involves giving active total care of the child's body, mind, and spirit as well as support to the family;
- Begins when illness is diagnosed and continues whether or not a child receives treatment directed at the disease;
- Requires that the healthcare provider evaluate and alleviate the child's physical, psychological, and social distress;
- Requires a broad multidisciplinary approach that includes the family and effectively uses available community resources;
- Can be provided in tertiary-care facilities, community health centers, and the child's home.

Who Are the Affected Children?

Typically, people think of children diagnosed with cancer and other life-limiting illnesses as the exclusive recipients of PPC. However, their siblings are also important beneficiaries, as are the child's community of friends, peers, and classmates and children of adult cancer patients, an expanding group due to childbirth into later years.

Affected siblings are often overlooked by healthcare professionals and receive less attention from their parents than the ill child in part because of the care-giving needs and the emotional distress associated with parenting a seriously ill child.

Clinical Pearl

- Pediatric palliative care is not limited to child and adolescent patients. All children whose lives are affected by serious medical illness in a loved one are potential beneficiaries: pediatric patients, their siblings and peers, as well as children and grandchildren of adult patients.

Box 27.1 Pediatric Palliative Care: Differences from Care of Adult Patients

- Child's developmental stage
- Family life cycle stage
- Disease spectrum
- Illness trajectories

Differences from Palliative Care for Adults

While the overall approach to palliative care for children is similar to that provided for adults, there are several differences that influence the provision of care (Box 27.1).[2]

Child's Developmental Stage

In addition to physiological and pharmacokinetic differences that influence pharmacotherapy, developmental factors that impact communication, as well as the understanding of illness and death, distinguish care of the child from that of adults. Healthcare providers must be familiar with these differences in order to provide effective and compassionate care.

Family Life Cycle

Parents or adult siblings function as proxy reporters and decision-makers. When children are very young or ill, these proxies may be the only source of input. Assuming these new roles and responsibilities is emotionally taxing on parents and siblings, and they need additional emotional support.

For older children who are healthy enough to provide self-report and participate in decision-making, both parents and patients often participate in reporting and decision-making. Differences in parent and patient wishes may result in ethical dilemmas.

Disease Spectrum

Death is an uncommon phenomenon in children. In 2010, 29,138 deaths occurred during the first year of life, with congenital defects, prematurity, and sudden infant death syndrome representing the most common causes.[3] Somewhat less than this number occurred from ages 1–19, where the overwhelming causes of death result from traumatic accidents and injuries. This type of death raises the need for acute palliative care for bereaved families that may have no or very little time to adjust to the threat of premature mortality.[3]

In the 1–19-year-old group, cancer is the most common medical cause of death at 2,000 annually in the United States,[4] followed by cardiac diseases, congenital anomalies, and multiple other uncommon diseases. The relative rarity of pediatric death and the limited availability of disease-specific expertise often require medical care in locations distant from the family's home.[3]

Illness Trajectories

The spectrum of illness trajectories that accompany life-limiting illness is different from those associated with adult causes of mortality, some without the predictable decline that is common to adults:[5]

- Potentially curable conditions, such as cancer (over 70% of children with cancer are cured)
- Progressive conditions for which intensive therapy prolongs and enhances life, such as cystic fibrosis
- Progressive conditions for which curative or disease-altering therapy is not available, such as a variety of neurodegenerative conditions
- Nonprogressive conditions for which death before adulthood is likely from complications, such as prolonged seizures or respiratory failure with cerebral palsy.

The Role of Family-Centered Care

Family-centered care, integral to the definition of palliative care in general, plays an especially strong role in caring for children living with life-limiting illness and their families. In pediatrics, family-centered care recognizes that parents are the true experts regarding their own children and that they are the primary source of information, strength, and support for each child.[6]

To provide for a true partnership, healthcare professionals must step back from their customary roles as experts to realize that families are experts in their own right and must be involved at all levels of healthcare delivery, including development and execution of treatment plans.

Symptom Assessment and Management

Symptom Epidemiology

Available data, while limited, suggest that children living with life-limiting illnesses experience a high symptom burden. The data are best described in cancer patients.[7,8]

Almost two-thirds of children with non-CNS tumors have symptoms at diagnosis, which typically resolve with initiation of treatment. However, multiple symptoms are common throughout the course, with inpatients and those receiving chemotherapy reporting more symptoms than outpatients.[9,10]

Unrelieved symptoms are also prevalent at the end of life, with pain, fatigue, dyspnea, and anorexia being the most common. In addition to the cancer, symptoms may occur as a result of the treatment or procedures or from noncancer etiologies.

Causes of treatment- and procedure-related pain are noted in Table 27.1 and Box 27.2. These can often be anticipated and prevented. In noncancer illnesses, symptoms vary depending on the diagnosis, but often reflect respiratory, neurological, or feeding problems.

Paradigm for Symptom Assessment and Management

As for adults, optimal management of pain and other disease-associated symptoms is predicated on an understanding of the multidimensional nature of the symptom experience. Contributing to symptom expression are medical factors, including underlying pathophysiological mechanisms and comorbid medical conditions, as well as psychological, social, and spiritual factors.

Table 27.1 Treatment-Related Pain in Children with Cancer

Chemotherapy	Surgery
Myalgias	Postoperative
Mucositis	Phantom limb
Extravasation	(preoperative analgesia)
Neuropathy	**Radiation**
GVHD (allogeneic BMT)	Mucositis
	Dermatitis

BMT = bone marrow transplantation; GVHD = graft-versus-host disease.

Box 27.2 Procedure-Related Pain in Children with Cancer

- Needles
- Bone marrow
- Aspiration and biopsy
- Central line removal
- Diagnostic procedures

Symptom assessment includes a systematic symptom survey, a symptom-specific history, oncological history, including disease-directed therapies, general medical history, spiritual review, and psychosocial and family history that includes screening for substance abuse. When available, validated age- and developmentally appropriate symptom screening batteries such as the pediatric versions of the Memorial Symptom Assessment Scale[9,10] and symptom-specific scales should routinely be incorporated into the clinical history.

Optimal management is contingent upon ongoing assessment of the symptom experience, physical examination, and indicated diagnostic testing, as expert assessment is the basis for a working diagnosis and treatment plan in keeping with the goals of care.

Pain Assessment Tools

Types of assessment tools include behavioral, numeric rating, categorical, and visual analog scales. For pain, behavioral observation scales are the primary assessment method for neonates, infants, children under 4 years of age, and those with developmental disabilities.

Children aged 3–8 years are usually able to use faces scales, with a series of photographs or drawings depicting varying degrees of distress. Children aged 8 years and older can generally also use verbal rating scales (no pain, mild, moderate, severe) and horizontal versions of adult visual analog scales, for example, measuring pain against a horizontal ruler.[11]

Examples of age-appropriate pain assessment scales are noted in Box 27.3.

Assessment of Psychological Distress

Assessment of psychological distress should be an early and ongoing component of care for persons with a life-threatening illness. Learning of and

---

Box 27.3 Pain Assessment: Examples of Age- and Developmentally Appropriate Scales

Children < 4 Years or with Developmental Disabilities
- Behavioral observation scales
- FLACCS (Face, Legs, Activity, Cry, Consolability)
- Children's Hospital of Eastern Ontario Pain Scale (CHEOPS)
- Gustave Roussy pain scale

Children 3–7 Years
- Faces scales (e.g., Oucher, revised Bieri, Baker–Wong)
- Color analog scale (e.g., pain thermometer)
- Poker chip tool
- Body maps

Children ≥ 8 Years
- Verbal rating scales
- Numeric rating scales
- Visual analog scales (horizontal)

living with the illness are both initially and intermittently distressing and often relate to losses.

Acutely, losses may include disruption of daily life and loss of physical well-being. Progressive losses may include deaths of friends at the same treatment center and health decline from advanced disease or treatment side effects. Examples of anticipated losses include independence from caregiver or career options.

With most life-threatening or life-limiting illnesses, persons are at risk for symptoms of depression and anxiety, including traumatic stress. A source for reviewing the symptoms of possible diagnoses is the *Diagnostic and Statistical Manual of Mental Disorders (DSM)*, published by the American Psychiatric Association. Portions of the *DSM* are available online at www. psyweb.com.

Given that depression, anxiety, and traumatic stress need to be evaluated, assessing sleep quality is a nonthreatening way to begin screening for these conditions. Sleep has behavioral qualities and concrete descriptors, is usually not stigmatizing to discuss, and involves personal disclosure. Easily disrupted by emotional distress, sleep patterns provide some transparency regarding a person's emotional state.

A possible questioning sequence may be "How have you been sleeping? How long do you take to fall asleep? Once you are asleep, do you awaken prematurely? If so, what causes you to awaken? What is on your mind when you awaken? How are you feeling when you awaken?"

Questions about feeling states such as worry and sadness are a natural progression. When assessing concerns, normalizing the experience is important before asking questions: "Many people have new worries and concerns when they are feeling sick. Some people have never been to a hospital before, and others have never spent a night away from home before. I would like to know how you feel."

The fear thermometer is a single-item numeric rating scale that can be used to simplify assessment of worry.[12,13] Similar to a pain thermometer, it is a type of tool with which many children are already familiar.

Online screening tools and resources developed for assessing depression and anxiety are available from the International Psycho-oncology Society (www.ipos-society.org), the American Psychosocial Oncology Society (www. apos-society.org), and the National Child Traumatic Stress Network (www. NCTSNet.org).

Clinical Pearl

- Asking about sleep is a nonthreatening way to begin screening for depression and anxiety.

Synthesis of Symptom Diagnosis and Management Plan

Once a working diagnosis is established, treatment is directed at modifying the underlying causes as well as palliation of the symptom itself. Symptom-directed therapy (i.e., analgesics for pain) is often an integral component of the treatment plan while awaiting the benefit of disease-directed therapy or when primary therapy is ineffective.

Psychological, social, and spiritual concerns often exacerbate the symptom and necessitate corresponding interventions for optimal symptom management and to avoid unnecessary drug toxicity.

Modalities of Symptom Control

Modalities of symptom control, reviewed elsewhere in this book, are numerous and include disease-specific, pharmacological, anesthetic, surgical, psychiatric, psychological, spiritual, and integrative-medicine interventions.

Optimal management is often multimodal and is best configured with the interdisciplinary input of team members working closely together. Understanding the impact of illness and associated symptoms on the child is essential. If barriers are present, psychosocial staff, including a child-life specialist when available, can foster communication about these issues.

Principles of Pharmacotherapy

Pharmacotherapy is a mainstay of treatment for most children. There is a paucity of studies conducted in children; thus use is largely based on clinical experience. The principles of management are noted in Box 27.4.

Indications for most medications and medication side effects are similar to those for adults in most cases.

Given the variation in starting doses and dose range due to developmental issues (see the following section, "Developmental Issues in Drug Use"), specific dose recommendations are beyond the scope of this text.

Developmental Issues in Drug Use

Factors that influence drug management include ratio of body compartments, differences in plasma protein binding, development of hepatic enzyme systems for drug metabolism, extent of renal filtration and excretion of drugs and their metabolites, metabolic rate, oxygen consumption, and degree of maturation of respiratory function.[11]

For individuals not experienced in working with premature infants or children of different developmental stages, close coordination with pediatricians and pediatric pharmacists is essential to providing safe and expert pharmacotherapy, and use of pediatric-specific resources is advised.

Box 27.4 Principles of Pharmacotherapy for Symptom Management

- Start one drug at a time and allow an adequate trial to assess benefit and side effects.
- Choose the appropriate route of administration.
- Use the oral route whenever possible.
- Avoid the intramuscular route.
- Provide regularly scheduled medication for continuous pain.
- Use PRN or "breakthrough" doses for prevention of predictable incident pain and treatment of pain exacerbations.
- Anticipate and manage side effects, for example, bowel management with opioids.

Communication Issues in Pediatric Palliative Care

Communication: The Principal Determinant of High-Quality Care

The literature consistently demonstrates that parents value direct, clear, and caring communication about what to expect, and that this is the principal determinant of quality pediatric palliative care.[14] Involvement of the child, when considered age- and culturally appropriate by the parents, is key to satisfaction with care.

Furthermore, most children adjust best to death, be it their own, their sibling's, or their parent's, when provided with a safe and permissive environment in which they are allowed to openly ask questions, voice concerns, and participate in care.

Clinical Pearl

- Parents value direct, clear, and caring communication about what to expect; this is the principal determinant of quality of care.
- Involvement of the child in discussions about the illness and care plans, when considered age- and culturally appropriate by the parents, is key to parents' satisfaction with care.

Formats for Medical Conversations

The format of medical conversations may be (1) patient only; (2) patient and parent simultaneously; (3) parent first, followed by parent and patient simultaneously; or (4) parent only. Problems commonly arise when negotiation of the format does not occur, for example:

- Patient: "The worst part was waiting in the lobby when my parents and doctor were talking about me."
- Parent: "The doctor just said the diagnosis. I was not prepared. I was so upset. I wished I had been able to support my child."

The medical-conversation formats used in these examples are reasonable but not suited to the participants' needs. Once the conversations have taken place, fit of the conversation should be reassessed: What about the format worked? What did not work? What modifications should be made?

As participants gain treatment experience, the format may need to be changed. Optimally initiated at the beginning of the patient–professional caregiver relationship, these conversations should continue throughout the course of care and provide the opportunity for the medical professional to learn what is important to both the parent and child.

Empathic Listening

Communication requires both an empathic listening component and a treatment leadership component. Most often, the empathic listening component is omitted and communication is limited to biomedical information.

The patient needs permission and invitation to be heard; the medical professional can extend this invitation by asking open-ended questions. Open-ended questions are an invitation for the recipient to reflect, feel, and self-disclose.

Mack and Wolfe offer suggestions for best practice in this area, including how to initiate medical conversations, introduce the possibility of death, elicit care goals, introduce palliation, talk about expectations, and address children directly.[15]

Transitioning Between or Participating in Simultaneous Curative and Palliative Care Services

Communicating during transitions in care can be challenging. Language may become vague, euphemistic, autocratic, and/or complex biomedical speak, resulting in confusing communications.

Clear language, support, and commitment from the medical team, along with active engagement with the family in decision-making, are the ideal; for example: "It is time to rethink our goals and plans. We had each hoped that the treatment would cure the disease, but we now know the disease is worsening. Our goal is to help you in the best way possible. Do you have ideas regarding what is best for you? Would examples of goals, options, or plans help us start the conversation?"

Core Concepts to Complete Understanding of Death

Core concepts to a mature understanding of illness and death develop during childhood.[16] The first concept to develop is the *irreversibility* of death. Dead people do not come back to life the way that cartoon characters do.

Finality signifies that all body functions cease. When the concept of finality has not yet been grasped, children will ask how the deceased will eat or breathe, once buried. Failure to address these developmentally appropriate concerns can lead to misperceptions, which can be traumatic if not corrected.

Universality implies that death happens to all living things and that, one day, death will happen to the child.

Causality is the understanding that death occurs for a proximate reason independent of oneself. Younger children commonly blame themselves for the death, rather than a cause independent of themselves. This misattribution of cause and effect is labeled "magical thinking." Young children may believe that they have "wished" somebody dead; their misbehavior caused the death; or that death is contagious. Given the likelihood that these beliefs will occur, it is important to identify and rectify misattributions.

Age-Specific Recommendations Regarding Care of Children Exposed to Life-Threatening Illness and Death

Preschool-age children understand physical discomfort. Parents' presence and soothing of the child are the focal parenting tasks. Preschool-age children live in the present. They do not have "issues" to resolve or need "closure" before death.

Young school-age children need help with magical thinking, as discussed in the preceding section. A sample script is as follows: "The (name of illness) is stronger, and the medicines are not able to help as much as they had. You worked hard and followed the prescriptions. We are very proud of you. You did not cause the (illness), nor did you do anything to make it stronger. No one knows why this happened. We will do everything possible to help you and one another."

Older school-age children and adolescents have a broad range of concerns and need for information. Commonly reported concerns include the following:

- What dying feels like, including whether dying will be painful
- Separation from loved ones
- How others will fare after the child dies
- What happens to the child after death.

School-age children and adolescents need permission to voice concerns. Some may need to hear examples of commonly experienced concerns, as most are apprehensive to disclose private thoughts about death. They may need a neutral party with whom to disclose concerns, wanting to protect loved ones from sadness.

Grief and Bereavement in Pediatric Palliative Care

Children may cross many milestones during the course of an illness. Normalizing life as much as possible by facilitating participation in milestones important to the child is necessary. If this is not done, treatment adherence and psychological adjustment may both deteriorate.

The Child Patient: Disclosure of Impending Death

Parental Grief

Parents may need to grieve the anticipated death of their child, spouse, or other beloved individual before they are able to assist their child or children in the grieving process. This timing may conflict with the healthcare professional's readiness to discuss dying with the child. The healthcare professional should discuss timing of disclosure with the parent.

Negotiating a balance between the parents' needs and the child's needs is the goal. In addition to reflective listening and empathic responses from the medical professional, the parent(s) may benefit from additional services to work through their grief.

Describing the role and accessibility of expert assistance and offering to facilitate the connection are ideal. If such an expert is not available within the institution, a member of the treatment team should assume the responsibility of making a community-based referral.

A national locator for licensed psychologists is provided by the National Registry of Health Service Providers at www.findapsychologist.org. State licensing boards provide online rosters of licensees by city or zip code. The key search words are "state board of examiners of (psychologists, psychiatrists, licensed professional counselors, or social workers)."

Parental Role in Protecting the Child from Harm

Parents' jobs involve protection of their child from harm; accordingly, they may want to protect their child by avoiding discussion of death. However, one cannot be protected from one's own death. Parents may need input, discussion, and suggestions as to how to help their dying child with developmentally appropriate information.

When a child does not have adequate, age-appropriate information, what the child imagines is likely worse than the truth. With information, the child can trust in others, know what to expect, and be part of the family experience. By modeling how persons are helped, regardless of circumstances, death need not be feared.

Parents may benefit from opportunities to plan and rehearse ways to discuss the possibility and likelihood of the child's dying with the treatment team or community experts.

Clinical Pearl

- Giving children permission to talk about the impending death of themselves or of a loved one is important, as it demonstrates confidence in their ability to cope and allows for correction of potentially distressing misperceptions.

Psychosocial Support of Parents and Siblings of a Child with Life-Limiting Illness

During Illness

Healthy siblings need to maintain normalcy. Maintaining contact with the familiar is important. Routines such as school- and peer-based activities need to continue. When parents are unable to sustain these routines, surrogate caregivers should be identified to help.

In addition, the healthy sibling needs consistent, trustworthy information regarding the ill sibling, as well as contact with parents and the ill sibling during the course of medical care. To foster contact, sibling-oriented services are often available, for example, sibling support groups and summer camps that include healthy and ill sibling groups.

Parents may need suggestions of how best to parent a healthy child when another child in the family is ill. National organizations, such as American Childhood Cancer Organization (www.acco.org), provide parent support, and Supersibs (www.alexslemonade.org) provides sibling support and parenting information.

During Bereavement

Psychosocial support and intervention subsequent to the death of a patient is also an important and often neglected aspect of care. Brief contact by phone or mail by the primary medical team members provides both the opportunity for the shared loss to be recognized and an offer to locate local bereavement resources.

Bereaved parents often do not fit into generic, community grief support groups because of the rarity of and aspects unique to a child's death.

National organizations available to facilitate identification of local bereavement resources include the following:

- *Compassionate Friends* (www.compassionatefriends.org) is a national organization for bereaved parents, with local chapters that provide parent support groups.
- *Dougy Center* (www.dougy.org) provides sibling bereavement services and an international listing of similar organizations.

Palliative Care for the Child Whose Parent Is Dying

A child whose parent is at the end of life can be an important beneficiary of palliative care services, either directly or through the proxy of his or her parent. Like parents of seriously ill children, parents affected by a terminal illness may need help in learning how to talk with a child about their own or the other parent's illness.

Assistance in talking with their children about the illness should be offered at the beginning of treatment and whenever health status changes significantly. Parents are encouraged to do the following:

- Openly discuss the illness
- Involve the treatment team expert as needed
- Use the proper name of the illness
- Clarify whether or not the illness is contagious
- Dispel magical thinking regarding causality
- Bring the child to an appointment

- Encourage visitation during hospitalizations; though most children wish to visit, visitation is the child's choice
- Prepare the child before the visit; explain the parent's status, the medical equipment being used, treatment of the disease, and treatment for comfort
- Foster discussions about dying; ensure an age-appropriate understanding of what dying means, e.g., the body stops working
- Reassure the child regarding who and how the child will be cared for during end of life and after the parent's death
- Inform and update school counselors and other involved adults
- Maintain normalcy as much as possible

Kathleen McCue provides more detailed guidance in her book *How to Help Children Through a Parent's Serious Illness* (1994), published by St. Martin's Press, New York.

Grieving Children: How Do They Differ from Adults?

Whenever possible, children should be offered the opportunity to be present with the ill individual and to participate in death rituals such as funerals to the extent that they would like. Explanations of what to expect and provision of an adult dedicated to that child in the event that the child's needs change is integral to a successful bereavement outcome.

Unlike most adults, children do not exhibit intense emotional and behavioral expressions of grief in a continuous fashion. For example, a typical developmental response for a school-age child might be to exhibit intense signs of grief, followed by a request to play at the neighbor's house. While grief may not be continuous, it can last longer than the grief of adults, with the need to repeat the work of mourning at developmental and chronological milestones.

The bereavement process itself is affected by many factors, including closeness of relationship with the deceased, family functioning, and family style of communication.

Pediatric Palliative Care: What Do Parents Need?

Consistent themes include:
- Effective pain and symptom control for their child
- Direct, sensitive, and clear communication, as influenced by culture and personal preferences
- Collaborative, caring relationships between the child, family, and healthcare team members
- Parent and child involvement in treatment and end of life decision-making, as suited to the child's age and health status
- Readily available healthcare services, which may be continuous proximal to the end of the child's life
- Continued relationships with healthcare professionals in the form of bereavement services

References

1. World Health Organization (2002). *National Cancer Control Programmes: Policies and Managerial Guidelines*, 2nd ed. Geneva: World Health Organization.

2. Field JM, Behrman RE (eds.) (2003). *When Children Die: Improving Palliative and End-of-Life Care for Children and Their Families*. Washington, DC: National Academies Press, pp. 41–71.

3. Health Status Pages. (2012). Child Health USA website. Retrieved May 12, 2014, from http:// mchb.hrsa.gov/chusa12/hs/hsa.html.

4. United States Cancer Statistics (2009). Centers for Disease Control and Prevention website. *2009: By Age (0–14, 0–19) and Cancer Type*. Retrieved May 12, 2014, from https://apps.nccd. cdc.gov/uscs/childhoodcancerbyprimarysite.aspx.

5. Hynson JL, Sawyer SM (2001). Paediatric palliative care: distinctive needs and emerging issues. *J Paediatr Child Health* 37:323–5.

6. Academy of Pediatrics (2014). Patient-and family-centered care coordination: a framework for integrating care for children and youth across multiple systems. *Pediatrics* 133:e1451–60.

7. Baggott C, Dodd M, Kennedy C, Marina N, Miaskowski C. (2009). Multiple symptoms in pediatric oncology patients: a systematic review. *J Pediatr Oncol Nurs* 26:325–39.

8. Wolfe J, Grier HE, Klar N, et al. (2000). Symptoms and suffering at the end of life in children with cancer. *N Engl J Med* 342:326–33.

9. Collins JJ, Byrnes ME, Dunkel IJ, et al. (2000). The measurement of symptoms in children with cancer. *J Pain Symptom Manage* 19:363–77.

10. Collins JJ, Devine TD, Dick GS, et al. (2002). The measurement of symptoms in young children with cancer: the validation of the Memorial Symptom Assessment Scale in children aged 7–12. *J Pain Symptom Manage* 23:10–6.

11. Berde CB, Sethna NF (2002). Analgesics for the treatment of pain in children. *N Engl J Med* 347(14):1094–103.

12. Silverman W, Kurtines W (1996). *Anxiety and Phobic Disorders: A Pragmatic Approach*. New York: Plenum Press.

13. Walk RD (1956). Self-ratings of fear in a fear-invoking situation. *J Abnorm Social Psychol* 52:171–8.

14. Mack JW, Hilden JM, Watternson J, et al. (2005). Parent and physician perspectives on quality of care at the end of life in children with cancer. *J Clin Oncol* 23:9155–61.

15. Mack J, Wolfe J (2006). Early integration of pediatric palliative care: for some children, palliative care starts at diagnosis. *Curr Opin Pediatr* 18:10–4.

16. Himelstein BP, Hilden JM, Boldt AM, Weissman D (2004). Pediatric palliative care. *N Engl J Med* 350:1752–62.

Palliative Care in Older Adults

Brook A. Calton and Christine S. Ritchie

Aging with Chronic Disease

Older adults are living longer with multiple chronic conditions. The number of adults over the age of 65 numbered 43.1 million in 2012, representing 13.7% of the US population. Persons reaching age 65 in the United States have an average life expectancy of an additional 19.2 years (20.4 years for females and 17.8 years for males.[1] Also in 2011, approximately two-thirds (67.3%) of Medicare beneficiaries had two or more chronic conditions (MCC2+), and 14% had six or more.[2]

Given that older adults are surviving into advanced age, many with chronic disease, the majority of hospice diagnoses are now non-cancer-related, for example, congestive heart failure (CHF), chronic obstructive pulmonary disease (COPD), or dementia.

Primary care and palliative care providers need to become familiar with managing the symptoms of chronic disease, as well as prognosticating in the setting of variable chronic disease courses.

Palliative Care Needs in Older Adults

The symptom burden of chronic serious illness is frequently under-recognized and undertreated. In a study of community-dwelling elders age 60 or older with advanced COPD, heart failure, or cancer, 86% reported at least one symptom rated as moderate or severe, and 69% had at least two such symptoms. The most commonly reported symptoms were limited activity (61%), fatigue (47%), and physical discomfort (38%).[3]

Cognitive, motor, visual, or auditory impairments can complicate symptom ascertainment and decision-making in older adults. Furthermore, functional and mobility decline may complicate symptom management in this population—for example, ambulatory function and the ability to get to the bathroom while using diuretics or laxatives, or fall-risk management for frail elders on psychoactive medication who live in multistory housing.

Psychosocial and caregiver support can be tenuous because of spousal loss, social isolation, and geographically dispersed extended families.

Generational and cultural factors may affect a patient's comfort level with caregiving dependence on others. This can be very challenging for patients who embrace a traditionally Western approach to autonomy and independence but are no longer able to function independently because of illness and physical decline.

Settings of Palliative Care and Hospice

Palliative care services, including but not limited to hospice, can be provided in multiple settings, including inpatient, outpatient, and long-term care facilities (Table 28.1). The range and breath of palliative care services in the United States are expanding as our healthcare delivery system and financing evolve.

Outpatient palliative care, including clinic- and home-based palliative care, are covered by Medicare Part B and private insurance companies. Medicare Part A covers the hospice benefit for hospice-eligible patients.

Increasingly, nursing homes have become the site of death for frail, older adults. Unfortunately, older adults who may benefit from both skilled nursing home care for rehabilitation or a skilled need (as opposed to nonskilled institutional care) and hospice care are typically unable to receive both services simultaneously. Medicare Part A will only cover one of these services at a time. Perhaps in part for this reason, there is great opportunity for improving palliative care in nursing homes.

Table 28.1 Settings of Palliative Care and Hospice for Older Adults

Benefit	Goals	Location	Services	Services Excluded	Eligibility	Payer
Inpatient palliative care	Provides palliation of symptoms, spiritual and psychosocial support during a hospitalization with expectation for survival or at the end of life	Hospital	Interprofessional palliative care team including medicine, nursing, social work, and spiritual care		Anyone hospitalized with palliative care needs	Medicare Part A or private insurance
Community-based palliative care	Provides palliation of symptoms, spiritual and psychosocial support in a clinic setting or in the patient's home	Clinic or patient's home	Medical and/or nursing care; team composition is variable		Anyone in the community with palliative care needs	Medicare Part B or private insurance
Skilled nursing facilities	Rehabilitation of physical deconditioning to achieve optimal health and functional autonomy	Long-term care facilities	Physical therapy, occupational therapy, speech therapy, and skilled nursing care. Room and board, medications, and medical supplies are covered.	Prohibits simultaneous enrollment in hospice	Meet skill needs in 3 therapy areas, or have at least one skilled nursing need (e.g., wound care, IV antibiotics, tube feeding, catheter care)	Medicare Part A or private insurance (if under 65 years of age)

Hospice	Provides palliation of symptoms, spiritual and psychosocial support at the end of life	Can provide services at long-term care facilities, residential hospices, inpatient hospices, and at home	Nursing care, medications, supplies, durable medical equipment, pastoral care, social work, personal aid and attendance, bereavement support	Does not pay for room and board in long-term care facilities. Cannot receive Medicare-reimbursed rehabilitation services simultaneously while on hospice	Physician-documented life-limiting illness with a prognosis of 6 months or less	Medicare Part A or private insurance

Barriers to Hospice for Older Adults

The number of adults over age 65 who enroll in hospice services has been rising over time.[4] However, a number of barriers that prevent older adults from accessing hospice services still exist, including the following:

- Absence of caregiver support at home, especially for widowed, older females
- Inability of patient or family to pay for custodial care at a long-term care facility
- Patients' fears of medical abandonment once on hospice.

Goals of Care Discussions

Key considerations when having goals of care discussions with older adults and their families include the following:

- Ageism bias occurs when healthcare providers withhold more aggressive treatments or interventions because of consideration of age alone rather than patient preferences, functional and cognitive abilities, or anticipated survival. People desire prolonged life at all ages. We cannot assume that people of advanced age will necessarily choose against life-prolonging therapy.
- Quality of life, even in the cognitively impaired, is best assessed by the patient, not by proxies or healthcare providers.[5,6] A person's functional capacity and quality of life influence the decision to endure procedures or treatments.[7]
- Prognostication can be challenging as the population lives longer with chronic diseases with variable survival courses (e.g., CHF, COPD, and Alzheimer's disease).
- Patients and families may feel strongly about the continued use of medications for chronic conditions unrelated to terminal illness (e.g., cholesterol medication). The healthcare provider needs to balance the need for rapport-building and trust with reducing unnecessary medications.
- Despite the tendency to approach dementia as if it were a single entity, it is important to recognize that different types of dementia present with different symptoms, clinical courses, and prognoses. Lewy body, vascular, and Alzheimer's dementia all have different clinical presentations and prognoses, necessitating nuanced, disease-specific care planning.

Clinical Pearl

- Age alone should not dictate treatment choices; rather, functional status, expected survival, and patient preferences should be the determining factors.

Biology of Aging and Pharmacokinetics

Decreased renal function, liver size, and hepatic blood flow occur with aging, leading to altered drug metabolism. Body composition also changes with aging, with a greater proportion of body mass composed of fat mass than fat-free mass.

Hydrophilic drugs have a lower volume of distribution due to decreased total body water (fat-free mass) in geriatric patients, leading to an increased risk of toxicity secondary to increased concentration of these medications. Such drugs include ethanol, lithium, and digoxin.

Lipophilic drugs (e.g. benzodiazepines, barbiturates, trazodone) take longer to reach steady state and eliminate because of increased fat stores.

Decreased albumin levels commonly seen in older adults cause increased unbound drug fractions, risking greater drug toxicity, for example, with phenytoin, valproate, benzodiazepines, and warfarin.

Drugs using hepatic phase I pathways (diazepam, propoxyphene, miperidine, tricyclic antidepressants, carisoprodol) produce active metabolites that result in prolonged clinical effects and toxicity. Drugs using phase II pathways (lorazepam) result in inactive metabolites and are preferred in geriatric care.

Given age-related changes in drug metabolism and excretion, psychoactive medications (opioids, sedatives, tricyclic antidepressants) can cause central nervous system toxicity and delirium in older adults.

The general guideline when starting a medication in an older adult is to "start low and go slow," with frequent reassessments for efficacy and side effects.

Clinical Pearl

- Psychoactive medications commonly used in palliative care increase risk for delirium in older adults.

Symptom Management in Geriatric Populations

As noted previously, cognitive, motor, visual, or auditory impairments in older adults can make symptom assessment and management challenging. The side effects from medications and drug–drug/drug–disease interactions in older adults can further complicate this important task.

Infection

Prolonged or recurrent antibiotic use can cause side effects (nausea, decreased appetite, diarrhea, infectious colitis, yeast infections) and drug resistance. However, antibiotic use at the end of life may decrease symptom burden and therefore improve quality of life, even when it does not prolong survival.[8]

Pressure Ulcers

Despite excellent skin care and pressure relief, pressure ulcers can be difficult to avoid at the end of life. Pressures ulcers tend to heal poorly in malnourished, frail older adults, particularly those with mobility limitations and incontinence.

Pressure ulcers are easier to prevent than to heal. Prevention measures include pressure-relieving mattresses, frequent turning, and good perineal hygiene.

In patients who are actively dying, the goal is to effectively manage symptoms. Metronidazole gel and frequent dressing changes help odor control and drainage. Patients should be premedicated as needed for incident pain from dressing changes.

Pain

Many providers erroneously assume that older adults do not experience pain as intensely as younger patient populations.

Pain from a terminal illness may be complicated by pain from chronic underlying conditions, such as osteoarthritis, which are frequently unrecognized and undertreated.

Pain assessment in cognitively impaired adults may require observation for nonverbal pain behaviors (grimacing, crying, withdrawing, behavioral and sleep disturbances, diminished appetite).

Acetaminophen is a good first-line agent for mild to moderate pain in older adults, at appropriate dosing for liver function.

Any pain complaint that affects physical function or quality of life should be recognized as a significant problem. Pharmacologic therapy, including but not limited to carefully titrated opioids, should be considered for patients who experience functional impairment or a reduction in quality of life from their pain.

Avoid use of medications such as NSAIDs (risk of GI upset, GI bleeding, and renal toxicity), opioids with toxic metabolites (miperidine, propoxyphene), and tricyclic antidepressants for neuropathic pain.

Exercise caution with sustained-release opioid preparations in patients with renal impairment because of the risk of increased neurotoxicity. In such circumstances, it is safer to use cleaner metabolizing, short-acting opioids, such as oxycodone.

Nausea and Vomiting

Use caution when initiating antiemetics in older adults.

- Metoclopramide can cause extrapyramidal side effects.
- Promethazine and benzodiazepines increase the risk of falls and can cause delirium.
- Steroids can precipitate delirium.
- Anti-emetics, including ondansetron and prochlorperazine, can worsen constipation.

Constipation

Many geriatric patients do not drink adequate fluids or have fluid restrictions placed for cardiac or renal conditions.

Ensure adequate fluid intake—a mainstay of constipation management.

Older patients should avoid fiber and bulking agents in opioid-induced constipation because of prolonged gut transit time, resulting in increased water reabsorption and risk for obstruction.

Anticholinergic medications (bladder antispasmodics, antihistamines, tricyclic antidepressants) and calcium channel blockers all worsen constipation. Bowel stimulants and osmotic agents are both effective in the treatment of constipation in older adults.

Diarrhea

Consider medication-induced causes (recent antibiotic use, chemotherapy) or infectious causes (*Clostridium difficile* colitis) of diarrhea.

Rule out infection before empirically using an antidiarrheal agent in patients who have recently taken antibiotics or who live in an institutional facility.

Consider using loperamide rather than diphenoxylate as it crosses the blood-brain barrier less and therefore induces fewer CNS side effects.

Cough

Some medications, such as calcium channel blockers and angiotensin-converting enzyme (ACE) inhibitors, can induce chronic cough weeks to months after initiation of the medication.

Gastric reflux can cause coughing and should be considered in patients who are tube fed.

Oral Complaints

Poor dentition, ill-fitting dentures from weight loss, oral candidiasis, and oral ulcerations can cause discomfort, resulting in decreased oral intake. A careful oral examination can identify these conditions and foster appropriate management.

Depression and Anxiety

Depression is often under-recognized in older adults, as they may not acknowledge "feeling depressed" because of perceived social stigmas associated with depression. The Geriatric Depression Scale (GDS) is a good clinical tool for capturing unrecognized depressive behaviors.

Stimulants, such as methylphenidate, can quickly improve depressive symptoms in advanced terminal illness. Guided by the patient's goals of care, the decision to prescribe stimulants should be considered carefully in patients with a history of cardiac arrhythmia, coronary artery disease, CHF, or stroke.

SSRIs, such as citalopram and sertraline, are generally well tolerated in older adults. They can, however, contribute to hyponatremia, particularly in patients who are at risk for hyponatremia from volume overload conditions.

Incontinence

Fecal and urinary incontinence are common in older adults with mobility, cognitive, and neurogenic impairments. Incontinence is an important cause of institutionalization.

Strategies for treating functional urinary incontinence include rearranging furniture to optimize safe navigation to the toilet, arranging for assistance, bedside commodes, eliminating restraints, scheduling voids, limiting fluid intake before bed, and treating depression.

Kegel exercises, timed voiding, and, after these strategies are tried, anticholinergics can help with urge incontinence. Of note, anticholinergics can cause delirium, severe bladder retention, constipation, and dry mouth, requiring close monitoring for tolerance.

Long-term in-dwelling Foley catheters promote recurrent urinary tract infection and antibiotic resistance, so risks and benefits should be carefully considered.

Long-term use of rectal tubes is not advised.

Mobility and Sensory Impairment

Both mobility and sensory impairment increase the risk of falls, particularly if psychoactive medications are being used.

Decreased proprioception and hand coordination make self-care and medication administration difficult (e.g., glucose monitoring, shot administration, and opening pill bottles). Such impairments challenge patients and caregivers, contributing to the decision to institutionalize.

Insomnia

Insomnia results from sleep-cycle changes, medication use (some antidepressants, chemotherapy, steroids, sedatives/somniferents), day and nighttime inversion in dementia, occult alcohol use, and poor sleep hygiene.

A thorough assessment for the cause of insomnia should be undertaken, including addressing behavioral issues and uncontrolled symptoms. If medication is needed, low-dose trazodone is recommended as a safe first choice. Low-dose mirtazapine may improve both insomnia and appetite stimulation in patients suffering from anorexia.

Tricyclic antidepressants should be avoided because of anticholinergic side effects, causing delirium and falls.

Use caution when prescribing benzodiazepines and zolpidem because of the risk of delirium and falls. In geriatric populations, lorazepam is the preferred benzodiazepine.

Nutrition

Taste and smell diminish as we age, lowering appetite. In dementia, dietary modification using salty, sweet, and sour flavors can improve appetite, as can temperature adjustment (hot instead of cold dishes).

Modified consistencies, such as pureed foods, and tube feeding are often less appealing to patients, even though they may be safer in the setting of dysphagia. Value judgments weighing quality of life versus swallowing safety need to be assessed by the care team, patient, and family.

Cognitive Impairment and Delirium

Regardless of whether cognitive impairment is mild or severe, patients are at increased risk for delirium. Delirium in cognitively impaired individuals may last as long as weeks to months following the precipitating event(s).

Delirium is often multifactorial, resulting from the underlying terminal illness, drugs, infection, dehydration, or change in environmental circumstances (e.g., hospitalization).

In addition to treating the underlying causes, short-term use of haloperidol for behavioral disturbances is helpful.

If antipsychotic use is anticipated to last for months, atypical neuroleptics (quetiapine, risperdal, olanzapine) usually result in fewer extrapyramidal side effects. However, the practitioner must weigh the increased risk of cerebrovascular events and mortality in patients with dementia who take these medications for extended periods of time.[9]

Quetiapine is usually the antipsychotic of choice in the setting of Parkinsonism.

Ethical and Social Issues

Artificial Hydration and Nutrition

There is no clear evidence that tube feeding of institutionalized patients with dementia prolongs survival. Since different types of dementia have different clinical presentations and survival courses, we cannot assume that tube feeding uniformly provides the same survival benefits.[10]

The American Geriatrics Society (AGS) recommends careful hand feeding for older adults with advanced dementia who can no longer feed themselves over feeding tube placement.[11]

Proxy and Decision-Making

Patients with mild to moderate cognitive impairment are able to express preferences for treatments and interventions, even when they cannot provide formal consent. A common dilemma is when a patient's prior living will or advance directive does not coincide with expressed preferences once the person is cognitively impaired.

While this predicament involves value judgments, it is important for patient proxies and healthcare providers to be sensitive to the patient's preferences, since cooperation is necessary for successful treatment and care planning.

Financial Interdependence

It is not uncommon for spouses and family members to resist the institutionalization of a loved one if they are still dependent on the patient for housing or financial support.

Medicaid protects spouses against losing their homes in the setting of a Medicaid spend-down but does not extend the same benefit to adult children or other family members living in the patient's home. This dilemma is ethically challenging if the healthcare provider feels that the patient is not getting adequate care or supervision at home and needs institutionalization.

Existential Suffering

Many older adults endure the loss of a spouse, face marginal caregiving support, and shoulder economic worries due to constrained income. Autonomy may be tenuous at best, only to become logistically and functionally compromised after the diagnosis of a life-limiting illness.

The way in which older adults face these challenges is often framed through cultural and religious lenses. These concerns lead to fears of institutionalization and abandonment for many elders. Such fears can compromise the fluid communication of needs between patients and healthcare providers, underscoring the importance of a "whole-patient assessment" of needs.

Proper use of the interdisciplinary team model, through social work assistance, pastoral care, and psychology support services, can improve resource access and help patients cope with anxiety and stress.

Care of the Caregiver

Compared to younger patients, older patients are frequently more dependent in activities of daily living (bathing, dressing, toileting, eating, transferring) and instrumental activities of daily living (banking, shopping, cleaning). This dependency may be physically and emotionally challenging for caregivers of all ages.

Older, frail spouses or siblings often care for their loved ones at home, potentially jeopardizing caregiver well-being. This makes the patient vulnerable to institutionalization if the caregiver falls ill or dies.

Working-age caregivers frequently forego employment to provide informal care for a loved one, resulting in economic losses for the caregiver. In 2010, in the United States, the individual economic losses of caregiving were estimated to be $324,044 for women, and $283,716 for men.[1,2] Social work services can help families identify and maximize available resources to help reduce caregiving strain.

When institutionalization does occur, it can produce feelings of guilt in caregivers of all ages.

When an older spouse, sibling, or adult child cares for a patient during a protracted illness, the caregiver is at risk for complicated grief and depression after the caregiving role is lost, particularly in families with enmeshed emotional dynamics. The risk for complicated grief should be explored by the interdisciplinary team prior to the patient's death. Team members should probe for suicidal ideation.

Palliative psychology support services and contact with caregiver support groups can help surviving family members cope with loss.

Clinical Pearl

- Caregivers are at higher risk for depression, mortality, and complicated grief when their care recipient dies.

References

1. Administration on Aging, Administration for Community Living, Department of Health and Human Services (2013). *A Profile of Older Americans, 2013.*
2. Lochner KA, Goodman RA, Posner S, Parekh A. (2013). Multiple chronic conditions among Medicare beneficiaries: state-level variations in prevalence, utilization, and cost, 2011. *Medicare Medicaid Res Rev* 23(3):3.
3. Walke LM, Gallo WT, Tinetti ME, Fried TR (2004). The burden of symptoms among community-dwelling older persons with advanced chronic disease. *Arch Intern Med* 164(21):2321–4.
4. National Hospice and Palliative Care Organization (2015). *NHPCO's Facts and Figures: Hospice Care in America.*
5. Hoe J, Katona C, Orrell M, Livingston G (2007). Quality of life in dementia: care recipient and caregiver perceptions of quality of life in dementia: the LASER-AD study. *Int J Geriatr Psychiatry* 22(10):1031–6.
6. Berlowitz DR, Du W, Kazis L, Lewis S (1995). Health-related quality of life of nursing home residents: differences in patient and provider perceptions. *J Am Geriatr Soc* 43(7):799–802.
7. McCarthy EP, Pencina MJ, Kelly-Hayes M, et al. (2008). Advance care planning and health care preferences of community-dwelling elders: the Framingham Heart Study. *J Gerontol A Biol Sci Med Sci* 63(9):951–9.
8. Van der Steen JT, Ooms ME, van der Wal G, Ribbe MW (2002). Pneumonia: the demented patient's best friend? Discomfort after starting or withholding antibiotic treatment. *J Am Geriatr Soc* 50(10):1681–8.
9. Schneider LS, Dagerman KS, Insel P (2005). Risk of death with atypical antipsychotic drug treatment for dementia: meta-analysis of randomized placebo-controlled tirals. *JAMA* 294(15):1934–43.

10. Casarett D, Kapo J, Caplan A (2005). Appropriate use of artificial nutrition and hydration: funda-mental principles and recommendations. *N Engl J Med* 353(24):2607–12.
11. American Geriatrics Society (2013). *Feeding Tubes in Advanced Dementia Position Statement*.
12. MetLife Mature Market Group, National Alliance for Caregiving (2011). *Study of Working Caregivers and Employer Health Costs: Double Jeopardy for Baby Boomers Caring for Their Parents*. New York: Metropolitan Life Insurance Company.

Further Reading

Brown JA, Von Roenn JH (2004). Symptom management in the older adult. *Clin Geriatr Med* 20(4):621–40.
Duncan JG, Forbes-Thompson S, Bott MJ (2008). Unmet symptom management needs of nursing home residents with cancer. *Cancer Nurs* 31(4):265–73.
Evers MM, Meier DE, Morrison RS (2002). Assessing differences in care needs and service utiliza-tion in geriatric palliative care patients. *J Pain Symptom Manage* 23(5):424–32.
Meier D, Monias A (2004). Palliative medicine and care of the elderly. In: Doyle D, Hanks G, Cherny N, Calman KC (eds.), *Oxford Textbook of Palliative Medicine*, 3rd ed. Oxford: Oxford University Press, pp. 935–44.
Schwartz CE, Wheeler HB, Hammes B, et al. (2002) Early intervention in planning end-of-life care with ambulatory geriatric patients: results of a pilot trial. *Arch Intern Med* 162(14):1611–8.
Wijnia JW, Corstiaensen IJ (2008). A poor prognosis: guide or misleading? *Am J Hosp Palliat Care* 25(1):5–8.

Palliative Care in End-Stage Heart Failure

José L. Ramos and Marieberta Vidal

Introduction

The syndrome of heart failure is one of the most common constellation findings encountered in medicine today. It accounts for at least 20% of medical admissions to all hospitals for patients older than 65 years of age. It is, of course, quite prevalent in terminally ill patients, not only as a primary diagnosis but also as a complication of other disease processes. It is important to recognize this syndrome and some of its most common causes in order to be an effective palliative care team.

The definition of heart failure can be summarized as (1) the inability of the heart to deal with the metabolic demands of the body, and (2) the constellation of symptoms associated with this phenomena. In essence, this syndrome has different stages that can roughly be divided into acute decompensation and chronic disease.

The *acute* syndrome of heart failure, better known as congestive heart failure (CHF), is not a specific disease but rather a collection of symptoms, physical findings, and classic laboratory findings that help the clinician develop a differential diagnosis of more specific disease entities.

Very much like a fever, which can help the clinician narrow the differential diagnosis, it is best to think of the phenomena of CHF as a symptom or problem, rather than a specific disease process. In contrast, the patient with *chronic* heart failure has some, but certainly not all, of the many characteristic findings of congestive heart failure.

One of the most challenging aspects is diagnosis, as many other diseases can mimic the syndrome.

Epidemiology

Cardiac disease was listed as the most common cause of death in the United States in 2010. With life expectancy hitting a record high in 2010 and Centers for Disease Prevention and Control (CDC) data showing the average life expectancy of white males to be 76.5 years, black males 71.8 years, white females 81.3 years, and black females 78.0 years, it is likely that most of us will develop some sort of cardiac issues before our death. In 2010, 57,757 deaths were caused by heart failure in the United States.

The physical and psychological symptom burden in patients dying from heart failure is similar to that in patients dying from terminal cancer. Table 29.1 illustrates some of the common symptomatology suffered by patients with heart failure.

Fatigue, difficulty ambulating, and edema are other common symptoms that can at times be alleviated with maximal medical management, which should be continued until the burden of administration outweighs the benefits.

Table 29.1 Common Symptoms Experienced by Patients with Heart Failure and Common Interventions

Symptom	Affected	Intervention
Pain	78%	Identify etiology, if possible
		Consider opioids for angina
Dyspnea	61%	Optimize medication
		Treat reversible causes—effusions, dysrhythmias, COPD
Depression	59%	Screen for hypoactive delirium, screen for chemical coping, CAGE*
		Consider SSRI, use psychostimulants with caution**
Insomnia	45%	Screen for delirium
		Screen for depression
		Treat reversible causes, i.e., pain or dyspnea
Anorexia	43%	Screen for treatable causes—depression, delirium, constipation
Anxiety	30%	Screen for delirium, depression, spiritual, or emotional suffering
		Consider SSRI
Constipation	37%	Monitor fluid balance
Nausea/ Vomiting	32%	Appropriate bowel program when using opioids Optimize anti-emetic regimen Naso-gastric tube for decompression

* CAGE = Cut back, Annoyed, Guilt, Eye opener.

** The drugs of choice are still the SSRIs because they preserve ejection fraction, lack hypotensive and dysrhythmogenic effects, and have few drug interactions. There are no data documenting the safety of psychostimulants in heart failure, thus they should be initiated with caution.

Medical Management

Medical management of CHF has been refined over the past 10 years. The efforts at medical management are to improve the symptoms suffered by those with the disease. In palliative care, all efforts should be made to ensure that patients are receiving evidence-based medical management.

Systolic Dysfunction versus Diastolic Dysfunction

The causes of heart failure are many, and an exhaustive list is beyond the scope of this chapter. The palliative care team should be aware of the most common types of heart failure.

Roughly, patients should be divided into two groups: those with systolic dysfunction and those with diastolic dysfunction (sometimes referred to a congestive heart failure with normal left ventricular systolic function). The 2D echocardiogram is the most reliable and widely available diagnostic test used for this purpose. Most patients will have this information available before a palliative medicine consult is called.

Patients with predominantly diastolic heart failure are typically less complicated to treat. Most of these patients will have hypertensive heart disease. Treatment for these patients is usually directed at blood pressure management with a variety of agents (i.e., β-blockers, ACE inhibitors, angiotensin II receptor blockers [ARBs], calcium channel blockers, hydralazine, nitroglycerin [NTG], etc.). However, diuretics are also frequently employed in the management of this syndrome.

In the patient whose pain is being managed, careful review of medications must be done to identify medications that may antagonize the effects of diuretics or affect renal function (e.g., NSAIDs).

Patients with systolic dysfunction usually present a more difficult task to the clinician. While the mainstay of treatment is with similar agents, as with the previous syndrome, symptoms can be significantly more refractory to treatment. These patients tend to have multi-organ failure by the time they are referred to palliative care, so special care must be taken with the use of certain drugs that may exacerbate end-organ damage.

Changing oral diuretics to the intravenous or subcutaneous route can produce symptom relief within minutes. Furosemide is the mainstay of treatment and usually is used in incremental doses until symptoms subside or improve. Significant renal toxicity can result from aggressive use of these agents.

Because of this risk of renal toxicity and, ultimately, failure, patients on opioids, particularly morphine, should be opioid rotated to an agent that is not primarily cleared by the kidneys.

Intravenous Inotrope Therapy

Agents such as dobutamine, milrinone, and dopamine have a substantial record of use but lack data on their use in the home setting. While these agents may help to improve symptoms, the data show an increased risk of death. Intravenous inotrope therapy may allow hospitalized inotrope-dependent heart failure patients to be transferred to die at home.

The cost of these agents may be prohibitive to some hospices because of the capitated reimbursement system. They may be more feasible in the home health setting with the addition of hospice once the infusions are stopped.

Device Therapies

Cardiac Pacemakers in Advanced Heart Failure and at End of Life

Patients with congestive heart failure have been known to benefit from biventricular pacemakers for palliating and improving symptoms. This section will focus not on the selection of patients for a pacemaker but rather on the pacer's function at the time of death, indications for deactivation, and other end-of-life issues.

Each year over 1 million new pacemakers are implanted, and the majority are implanted in the United States (> 235,000 implants) and in patients over the age of 60.

Do Pacemakers Prolong the Dying Process?

Pacemakers do not prolong the dying process, as they are not resuscitative devices. When the patient is in the active stages of dying, the myocardium is usually too sick to respond to the pacemaker-generated signals.

When Is Pacer Deactivation Indicated?

Most patients are not pacer-dependent, particularly during the active stages of dying, when the most common rhythm is tachycardia. When a pacemaker's role is not meeting the goals of care, a family meeting to discuss expectations on its role should take place with the patient, family, primary medical team, and interdisciplinary team.

Routine deactivation is not recommended, as this can lead to bradycardia, which can produce worsening symptoms of heart failure such as dyspnea and fatigue. Family education should focus on what the pacemaker does *not* do, which is to prolong the dying stage and thus prolong suffering.

If an interdisciplinary discussion leads to the decision to deactivate the pacemaker, the cardiology team and pacemaker service should be informed of the decision. A patient's right to request withdrawal of life-sustaining medical interventions, including pacemakers, is legal and ethical.

During this time, advance directives and code status should be discussed with the patient and family and documented.

Implantable Cardioverter Defibrillator (ICD) at the End of Life

The purpose of an implantable cardioverter defibrillator (ICD) is to monitor cardiac rhythm and deliver electric cardioversion when ventricular tachycardias are detected. It has been shown that ICD therapy significantly prolongs life in patients at increased risk for sudden cardiac death from depressed left ventricular function. However, whether this increased longevity is accompanied by deterioration in the quality of life is unclear.

ICDs can also deliver pacing therapy aimed at increasing the heart rate when slow rhythms are detected by the device. The pacing and shocking capabilities of an ICD can be managed independently of each other.

ICDs and Quality of Life

In a randomized trial, ICD therapy or amiodarone was compared with state-of-the-art medical therapy alone in 2521 patients who had stable heart failure with depressed left ventricular function. Quality of life was retrospectively measured at baseline and at 3, 12, and 30 months after the ICD was implanted. No clinically or statistically significant differences in physical functioning between the study groups were observed.

Psychological well-being in the ICD group, as compared with medical therapy alone, was significantly improved at 3 months ($p = 0.01$) and at 12 months ($p = 0.003$) but not at 30 months. Additional quality-of-life measures were improved in the ICD group at 3 months, 12 months, or both, but there was no significant difference at 30 months. ICD shocks in the month preceding a scheduled assessment were associated with a decreased quality of life.

The use of amiodarone had no significant effects on the primary quality-of-life outcomes.

Turning Off an ICD

Indications

When a patient or family requests the deactivation of an ICD, this is acceptable both legally and ethically. This is done when an ICD is inconsistent with the patient's goals of care, when an antiarrhythmic medication is withdrawn and there is concern of impending arrhythmias, when death is imminent, or when the patient and family are concerned about the inconsistencies of having a functioning ICD and a DNR or AND (allow for natural death) directive. Turning off the ICD also prevents the patient from the discomfort of having unwanted therapeutic shocks whose therapeutic effects are not in line with the current goals of care, and saves the family from the distress of seeing their loved one convulsing in front of them.

Family and Patient Discussion

The physician primarily responsible for the ICD and the device company that has been monitoring the ICD should be informed of the patient's decision to deactivate the ICD. This can provide a level of comfort and closure for the patient and family and involve the ICD's primary medical team in the decision-making and goals of care.

At this point, it is important to discuss expectations once the ICD is deactivated and to answer any related questions or concerns. With an actively dying patient, families often expect that the patient will expire immediately after the ICD is deactivated. Families should be educated on what to expect; most patients do not expire immediately after deactivation. Rather, the disease must continue to follow its normal course. The majority of patients die within 1 month of device deactivation, and this may reflect the gravity of the underlying illness.

Deactivation

The cardiologist or electrophysiologist and device company are contacted, and arrangements are made for deactivation. Advance directives should be discussed and documented, and the patient and family must understand that the goal of deactivation is to allow for natural death.

If a patient and family expect heroics at the time of death, the goals of care must be discussed to clarify the purpose of deactivation of the ICD. It is important to note that most device manufacturers will not send representatives to a patient's home for the purpose of deactivating the device. These issues are best handled before the patient is discharged from the hospital.

Left Ventricular Assist Devices (LVADs)

Many types of LVADs have been developed to assist patients with advanced heart disease. Most devices consist of an axial flow pump that provides a significant amount of blood flow to the body in the setting of severe systolic left ventricular heart failure.

The original intent of these devices was to provide a bridge to transplant; however, with the advent of smaller, easier-to-insert devices, they are now used for a variety of purposes, from destination therapy to ultra high-risk percutaneous revascularization.

The lack of heart donors and the prolonged survival of heart failure patients have led to applications of LVADs that were not previously expected. Patients previously too sick to undergo revascularization can now be treated effectively with the aid of these devices.

The palliative care team must collaborate closely with the cardiovascular team and must be aware of this very dynamic area of medicine.

Mortality after LVAD Implantation

The 1-year survival after LVAD implantation was up to 85%. The in-hospital mortality after LVAD surgery has improved to 34.1% with a range of 16.9%–44.5% depending on the volume of experience of the care team. Main causes of death included sepsis, right heart failure, and multi-organ failure. The most important determinants of in-hospital mortality were poor nutrition, hematological abnormalities, markers of end-organ or right ventricular dysfunction, and lack of inotropic support.

The appropriate selection of candidates and the timing of LVAD implantation are critical for improved outcomes of destination therapy.

Quality of Life after LVAD Implantation

The overall quality of life of patients with LVAD implantation as a destination therapy can be adversely affected in some cases by serious infections, neurological complications, and device malfunction. LVADs alter end-of-life trajectories, and caregivers of recipients may experience significant caregiver burden and financial strain. Thus, appropriate informed consent is vital.

Ethical Challenges with LVADs as Destination Therapy

Because LVADs can prolong the survival of average recipients over that with optimal medical management of chronic end-stage heart failure, which affects quality of life and increases caregiver burden, it is vital that recipients and their caregivers receive adequate informed consent.

Early use of a palliative care approach is recommended when use of an LVAD as a destination therapy is being considered, as this approach will help make the process a well-informed one.

Recommendations regarding a palliative care approach to LVAD use include, but are not limited to, the following:

- Participation of a multidisciplinary care team, including palliative care specialists
- A concise plan of care for anticipated device-related complications
- Careful surveillance, counseling, and community support for caregivers, to minimize caregiver burden
- Advance care planning for anticipated end-of-life trajectories and timing of device deactivation when it no longer benefits or supports the patient's goals of care
- A plan to address the long-term financial burden on patients, families, and caregivers
- Appropriate spiritual and emotional support for recipients as their devices alter end-of-life trajectories.

Prognostication

Providing accurate prognostic data for 6- to 12-month morality in heart failure is nearly impossible. Many factors are involved, including the unpredictability of disease trajectory, high risk of sudden death, disparities in the application of evidence-based guidelines, and other issues.

Based on data from the SUPPORT study, Framingham study, and IMPROVEMENT, 1-year mortality estimates are as follows:

- Class II (mild symptoms): 5%–10% mortality
- Class III (moderate symptoms): 10%–15% mortality
- Class IV (severe symptoms): 30%–40% mortality.

Other factors associated with a limited prognosis are listed in Table 29.2.

Appropriate Referrals to Hospice

Given the difficulty in prognosticating the last 6 months of life in heart failure patients, hospice referrals are usually made very late in the course of the illness. The 1996 National Hospice and Palliative Care Organization (NHPCO) criteria are not predictors of a 6- to 12-month mortality. These criteria can, however, serve as guidelines to aid clinicians in identifying the decline of a patient and helping hospice staff focus their documentation when re-certifying a patient for hospice benefits.

A clinician should simply ask the question, "Would I be surprised if this patient died in the next 6 months?" If the answer is "no," the patient would be best served by being referred to hospice. This decision should also involve the cardiovascular specialist because of the complexity of therapies and prognostic trajectories.

NHPCO criteria include the following:

1. Symptoms of recurrent heart failure at rest NYHA class IV
2. Optimal medical management
3. Ejection fraction of < 20%
4. Treatment-resistant ventricular or supraventricular arrhythmias
5. History of cardiac arrest in any setting
6. History of unexplained syncope
7. Cardiogenic brain embolism
8. Concomitant HIV disease.

Table 29.2 Factors Associated with a Limited Prognosis in Heart Failure

Factor	Effect on Prognosis
Recent cardiac hospitalization	Triples 1-year mortality
SBP < 100 mmHG and/or pulse >100 bpm	Each doubles 1-year mortality
Hospitalized heart failure patient with acute decompensation BUN > 43 mg/dL Creatinine > 2.75 mg/dL SBP < 115 mmHg	*In-hospital mortality rates* 2% for 0/3 risk factors 20% for 3/3 risk factors
Anemia	Each 1 g/dL reduction associated with a 16% increase in mortality

Further Reading

1. Verma A, Solomon SD (2007). Optimizing care of heart failure after acute MI with an aldosterone receptor antagonist. *Curr Heart Fail Rep* 4(4): 183–9.

2. Mark DB, Anstrom KJ, Su JL, et al. (2008). Quality of life with defibrillator therapy or amiodarone in heart failure. *N Engl J Med* 359(10): 999–1008.

3. MacIver J, Rao V, Delgado DH (2008). Choices: a study of preferences for end-of-life treatments in patients with advanced heart failure. *J Heart Lung Transplant* 27(9):1002–7.

4. Powell LH, Calvin JE Jr, Mendes de Leon CF, et al. (2008). The Heart Failure Adherence and Retention Trial (HART): design and rationale. *Am Heart J* 156(3):452–60.

5. Holst M, Strömberg A, Lindholm M, Willenheimer R (2008). Description of self-reported fluid intake and its effects on body weight, symptoms, quality of life and physical capacity in patients with stable chronic heart failure. *J Clin Nurs* 17(17):2318–26.

6. Rizzieri AG, Verheijde JL, Rady MY, McGregor JL (2008). Ethical challenges with the left ventricular assist device as a destination therapy. *Philos Ethics Humanit Med* 3:20.

7. Lietz K, Long JW, Kfoury AD, et al. (2007). Outcomes of left ventricular assist device implantation as destination therapy in the post-REMATCH era: implications for patient selection. *Circulation* 116(5):497–505.

8. Bieniarz MC, Delgado R (2007). The financial burden of destination left ventricular assist device therapy: who and when? *Curr Cardiol Rep* 9(3):194–9.

9. Harrington MD, Luebke DL, Lewis WR, Aulisio MP, Johnson NJ (2004). Cardiac pacemakers at end of life. *Fast Facts and Concepts #111*. Retrieved December 28, 2010, from http://www.eperc.mcw.edu/fastfact/ff_111.htm.

10. Harrington MD, Luebke DL, Lewis WR, Aulisio MP, Johnson NJ (2004). Implantable cardioverter defibrillator (ICD) at end of life. *Fast Facts and Concepts #112*. Retrieved December 28, 2010, from http://www.eperc.mcw.edu/fastfact/ff_112.htm.

11. Reisfield GM, Wilson GR (2009). Prognostication in heart failure. *Fast Facts and Concepts #143*. Retrieved May 20, 2014, from http://www.eperc.mcw.edu/fastfact/ff_143.htm.

12. Reisfield GM, Wilson GR (2009). Palliative care issues in heart failure. *Fast Facts and Concepts #144*. Retrieved May 20, 2014, from http://www.eperc.mcw.edu/fastfact/ff_144.htm.

13. Murphy SL, Xu J, Kochanek KD (2013). Deaths: final data for 2010. *Natl Vital Stat Rep* 61(4). Retrieved May 20, 2014, from http://www.cdc.gov/nchs/data/nvsr/nvsr61/nvsr61_04.pdf.

14. Mond HG, Proclemer A (2011). The 11th World Survey of Cardiac Pacing and Implantable Cardioverter-Defibrillators: Calendar Year 2009–A World Society of Arrhythmia's Project. *PACE* 34:1013–27.

15. Buchhalter LC, Ottenberg AL, Webster TL, Swetz KM, Hayes DL, Mueller PS (2014). Features and outcomes of patients who underwent cardiac device deactivation. *JAMA Intern Med* 174(1):80–5.

16. Butler K, Puri S. (2014). Deathbed shock: causes and cures. *JAMA Intern Med* 174(1):88–9.

17. John R, Naka Y, Smedira NG, Starling R, Jorde U, Eckman P, Farrar DJ, Pagani FD. (2011). Continuous flow left ventricular assist device outcomes in commercial use compared with the prior clinical trial. *Ann Thorac Surg* 92(4):1406–13.

18. Shah N, Chothani A, Patel N, et al. (2014). Impact of annual operator volume on in-hospital mortality after left ventricular assist device (LVAD) implantation in advanced heart failure patients from 1998 to 2009: an analysis of 5,093 procedures. *J Am Coll Cardiol* 63(12_S). doi:10.1016/S0735-1097(14)60881-0.

Palliative Care in End-Stage Liver Disease

Valentina Medici and Frederick J. Meyers

End-stage liver disease (ESLD) is characterized by significant physical and emotional suffering. Patients with ESLD should receive intensive palliative care, to a degree that increases as the disease progresses; this care should be responsive to patient and family needs, and should include timely hospice referral. In addition, hospice referral and liver transplant evaluation should be considered simultaneously in patients with ESLD. When patients with ESLD are removed from the liver transplant waiting list, they often are not considered for palliative care, and the goals of care are infrequently discussed.[1]

Definition, Prevalence, and Consequences

End-stage liver disease (ESLD) is the final result of various pathophysiological disturbances that underlie chronic liver diseases (Table 30.1).

All of these chronic processes end in the histologic finding of cirrhosis, characterized by diffuse fibrosis and abnormal regenerative nodules of hepatocytes. This architecture leads to portal hypertension.

Signs of the increased portal pressure include esophageal and gastric varices, ascites, splenomegaly, and peripheral edema, whereas hepatocyte dysfunction leads to hepatic encephalopathy, coagulopathy, hypersplenism with pancytopenia, renal failure, malnutrition, and hepatocellular carcinoma.

Prevalence and Mortality

About 5.5 million people (2% of the US population) are affected by cirrhosis, with approximately 26,000 deaths each year, making this condition one of the leading cause of terminal illness among people aged 25–65.[2]

In the United States, 20,000 patients with advanced ESLD are waiting for liver transplantation, but with the scarcity of living and cadaveric donors (about 5000 yearly), most ESLD patients will not receive a graft and will need medical management (Table 30.2). All will require palliation.

Table 30.1 Etiologies of Chronic Liver Disease

Chronic hepatitis related to infectious agents	HCV
	HBV/HDV
	HIV-associated hepatobiliary disease
	Protozoan amoebiasis
	Malaria
	Toxoplasmosis
Toxic injury-related liver diseases	Alcohol
	Nonalcoholic fatty liver disease and nonalcoholic steatohepatitis
	Drug-induced liver diseases
Immune system-related diseases	Autoimmune hepatitis
	Primary biliary cirrhosis
	Primary sclerosis cholangitis
Genetic diseases	Hemochromatosis
	Wilson disease
	α_1-Antitrypsin deficiency
Other	Amyloidosis
	Budd–Chiari syndrome

Table 30.2 Management of the Most Common Signs and Symptoms of End-Stage Liver Disease

Sign/Symptom	Treatment	Dose	Note
Ascites	Sodium restriction (2 g/daily)		Increase the diuretics dose once a week, checking electrolytes levels.
	Spironolactone	50–400 mg daily	
	Fursomide	20–150 mg daily	
	Paracentesis	if > 4 liters with IV albumin	
	TIPS		TIPS frequently induces encephalopathy.
Spontaneous bacterial peritonitis (SBP)	Cefotaxime	2 g every 8 hours	After SBP resolution with IV antibiotics, prophylactic therapy with norfloxacin 400 mg daily for an indefinite time is recommended.
	Albumin	1.5 g/kg of body weight at diagnosis followed by 1 g/kg of body weight on day 3	Oral treatment can be considered in inpatients without vomiting, shock, encephalopathy ≥ grade 2, with creatinine < 3 mg/dL.
	Ofloxacin	400 mg twice daily	
Hyponatriemia	Recommend water restriction when Na⁺ ≤ 120 mmol/L		Volume expansion with colloid or saline might be recommended.
			Avoid increasing serum sodium by 12 mmol/L per 24 hours.
Hyperkaliemia	Stop spironolactone; start kayexalate	15 g 1–4 times daily	In case of severe hyperkalemia
Hepatic encephalopathy	Lactulose	Titrated to 3–4 bowel movements daily	Protein restriction is recommended only at the onset of severe hepatic encephalopathy.
	Rifaximin	550 mg two times daily	

Esophageal varices	β-blockers: Propranolol	20 mg twice daily	β-blockers can induce fatigue and dizziness. Relative contraindications are peripheral vasculopathy and insulin-dependent diabetes with recurrent hypoglycemia.
	Nadolol	40 mg daily	Nadolol might be associated with fewer side effects.
	Endoscopic variceal ligation TIPS		
Pruritus	Cholestyramine	4 g 3–4 times daily	
	Ursodiol	15–30 mg/kg daily	
	Rifampin	150–300 mg twice daily	
Hepatorenal syndrome	Octreotide	100–200 mg SC three times daily	Maximum of 2 months
	Midodrine	7.5–12.5 mg orally three times daily	
	Albumin 20%	20–40 g IV daily	
	Ornipressin	2–6 IU/h IV 3 days	3 days
	Albumin 20%	2–6 IU/h IV 3 days	
	Terlipressin	0.5–2 mg IV every 4 hours	Maximum of 15 days
	Albumin 20% 20–40 g IV daily		

TIPS = transjugular intrahepatic portosystemic shunt.

Complications of End-Stage Liver Disease

Ascites

Ascites, or fluid collection in the peritoneal cavity, is the most common complication of ESLD. Abdominal distension often leads to pain and dyspnea. The diagnosis is based on the physical examination or by abdominal ultrasound.

Primary management includes sodium restriction (maximum 2 g/day) and diuretic therapy, with the combination of spironolactone and furosemide achieving the best control of fluid retention and least electrolytes imbalances.

When diuretics are not sufficient, repeated paracentesis may be effective and safe, provided that it is associated with intravenous albumin infusion, 8 g/L removed, during or just after the end of any large-volume paracentesis (> 4 L).

The control of refractory ascites may also be accomplished using the transjugular intrahepaic portosystemic shunt (TIPS), which is superior to repeated paracentesis in controlling ascites but is complicated by worsening hepatic encephalopathy.[3]

Nevertheless, ascites often becomes refractory to medical management, and is an indication for opioids and sedatives to relieve the severe discomfort.

Spontaneous Bacterial Peritonitis

Spontaneous bacterial peritonitis (SBP), or ascitic fluid infection, possibly secondary to bacterial translocation from the intestinal lumen, is a common complication of ascites. The diagnosis is made when there is a positive ascitic fluid bacterial culture and/or an elevated ascitic fluid absolute PMN count (i.e., ≥ 250 cells/mm³) without an evident intra-abdominal source of infection.

IV cefotaxime or a similar third-generation cephalosporin is the first-line treatment for suspected SBP. Normally, the results of the ascitic fluid culture are not required to start the antibiotic treatment. The concomitant administration of intravenous albumin can prevent the development of hepatorenal syndrome and reduce mortality.[3]

Oral ofloxacin has been reported to be as effective as intravenous cefotaxime in patients without vomiting, shock, grade II (or higher) hepatic encephalopathy, or serum creatinine < 3 mg/dL.[4] After one episode of SBP, patients should receive long-term prophylaxis with daily norfloxacin or trimethoprim/sulfamethoxazole.

Electrolytes Imbalances

Most patients with ESLD develop and tolerate relatively low sodium levels. The best treatment when the sodium level is below 120 mmol/L is water restriction and temporary cessation of diuretics.

Hepatic Encephalopathy

Hepatic encephalopathy is characterized by several neuropsychiatric disturbances from insomnia and tremor to stupor and coma. The preferred treatment is a cathartic, nonabsorbable disaccharide, typically lactulose, which will acidify the luminal contents that promote the formation of ammonia, with consequent increased excretion with the stool. Rifaximin, a minimally absorbed antibiotic, has been shown to maintain remission of hepatic encephalopathy more effectively than placebo over a 6-month period.[5] Dietary protein restriction can worsen the risk of malnutrition.[6]

Esophageal Varices

A frequent complication, up to 50%, of portal hypertension is esophageal varices. Their rupture, often worsened by coagulopathy and thrombocytopenia, results in variceal hemorrhage.

Variceal hemorrhage occurs at a yearly rate of 5%–15%. The most important predictor of hemorrhage is the size of varices, which is determined by the esophagogastroduodenoscopy (EGD).

Pharmacological therapy consists of nonselective β-blockers (propranolol and nadolol) and endoscopic therapy using variceal banding ligation or sclerotherapy.[7] Of note, recent evidence points to the fact that propranolol should be stopped in the presence of refractory ascites, as it has been associated with reduced survival.[8]

Pruritus

Pruritus in ESLD is multifactorial. It is more frequently associated with cholestasis; opioids are also associated with pruritus. The most common but relatively ineffective treatment is oral antihistamines, which have a nonspecific sedating effect.

Cholestyramine is used for its effect in preventing bile acid uptake in the terminal ileum; however, it can interfere with the absorption of other medications. Other options in patients with ESLD are ursodiol and rifampin.

Hepatorenal Syndrome

Hepatorenal syndrome (HRS) is a marker of extremely poor prognosis and is irreversible in the absence of liver transplant. HRS is defined as renal failure associated with advanced hepatic failure and is characterized by impaired renal function and marked abnormalities in the arterial circulation and in the activation of the endogenous vasoactive systems. The major criteria for the diagnosis of the HRS are the following:

1. Low glomerular filtration rate < 40 ml/min or serum creatinine > 1.5 mg/dL
2. Absence of shock, ongoing bacterial infection, current treatment with nephrotoxic drugs, gastrointestinal fluid losses, renal fluid losses > 500 g/day
3. Proteinuria < 500 mg/dL
4. No ultrasonographic sign of primary renal disease.

In the palliative care setting, the administration of agonists of vasopressin receptors (ornipressin and terlipressin) may improve renal function. Octreotide and midodrine (an alpha-adrenergic agonist) have been used,[9,10] and are recommended in the treatment of HRS,[11] but no controlled randomized trials have ever shown increased survival. HRS is an absolute indication for intensive palliative care and referral to hospice.

Hepatocellular Carcinoma

Hepatocellular carcinoma (HCC) occurs at an estimate rate of 1%–6% per year in patients with ESLD. Potentially curative treatments for HCC are

Table 30.3 Therapeutic Options for Hepatocellular Carcinoma (HCC) Management and Their Indications

Surgical resection	Best option for patients without cirrhosis. Solitary HCC of the liver, without vascular invasion, no evidence of portal hypertension, and well-preserved hepatic function
Radiofrequency ablation (RFA)	Best outcomes are in patients with a single tumor < 4 cm in diameter. For cirrhotic patients, some clinicians restrict RFA to those with Child–Pugh class A or B.
Percutaneous ethanol injection (PEI)	PEI is often considered for patients with small HCCs who are not candidates for resection because of their poor functional hepatic reserve.
Transarterial chemoembolization (TACE)	Most often used for large unresectable HCCs that are not amenable to other treatments such as resection or RFA; sometimes it is used as a bridging therapy prior to transplant to down-stage the tumor.
Liver transplantation	Best option for unresectable patients who meet the Milan criteria (see Table 30.4)

Table 30.4 Milan Staging Criteria for Hepatocellular Carcinoma

Single Tumor	Multiple Tumors	
Single tumor maximum diameter	Maximum number	Largest tumor size
≤ 5 cm	3	≤ 3 cm

limited but include surgical resection, radiofrequency ablation (RFA), percutaneous ethanol injection (PEI), and liver transplantation (Table 30.3).[12]

The most commonly used criteria for liver transplantation for HCC are the Milan criteria (Table 30.4).

Palliative treatments for selected HCC include transarterial chemoembolization (TACE), which offers palliative benefits for patients with large and/or multifocal HCC without vascular invasion or extrahepatic metastasis, with 1- and 2-year survival rates of 82% and 63%, respectively.[12] This technique is based on the induction of embolization, which causes ischemic tumor necrosis, combined with selective intra-arterial chemotherapy.

Clinical trials of sorafenib, a small molecular inhibitor of several protein kinases, provide some modest prolongation of survival.

A large multicenter, randomized, placebo-controlled phase III trial studied the efficacy of sorafenib versus placebo in 602 patients with advanced HCC who had no prior systemic therapy. The median overall survival and the time to symptom progression was significantly longer for sorafenib than for placebo, and the disease control rate was higher in the sorafenib than in the placebo group.[13]

Malnutrition

Weight loss and muscle wasting are very frequent in ESLD and are related to increased metabolic needs as well as reduced caloric intake. Contributing factors are protein loss associated with paracentesis, early satiety and gastroesophageal reflux related to abdominal distention, and gastroparesis. We discourage families from force feeding patients, as the weight loss is a sign of advanced disease.

Pain Management in ESLD

The causes of pain in ESLD may be related to tense ascites, SBP, HCC with metastasis, or hepatic distension. Acetaminophen can be safely used in ESLD at the maximum dose of 2 gm daily.[14] If acetaminophen is not sufficient to control moderate to severe pain, opioids can be administered at the smallest indicated doses and more frequently to minimize possible side effects including constipation and encephalopathy. Steroid treatment to reduce pain from capsular distention is often effective in reducing pain. Opioids should be used and titrated to relief. Because the hepatic activation of opioids may be altered and the excretion of narcotic analgesics due to hepatic and renal function may be markedly altered, the usual half-lives of these drugs are significantly prolonged.[15] We recommend using rapid titration of the usual short-acting narcotic analgesics and then careful conversion to long-acting medications that may not be dependent upon hepatic activation, such as methadone.

Timely Hospice Referral for ESLD Patients

Patients with ESLD have significant physical and often unrecognized emotional suffering[16] and are thus excellent candidates for hospice care. The clinician must recognize the transition from chronic stable to end of life, must be prepared to have important conversations throughout the illness, and must use well-confirmed clinical indications, including a rising MELD score, as guides for patient and family to utilize hospice services.

Timely referral to hospice service should result in median length of stay on hospice of more than 2 months. While some patients and families may resist the acceptance of hospice, most do not. Physician delay in referral is the most common cause of delayed or nonreferral.

Hospice, which is regarded as the epitome of patient- and family-centered care, provides 24-hour on-call, regular nurse and social worker home visits; services related to the terminal illness, including medications, durable medical equipment, and volunteer and pastoral services; and bereavement services.

Hospice is associated with the highest rates of patient and family satisfaction in most medical systems and not only reduces the cost of care but can also prolong survival. The 2010 Supportive and Palliative Care Indicator Tool (SPICT) can support clinical judgment when identifying patients with any advanced illness who need earlier holistic assessment. However, the SPICT refers to a variety of terminal conditions, not only liver disease.[17]

A reliable tool to guide hospice referral is the Model of End Stage Liver Disease (MELD) score, which is calculated on the base of three laboratory values: PT-INR, creatinine, and bilirubin, and can be easily calculated using several websites (e.g., http://www.unos.org/resources/meldpeldcalculator.asp).[18]

We reported a negative correlation between MELD score and length of hospice stay. That is, as the MELD score increases, the average survival decreases.[18] Of course, this is why the MELD score is used to prioritize patients on the liver transplant list. However, as noted, relatively few patients receive transplant, and thus the MELD score is also a very useful guide to support a clinician's recommendation to families for hospice care, achieving one of the national benchmark goals of increasing hospice care duration beyond the current median of 2–3 weeks.[19] A higher MELD score should augment physician judgment regarding hospice referral. We strongly recommend hospice referral when the MELD score reaches 17–20.

How does one decide between liver transplantation and hospice in patients with increasing MELD scores? We are comfortable recommending that many patients receive consideration for both modalities, simultaneously.

Hospice care can be an important tool in the liver transplant setting. Patients on the liver transplant list suffer all of the chronic conditions that require close monitoring and continuous support when frequent hospitalizations are not indicated. Conversely, when potential candidates for liver transplantation are not considered for this option because of worsening medical condition and the occurrence of absolute contraindications to the procedure, they can be referred to hospice service (Figure 30.1).

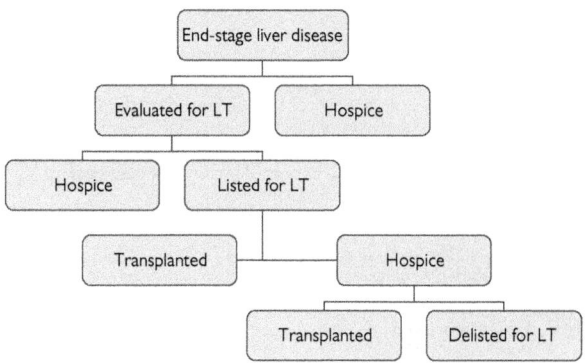

Figure 30.1. Integration model between hospice care and liver transplant (LT).

Clinical Pearls

- Na$^+$ restriction is the cornerstone of management of ascites and peripheral edema in ESLD.
- Patients with a previous episode of spontaneous bacterial peritonitis should receive long-term prophylaxis with daily norfloxacin or trimethoprim/sulfamethoxazole.
- Patients with ESLD should be considered for simultaneous hospice referral and liver transplant evaluation.

References

1. Poonja Z, Brisebois A, van Zanten SV, Tandon P, Meeberg G, Karvellas CJ (2014). Patients with cirrhosis and denied liver transplants rarely receive adequate palliative care or appropriate management. *Clin Gastroenterol Hepatol* 12:692–8.
2. Heron M (2013). Deaths: leading causes for 2010. *Natl Vital Stat Rep* 62:1–97.
3. Runyon BA (2004). Management of adult patients with ascites due to cirrhosis. *Hepatology* 39:841–56.
4. Navasa M, Follo A, Llovet JM, Clemente G, Vargas V, Rimola A, Marco F, Guarner C, Forné M, Planas R, Bañares R, Castells L, Jimenez De Anta MT, Arroyo V, Rodés J (1996). Randomized, comparative study of oral ofloxacin versus intravenous cefotaxime in spontaneous bacterial peritonitis. *Gastroenterology* 111:1011–17.
5. Bass NM, Mullen KD, Sanyal A, Poordad F, Neff G, Leevy CB, Sigal S, Sheikh MY, Beavers K, Frederick T, Teperman L, Hillebrand D, Huang S, Merchant K, Shaw A, Bortey E, Forbes WP (2010). Rifaximin treatment in hepatic encephalopathy. *N Engl J Med* 25;362:1071–81.
6. Blei AT, Córdoba J (2001). Practice Parameters Committee of the American College of Gastroenterology. Hepatic encephalopathy. *Am J Gastroenterol* 96:1968–76.
7. Garcia-Tsao G, Sanyal AJ, Grace ND, Carey W (2007). Prevention and management of gastro-esophageal varices and variceal hemorrhage in cirrhosis. *Hepatology* 46:922–38.
8. Serste T, Melot C, Francoz C, Durand F, Rautou P-E, Valla D, Moreau R, Lebrec D (2010). Deleterious effects of beta-blockers on survival in patients with cirrhosis and refractory ascites. *Hepatology* 52:1017–22.
9. Kashani A, Landaverde C, Medici V, Rossaro L (2008). Fluid retention in cirrhosis: pathophysiology and management. *QJM* 101:71–85.
10. Angeli P, Volpin R, Gerunda G, Craighero R, Roner P, Merenda R, Amodio P, Sticca A, Caregaro L, Maffei-Faccioli A, Gatta A (1999). Reversal of type 1 hepatorenal syndrome with the administration of midodrine and octreotide. *Hepatology* 29:1690–97.
11. Runyon BA (2013). Introduction to the revised American Association for the Study of Liver Diseases Practice Guideline management of adult patients with ascites due to cirrhosis 2012. *Hepatology* 57(4):1651–3.
12. El-Serag H, Marrearo JA, Rudolph L, Reddy KR (2008). Diagnosis and treatment of hepatocellular carcinoma. *Gastroenterology* 134:1752–63.
13. Llovet JM, Ricci S, Mazzaferro V, Hilgard P, Gane E, Blanc JF, de Oliveira AC, Santoro A, Raoul JL, Forner A, Schwartz M, Porta C, Zeuzem S, Bolondi L, Greten TF, Galle PR, Seitz JF, Borbath I, Häussinger D, Giannaris T, Shan M, Moscovici M, Voliotis D, Bruix J; SHARP Investigators Study Group (2008). Sorafenib in advanced hepatocellular carcinoma. *N Engl J Med* 24(4):378–90.
14. Benson GD, Koff RS, Tolman KG (2005). The therapeutic use of acetaminophen in patients with liver disease. *Am J Ther* 12:133–41.
15. Harris DG (2014). Management of pain in advanced disease. *Br Med Bull* 110:117–28.
16. Kimbell B, Murray SA (2015). What is the patient experience in advanced liver disease? A scoping review of the literature. *BMJ Support Palliat Care* 5(5):471–80.
17. Highet G, Crawford D, Murray SA, Boyd K (2014). Development and evaluation of the Supportive and Palliative Care Indicators Tool (SPICT): a mixed-methods study. *BMJ Support Palliat Care* 4(3):285–90.
18. Kamath PS, Kim WR (2007). Advanced Liver Disease Study Group. The Model for End-stage Liver Disease (MELD). *Hepatology* 45:797–805.
19. Medici V, Rossaro L, Wegelin JA, Kamboj A, Nakai J, Fisher K, Meyers FJ (2008). The utility of the Model for End-stage Liver Disease score: a reliable guide for liver transplant candidacy and, for select patients, simultaneous hospice referral. *Liver Transpl* 14:1100–6.

Kidney Palliative Care

Sara Davison and David Hui

Introduction

Chronic kidney disease (CKD) is defined as abnormalities of kidney structure or function, present for ≥ 3 months, and classified based on glomerular filtration rate (GFR) (Table 31.1). GFR category 5 (G5) CKD is also known as end-stage kidney disease (ESKD), in which patients will ultimately require kidney replacement therapy in the form of either dialysis or a kidney transplant to sustain life. CKD may develop as a result of chronic disorders such as diabetes and hypertension or from intrinsic kidney disease such as polycystic kidney disease, glomerulonephropathy and interstitial nephritis.

As kidney function declines, patients with CKD typically experience significant morbidity and mortality. Given that the annual mortality rate for dialysis patients approaches 25%,[1] early integration of palliative care into kidney care is essential. Specifically, palliative care can help optimize symptom control, facilitate advance care planning, and ease transitions at the end of life.[2]

In this chapter, prognosis, decision-making around the initiation and withdrawal of dialysis, and symptom management for patients with ESKD are discussed.

Clinical Pearl

- G5 CKD is associated with very high mortality, very high symptom burden, and for many a poor quality of life. Median survival of dialysis patients is 3–4 years. Early involvement of palliative care is essential.

Table 31.1 Kidney Disease: Improving Global Outcomes (KDIGO) Classification of CKD

GFR category	GFR (mL/min/1.73m²)*
G1	≥ 90, proteinuria
G2	60–89
G3a	45–59
G3b	30–44
G4	15–29
G5	< 15

*GFR is estimated (eGFR) from serum creatinine (Cr) using the 2012 CKD-EPI creatinine-cystatin C equation. eGFR can also be calculated by creatinine clearance (CrCl) using the Cockroft Gault formula:

$$CrCl = (140 - age) \times (weight~in~kg)/(72 \times serum~creatinine~in~mg/dL) \times 0.85~if~woman.$$

Adapted from KDIGO. Kidney International supplements (2013); 3:19–62.

Prognosis of Patients with End-Stage Kidney Disease

The life expectancy of patients on dialysis is approximately 20% of age-matched individuals without kidney disease (Table 31.2). Factors associated with poor prognosis include the following:

- Advanced age
- Poor nutritional status: low serum albumin < 3.5 g/dL is associated with a 50% 1-year mortality
- Low functional status
- Comorbidity: modified Charlson Comorbidity Index > 8 is associated with a 50% 1-year mortality
- "Surprise Question": "Would you be surprised if this patient were to die in the next 12 months?" Answering "no" is associated with a 3.5 times greater likelihood of death within one year.[3]

The ability to accurately estimate prognosis is of great importance to patients, families, and clinicians. Knowing what to expect can facilitate the process of advance care planning and can help give patients a sense of control. Prognostication is particularly important in decision-making around the appropriate initiation and withdrawal of dialysis, and timely referral to palliative care and hospice. A prognostic model, recently developed for predicting the survival of prevalent hemodialysis patients[4] is available online and as an application for handheld devices.[5] Further validation of this model is underway. (Chapter 25 provides a general approach to discussing prognosis.)

Table 31.2 Adjusted Survival Probabilities (%) for Incident Dialysis Patients

Age	1 year	2 years	3 years	5 years
20–44	91	84	78	67
45–64	84	74	64	47
65–74	74	59	48	30
75+	60.5	40.8	25.7	9.6

From US Renal Data System (2013). *USRDS 2013 Annual Data Report: Atlas of End-Stage Renal Disease in the United States*. Bethesda, MD: National Institutes of Health, National Institute of Diabetes and Digestive and Kidney Diseases.

Decision-Making Regarding Dialysis

Decision-making for the initiation and withdrawal of dialysis is a complicated process. Hemodialysis is required three times per week, whereas peritoneal dialysis necessities multiple exchanges every day. Patients on dialysis tend to experience multiple, complex symptoms as a result of their comorbidities, CKD, or the dialysis treatment itself. Potentially life-threatening acute complications such as infections and cardiovascular incidents are common.

Although dialysis is generally associated with survival and quality-of-life benefits, some patients (especially the frail with multiple comorbidities) have especially poor outcomes, with poor survival, functional decline, and poor quality of life following the initiation of dialysis. A retrospective study using administrative data reported that by 12 months after starting dialysis, 6 out of 8 long-term care residents ≥ 75 years had died, 1 in 8 had functional decline, and only 1 in 8 had maintained functional status.[6] For patients with limited benefit and considerable burden, conservative (non-dialysis) care pathways may result in improved survival with better preservation of physical function, cognition and quality of life, and therefore may be more appropriate and better aligned with patient-derived goals of care. These observations require us to determine carefully whether dialysis care is better care. Patients should be educated on the potential risks and benefits of dialysis prior to committing to this aggressive intervention.

For patients with acute, life-threatening illnesses who develop acute kidney injury (with or without preexisting kidney disease), the mortality rate is 50%–75%. Dialysis should be decided on a case-by-case basis.

Initiating Chronic Dialysis

General indications for starting dialysis in patients with G5 CKD include the following:
- Creatinine clearance typically ≤ 8mL/min/1.73 m² in combination with uremic symptoms
- Uremic symptoms including anorexia, nausea/vomiting, fatigue, restless legs, muscle cramps, paresthesias
- Uremic pericarditis or encephalopathy
- Persistent metabolic acidosis, hyperkalemia, or fluid overload despite optimal medical treatment.

Withdrawal of Dialysis

Once dialysis is initiated, the nephrology team works closely with patients to evaluate the ongoing utility of dialysis. It is now a widely accepted practice in most countries to stop dialysis when it is no longer achieving a meaningful goal for the patient.

Approximately 25% of deaths of dialysis patients in the United States are preceded by a decision to discontinue dialysis. Decreased functional status and overall loss of a meaningful quality of life are the most common reasons to stop dialysis for patients dying at home. Medical complications are the most common reasons for hospitalized patients.[1]

The palliative care team should work closely with the nephrology team to provide longitudinal counseling, optimal symptom control, and end-of-life preparations. Once dialysis is stopped, patients with no residual kidney function (i.e., those that make no urine) have an average survival of 8–10 days.

ESKD patients underuse hospice. Dialysis patients in the United States are eligible to receive hospice while receiving dialysis if they have a non-ESKD diagnosis that affords them a prognosis of less than 6 months. In some cases, this may be a "failure to thrive" diagnosis. Thus, the decision to continue dialysis should not defer hospice referral in the appropriate patient. If a dialysis patient withdraws from dialysis, he or she is immediately eligible to receive hospice care.

The clinical practice guideline *Shared Decision-Making in the Appropriate Initiation of and Withdrawal from Dialysis* was developed to assist nephrologists, patients, and families in reaching decisions on whether to initiate or stop dialysis.[7] This guideline recommends a shared decision-making process between clinicians and the patient, taking into account the patient's overall prognosis and goals of care. Criteria for withholding or withdrawing dialysis include patient- or surrogate-informed wishes, profound neurological impairment, or a medical condition that precludes the technical process of dialysis.

Clinical Pearl

- The decision to initiate, withhold, or withdraw dialysis should be highly individualized, taking into account patient preference, risks, and benefits, after extensive counseling.

Symptom Management for Chronic Kidney Disease

Excellent symptom management is important for patients with advanced CKD, as these patients are among the most symptomatic of any chronic disease group.[8]

Symptoms may be due to the primary kidney disease (e.g., polycystic kidney disease), comorbidity (e.g., diabetes, peripheral vascular disease), disease consequent upon kidney failure (e.g., bone pain from renal osteodystrophy, calcific uremic arteriolopathy, and nephrogenic systemic fibrosis—see later discussion), or from the dialysis procedure itself. Common symptoms include the following:

- Constitutional: fatigue, generalized weakness
- Neurological: decreased memory and concentration, myotonic jerks, seizures, altered smell and taste, peripheral neuropathy, sleep disturbances, restless leg syndrome
- Gastrointestinal: anorexia, nausea, vomiting
- Musculoskeletal: bone pain, arthropathy, muscle cramps
- Dermatological: pruritus
- Sexual: amenorrhea, sexual dysfunction, infertility
- Psychological: depression, anxiety

Symptoms often occur in complex clusters and significantly impact the quality of life of patients and their functional capacity. Dialysis is not effective in ameliorating many of these symptoms and sometimes contributes to them.

In this section, discussion is focused on pain, fatigue, pruritus, anorexia, and sleep disturbances.[9,10] (Discussion of the management of other symptoms common in CKD can be found in Chapter 16 of this Handbook.)

Pain

Over 58% of CKD patients experience chronic pain, and 49% of patients rate their pain as moderate or severe.[11] Pain appears to be predominantly musculoskeletal in origin, but neuropathic pain is also common, and chronic pain in CKD is often mixed nociceptive/neuropathic. Common causes include the following:

- Infections: osteomyelitis, cellulitis
- Procedures: needling of aterial venous fistulas
- Peripheral neuropathy: diabetic neuropathy, uremic neuropathy
- Peripheral vascular disease: diabetes, hypertension
- Musculoskeletal: renal osteodystrophy, osteoarthritis, osteoporosis

Calcific Uremic Arteriolopathy

Calcific uremic arteriolopathy (CUA), or "calciphylaxis," is a relatively rare but serious disorder seen almost exclusively in ESKD patients, and is characterized by tissue ischemia due to metastatic calcification of subcutaneous tissue and small arteries.

Patients develop painful violaceous mottling of the skin that can progress to extremely painful ulcers and eschar formation. Even with aggressive therapy, 60%–90% of patients with CUA die from sepsis. This condition may be related to secondary hyperparathyroidism, elevated serum calcium/phosphate levels, and the use of calcitriol.

No definitive treatment regimens are available. However, hyperbaric oxygen may cure the cutaneous ulcers of CUA, and most reports recommend normalization of serum calcium, phosphorous, and parathyroid levels. This often includes cessation of calcitriol and may require daily dialysis or surgical parathyroidectomy. Treatment may also include sodium thiosulfate.

Nephrogenic Systemic Fibrosis

Nephrogenic systemic fibrosis (NSF) may be related to the use of gadolinium-containing contrast agents for magnetic resonance imaging in patients with advanced CKD. NSF causes substantial pain and disability characterized by an acute onset of hardening of the skin of the extremities and trunk, nodules with hyperpigmentation, and flexion contractures. Patients typically describe pain and pruritus at the site of the fibrosis.

There is no consistently effective treatment, although physical therapy, steroids, thalidomide, methotrexate, and UVA light therapy have all been tried. (Principles of pain management can be found in Chapter 4.) Optimal use of analegsics in patients with CKD requires a good understanding of the pharmacokinetics of various medications.

Acetaminophen

Acetaminophen is metabolized by the liver and does not require dose adjustment in ESKD. It is considered the non-narcotic of choice for mild to moderate pain in patients with CKD. A typical dose is 325–650 mg PO q6h PRN and a maximum dose would be 3 g daily.

Nonsteroidal Anti-Inflammatory Drugs

Nonsteroidal anti-inflammatory drugs (NSAIDs) may increase the risk of gastrointestinal bleeding in patients with ESKD because of their effects on platelet function, and they have potential cardiovascular risks and may cause loss of residual kidney function. For these reasons, NSAIDs should be used for precise indications (e.g., gout) and for a limited time only in patients with ESKD.

Opioids

Methadone and fentanyl are opioids of choice for patients with ESKD.

- Methadone may be a safe, effective analgesic for use in CKD patients, by those familiar with its use and if monitored carefully, as it is excreted mainly in the stool in ESKD patients. A reasonable starting dose is 5 mg PO bid. Methadone does not appear to be dialyzable and thus does not require supplementation post-dialysis.
- Fentanyl is generally considered safe for patients with ESKD. However, up to 10%–25% of fentanyl is excreted in urine unchanged; thus dose reduction may be required.
- The active metabolites of hydromorphone and oxycodone are primarily renally excreted. Exercise caution when using these opioids in CKD patients, particularly at high doses, with long-term use or if GFR < 30 mL/min. The general principle is to start low (~25% dose if CrCl 10–50 mL/min, and 50% dose if CrCl < 10 mL/min), titrate slowly, and monitor patients closely for opioid toxicity.

- Because of reports of toxicity in ESKD, morphine is not recommended for chronic pain management. Even for acute pain management, a more appropriate opioid would be hydromorphone if available.
- Meperidine is not recommended in CKD patients, as it is associated with significant neurotoxicity and anticholinergic effects.

Gabapentin and Pregabalin

These are first-line drugs for the management of neuropathic pain in ESKD, although the maximum dose should be limited to 300 mg/day for gabapentin and 75 mg/day for pregabalin (given post-hemodialysis on dialysis days). Starting doses as low as 50 mg and 25 mg, respectively, given post-dialysis only (i.e., 3/week) may be beneficial in some patients with mild to moderate neuropathic pain.

Tricyclic Antidepressants

Tricyclic antidepressants (TCAs) are effective in the management of neuropathic pain, but are less well tolerated than the gabapentinoids in patients with ESKD because of anticholinergic, histaminergic, and adrenergic side effects, resulting in symptoms such as dry mouth, orthostatic hypotension, and somnolence. For these reasons, TCAs are considered second-line therapy for neuropathic pain in ESKD.

Although dose reduction is not necessarily required in ESKD, patients will often respond to lower doses. If TCAs are to be used, consider initiating at lower doses such as amitriptyline 25 mg daily.

Fatigue

Fatigue is one of the most common and distressing symptoms for dialysis patients, affecting 30%–97%, depending upon the study population. Causes include inadequate dialysis, dialysis-related hypotension, carnitine deficiency, electrolytes imbalances, sleep disturbances, malnutrition, anemia, medications, and depression.

The management of fatigue should be focused on treatment of any reversible causes, along with the optimization of dialysis. The target hemoglobin should be 9–11 g/dL. Higher targets have been associated with increased morbidity and mortality, without improvement in quality of life. Patients should also be encouraged to exercise regularly, if possible.

Pruritus

Pruritus is one of the most frustrating and challenging symptoms for CKD patients and moderate to severe pruritus is experienced by approximately 40% of ESKD patients.[12] The pathophysiology is not well understood. Evidence has not consistently substantiated prior hypotheses relating to hyperparathyroidism and abnormalities in calcium and phosphate deposition or mast cell secretion of histamine. The most recent hypotheses include the "immune hypothesis" in which pruritus is a dermatologic manifestation of chronic inflammation seen with advanced CKD. Reasonably successful use of topical immunomodulators (tacrolimus and thalidomide) and the lack of pruritus in kidney transplant patients with progressive CKD on immunosuppressant drugs support this theory. The "opioid hypothesis" began as an observation that mu-receptor agonists caused pruritus, while mu-receptor antagonists such as naltrexone had some success in treating dialysis-associated pruritus. Other contributors may include alterations in peripheral nerve perception from uremic toxins and very dry, atrophic skin often seen in ESKD patients.

A stepwise approach to treatment, beginning with optimization of dialysis adequacy and calcium and phosphorous levels, skin hydration, adequate nutrition, and avoidance of scratching, is recommended. If symptoms persist, nonpharmacologic options (UVB therapy, acupuncture), topical therapies (emollients or capsaicin cream), and systemic pharmacologic therapies (gabapentin, nalfurafine, naltrexone) are available.

Anorexia

Anorexia is common in patients with ESKD, with a reported prevalence ranging from 9% to 82% and a mean weighted average of 56%. It is frequently associated with malnutrition and cachexia, poor quality of life, greater hospitalization rates, and an increase in mortality. Many factors may contribute to anorexia, including inadequate dialysis, nausea, taste alterations, xerostomia, gastroparesis, pain, constipation, and depression.

There is limited evidence to guide the treatment of anorexia in ESKD. In addition to ensuring adequate dialysis, a number of strategies may be useful, including antiemetics for nausea; zinc 220 mg PO daily for taste change; artificial saliva every 1–2 hours or pilocarpine 5–10 mg PO tid for dry mouth; metoclopramide 10 mg PO q4h for early satiety; and megestrol acetate 100–400 mg PO daily and dronabinol 2.5–5 mg bid for appetite stimulation. (Further discussions on anorexia–cachexia can be found in Chapter 6.)

Sleep Disturbances

Approximately 60% of patients with ESKD report insomnia, which may be exacerbated by pain, pruritus, medications, and emotional distress. Poor sleep in ESKD is highly associated with fatigue, poor quality of life, and depression.

Other common sleep disturbances in ESKD include periodic leg movement syndrome (PLMS), restless leg syndrome (RLS), and sleep apnea.

RLS occurs in approximately 20% of long-term dialysis patients and can lead to premature withdrawal from dialysis and increased cardiovascular morbidity and mortality. The etiology of RLS in ESKD may be partially due to abnormalities in the dopamine pathways in the subcortical areas of the brain, as seen with idiopathic RLS. However, other factors, such as uremic toxins, iron deficiency, and alterations in parathyroid/calcium/phosphorous balance, may also play a role. It is characterized by an urge to move the legs, usually with unpleasant sensations in the legs, brought on by rest, particularly at night or during dialysis runs, and relieved with movements. Treatment options include correction of iron deficiency and parathyroid/calcium/phosphorous levels, dopamine agonists (pergolide, pramipexole or ropinirole), gabapentin, and clonazepam.

Clinical Pearl

- Patients with ESKD often experience a multitude of physical and psychosocial symptoms. Frequent assessments, early intervention, and involvement of the multiprofessional team are key to providing care for these patients.

References

1. US Renal Data System (2013). *USRDS 2013 Annual Data Report: Atlas of Chronic Kidney Disease and End-Stage Renal Disease in the United States*. Bethesda, MD: National Institutes of Health, National Institute of Diabetes and Digestive and Kidney Diseases.

2. Chambers EJ, Brown E, Germain M (2010). *Supportive Care for the Renal Patient*. Oxford: Oxford University Press.

3. Moss AH, Ganjoo J, Sharma S, Gansor J, Senft S, Weaner B, et al. (2008). Utility of the "surprise" question to identify dialysis patients with high mortality. *Clin J Am Soc Nephrol* 3(5):1379–84. PubMed PMID: 18596118. Pubmed Central PMCID: PMC2518805.

4. Cohen LM, Ruthazer R, Moss AH, Germain MJ (2010). Predicting six-month mortality for patients who are on maintenance hemodialysis. *Clin J Am Soc Nephrol* 5(1):72–9.

5. Cohen LM, Ruthazner R, Moss AH, Germain MJ (2014). *Predicting 6 Month Mortality on Hemodialysis*. http://www.qxmd.com/calculate-online/nephrology/predicting-6-month-mortality-on-hemodialysis.

6. Tamura MK, Covinsky KE, Chertow GM, Yaffe K, Landefeld CS, McCulloch CE (2009). Functional status of elderly adults before and after initiation of dialysis. *New Engl J Med* 361(16):1539–47.

7. Renal Physician Association (2010). Shared decision-making in the appropriate initiation of and withdrawal from dialysis. In Clinical Practice Guideline, 2nd ed. RPA Rockville, Maryland, USA. http://www.renalmd.org/page.aspx?id=2684 (Last accessed 12/1/2015)

8. Murtagh FEM, Weisbord S (2010). Symptoms in renal disease: their epidemiology, assessment and management. In: Chambers EJ, Germain M, Brown E (eds.), *Supportive Care for the Renal Patient*, 2nd ed. Oxford: Oxford University Press.

9. Moss AH, Holley JL, Davison SN, Dart RA, Germain MJ, Cohen L, et al. (2004). Palliative care. *Am J Kidney Dis* 43(1):172–3.

10. Davison SN (2003). Pain in hemodialysis patients: prevalence, cause, severity, and management. *Am J Kidney Dis* 42(6):1239–47.

11. Davison SN, Koncicki H, Brennan F (2014). Pain in chronic kidney disease: a scoping review. *Semin Dial* 27(2):188–204. PubMed PMID: 24517512.

12. Combs SA, Teixeira JP, Germain MJ. (2015). Pruritus in Kidney Disease. Semin Nephrol 35(4):383-91.

Palliative Care in Patients with AIDS

Kirsten Wentlandt and Camilla Zimmermann

Introduction

The human immunodeficiency virus (HIV) is a retrovirus that causes acquired immune deficiency syndrome (AIDS), a syndrome once considered rapidly fatal. Since the introduction of antiretroviral drugs, HIV has become a manageable chronic illness: over 35.3 million people across the globe are living with HIV, of whom 1.3 million are North Americans.[1]

Effective prevention strategies, earlier diagnosis, and the use of antiretroviral therapy (ART) have all improved survival rates. Despite this, there remain approximately 20,000 AIDS deaths per year in the United States alone.[1]

The purpose of this chapter is to review how clinicians can improve patient care by combining recent disease-specific therapies with palliative care practices.

Clinical Course and WHO Staging

HIV is transmitted by sexual contact, exposure to contaminated blood products and bodily fluids, or perinatal transmission from mother to child. The acute phase of HIV infection is characterized by a febrile illness, much like a typical flu.

This is followed by an asymptomatic second phase lasting 4–5 years, and then a more chronic symptomatic phase in which patients develop persistent lymphadenopathy and AIDS-defining malignancies.

The final stage is clinical AIDS, defined as a CD4 count < 200/μL or occurrence of AIDS-defining conditions.

The World Health Organization (WHO) has developed a clinical staging paradigm for HIV/AIDS, which enables a clinician to stage patients on the basis of clinical features, rather than laboratory values (Table 32.1).

The impact of antiretrovirals on survival has made it difficult to use traditional prognostic indicators. For many patients, mortality results not from end-stage HIV disease but from other comorbidities, such as hepatitis C or B (cirrhosis and liver failure) or HIV-related malignancies.

Overall, the clinical course of HIV/AIDS is fluctuating, with considerable variation among patients, and is marked by a number of opportunistic infections requiring treatment. Specific guidelines have been developed to prevent opportunistic infections, including tuberculosis, *Pneumocystis carinii*, toxoplasmosis, *Mycobacterium avium* complex, and varicella (Table 32.2).

Clinical Pearls

- *AIDS* is defined as a CD4 count < 200/μL or occurrence of AIDS-defining conditions.

Table 32.1 Revised WHO Clinical Staging of HIV/AIDS for Adults and Adolescents

Primary HIV infection
- Asymptomatic
- Acute retroviral syndrome

Clinical stage 1
- Asymptomatic
- Persistent generalized lymphadenopathy

Clinical stage 2
- Moderate unexplained weight loss
- Recurrent respiratory tract infections
- Herpes zoster
- Angular cheilitis
- Recurrent oral ulcerations
- Papular pruritic eruptions
- Fungal nail infections
- Seborrhoeic dermatitis

Clinical stage 3
- Severe weight loss (> 10% of presumed or measured body weight)
- Unexplained chronic diarrhea for longer than 1 month
- Unexplained persistent fever (intermittent or constant for longer than 1 month)
- Persistent oral candidiasis
- Oral hairy leukoplakia
- Pulmonary tuberculosis (TB)
- Severe presumed bacterial infections (e.g., pneumonia, empyema, pyomyositis, bone or joint infection, meningitis, bacteremia)
- Acute necrotizing ulcerative stomatitis, gingivitis, or periodontitis
- Unexplained anemia (< 8 g/dL), neutropenia (< 500/mm^3) and/or chronic thrombocytopenia (< 50,000/mm^3)

Clinical stage 4
- HIV wasting syndrome
- Pneumocystis pneumonia
- Recurrent severe bacterial pneumonia
- Chronic herpes simplex infection (>1 month's duration or visceral at any site)
- Esophageal candidiasis
- Extrapulmonary TB
- Kaposi's sarcoma
- Cytomegalovirus (CMV) infection
- Central nervous system toxoplasmosis
- HIV encephalopathy
- Extrapulmonary cryptococcosis (including meningitis)
- Disseminated non-tuberculous mycobacterial infection
- Progressive multifocal leukoencephalopathy
- Chronic cryptosporidiosis
- Chronic isosporiasis
- Visceral herpes simplex infection
- Disseminated mycosis (extrapulmonary, histoplasmosis, coccidiomycosis)
- Lymphoma (cerebral or B-cell non-Hodgkin)
- Symptomatic HIV-associated nephropathy or cardiomyopathy
- Recurrent septicemia (including non-typhoidal salmonella)
- Invasive cervical carcinoma
- Atypical disseminated leishmaniasis

Consolidated guidelines on the use of antiretroviral drugs for treating and preventing HIV infection: recommendations for a public health approach (June 2013). Publications of the World Health Organization are available at www.who.int.

Table 32.2 Opportunistic Infection Prevention and Prophylaxis

	Indications for Prophylaxis	Prophylaxis
P. carinii pneumonia	CD4 < 200	Trimethoprim 160 mg/sulfamethoxazole 800 mg PO od
Toxoplasmosis	CD4 < 100	Trimethoprim 160 mg/sulfamethoxazole 800 mg PO od
M. avium complex	CD4 < 50	Clarithromycin 500 mg PO bid or Azithromycin 1200 mg every week
Tuberculosis	PPD + High-risk exposure	Izoniazid 300 mg PO od + Pyridoxine 50 mg PO od for 6–12 months
Varicella	Exposure with no history	Varicella immune globulin (VZIG) 125 UI/10kg, max 625 IU IM < 10 days post-exposure

From World Health Organization, *HIV/AIDS Treatment and Care*. Copenhagen: WHO Regional Office for Europe and Panel on Opportunistic Infections in HIV-Infected Adults and Adolescents (2015). Guidelines for the prevention and treatment of opportunistic infections in HIV-infected adults and adolescents: recommendations from the Centers for Disease Control and Prevention, the National Institutes of Health, and the HIV Medicine Association of the Infectious Diseases Society of America. Available at https://aidsinfo.nih.gov/contentfiles/lvguidelines/adult_oi.pdf.

Antiretroviral Therapy

Antiretroviral therapy (ART) has had a profound effect on the clinical course of HIV/AIDS. Since the introduction of zidovudine in the 1980s, several new classes of HIV medications have been developed that have differing mechanisms of action and are used together to produce durable suppression of HIV. The combinations of these drugs were initially known as highly active antiretroviral therapy (HAART) and are now commonly termed ART.

The introduction of ART has dramatically changed the clinical features of HIV/AIDS. As a result of suppressing the virus, ART is associated with symptom improvement (e.g., reducing weight loss, fatigue, and dementia) and a decrease in opportunistic infections. There has also been a decrease in AIDS-defining malignancies, including Kaposi's sarcoma and cerebral lymphoma.

Unfortunately, ART is associated with substantial side effects. These result mainly from mitochondrial toxicity, hypersensitivity reactions, and lipodystrophy, which commonly result in anorexia, diarrhea, nausea, vomiting, and pain. Side effects contribute heavily to nonadherence to ART but can be minimized by proper symptom management and palliative care.

There are many potential drug interactions when using ART. Most are related to the liver's cytochrome P-450 system, and many involve medications central to palliative care and pain management (e.g., benzodiazepines, opioids, anticonvulsants, and antidepressants).

Table 32.3 shows a list of potential drug interactions with medications commonly used in palliative care. Methadone levels are decreased by several non-nucleocide reverse transcriptase inhibitors (i.e., nevirapine and efavirenz), requiring dosage adjustments. In some cases, medications may be contraindicated; for instance, midazolam is contraindicated with the use of most protease inhibitors.

A useful online resource for HIV drug interactions has been designed by the University of Liverpool and can be found at http://www.hiv-druginteractions.org/.

Clinical Pearls
- Potential interactions with antiretroviral therapy should be checked before prescribing medications for symptoms.

Table 32.3 Possible HIV and Palliative Care Drug Interactions

HIV Medications	Palliative Care Medication
Protease inhibitor interactions	
Atazanavir, darunavir, fosamprenavir, indinavir, lopinavir, nelfinavir, ritonavir, saquinavir, tipranavir	**Analgesics:** most opioids **Anticonvulsants:** carbamazepine, clonazepam, phenobarbital, phenytoin **Antidepressants:** all classes **Antipsychotics:** chlorpromazine, clozapine, haloperidol, olanzapine, quetiapine, respiridone **Anxiolytics:** most anxiolytics except for lorazepam, oxazepam and temazepam **Gastrointestinal agents:** domperidone, cisapride, ondansetron, prochlorperazine **Steroids:** dexamethasone, prednisone, testosterone
Non-nucleoside reverse transcriptase inhibitor interactions	
Group 1 Delavirdine, efavrenz, etravirine, nevirapine, rilpirvirine *Group 2* Abacavir, didanosine, emtricitabine, lamivudine, stavudine, tenofovir, zidovudine	**Analgesics:** most opioids **Anticonvulsants:** clonazepam Carbamazepine, phenobarbital, and phenytoin are contraindicated with use of delavirdine, rilpirvirine, and etravirine **Antidepressants:** most antidepressants except for desipramine, amitriptyline, nortriptyline, and paroxetine **Antipsychotics:** olanzapine, quetiapine, risperidone, haloperidol, clozapine **Anxiolytics:** most anxiolytics except for lorazepam, oxazepam, and temazepam **Gastrointestinal agents:** cisapride, domperidone, proton pump inhibitors with the use of rilpivrine and delavirdine **Steroids:** dexamethasone, prednisone, testosterone **Analgesics:** methadone; tenofovir has possible interactions with NSAIDs **Anticonvulsants:** phenobarbital, and phenytoin with the use of abacavir and zidovudine
Entry and integrase inhibitor interactions	
Maraviroc, raltegravir, dolutegravir, elvitegravir + cobicistat	**Analgesics:** all opioids with the use of elvitegravir + cobicistat **Anticonvulsants:** carbamazepine, phenobarbital, phenytoin, clonazepam **Antidepressants:** elvitegravir + cobicistat have possible interaction with all classes **Anxiolytics:** elvitegravir + cobicistat have possible interaction with all classes of anxiolytics **Gastrointestinal agents:** antacids, cisapride, elvitegravir + cobicistat have possible interaction with all classes of anti-emetics (except metoclopramide)

Always check for the most up-to-date information on drug interactions before prescribing additional medications. For more details on HIV drug interactions, see the website http://www.hiv-druginteractions.org/.

HIV-Related Cancer

Approximately 25% of patients with HIV/AIDS will develop cancer. Kaposi's sarcoma and cerebral non-Hodgkin's lymphoma occur more frequently as the disease progresses and are thought to be directly related to immunosuppression by HIV. Consequently, the introduction of ART has greatly reduced the incidence of these malignancies.

Several other cancers occur with a higher frequency in the HIV population. Non-AIDS-defining malignancies that occur in greater frequency in patients with HIV/AIDS include multiple myeloma and cancers of the head and neck, lung, and gastrointestinal tract.

There is a greater incidence of human papilloma virus (HPV)–associated anal and cervical cancers, but this is likely related to the sexual transmission of both HIV and HPV.[2]

Common Symptoms

Patients with HIV/AIDS present with a spectrum of symptoms and medical issues. Symptom management generally follows the same basic principles as those for the oncological population, but in some instances the best treatment may be HIV/AIDS specific. Pain is a good example of this. Pain may be directly related to HIV (e.g., neuropathy, opportunistic infection, HIV-related malignancy), associated with treatment (e.g., procedures, ART, radiotherapy), or related to chronic illness (pressure sores, constipation). An overview of symptom causes and suggested treatment regimes (for both HIV- and non-HIV-specific causes) is given in Table 32.4.[3,4,5]

Most pain syndromes in patients with HIV are neuropathic rather than nociceptive. There are a wide range of common neuropathic syndromes in

Table 32.4 Common Symptoms and Possible Treatments in HIV/AIDS

Symptom	Causes	HIV-Related and General Treatment Options
Fatigue	AIDS Opportunistic infection Anemia Nonspecific	ART Antibiotics Transfusion/erythropoietin Corticosteroids, stimulants Dexamethasone 4–16 mg PO/IV od Methylphenidate 2.5–5 mg PO bid (max 60 mg/day) Modafinil 50 mg PO od/bid (increased weekly to effect, max 400 mg/day) Testosterone patch
Depression	Nonspecific	SSRIs Psychotherapy Mirtazapine, bupropion, venlafaxine
Constipation	Dehydration Malignancy Medications	Hydration Radiation/chemotherapy Change medications Activity/diet changes Lactulose 15–30 mL PO od/bid Senna 2–4 tabs PO od/bid
Diarrhea	Infections ART Malabsorption	Antibiotics/antifungals/antivirals Discontinue ART or change regime Loperamide 4 mg PO, then 2 mg PO after each loose stool (maximum dose 16 mg/day)
Dyspnea	P carinii pneumonia Anemia Tuberculosis Pleural effusion	Trimethoprim 320 mg/sulfamethoxazole 1600 mg PO qid Transfusion/erythropoietin TB treatment/antibiotics Oxygen supplementation, bronchodilators Opioids: morphine 2.5–5 mg PO q4hr

Table 32.4 (Continued)

Symptom	Causes	HIV-Related and General Treatment Options
Nausea/Vomiting	Candidiasis CMV HAART Nonspecific	Antifungals: nystatin susp 4–6 mL qid or Fluconazole 100 mg PO od Antivirals: ganciclovir, acyclovir; Discontinue ART or change regime Dopamine antagonists, prokinetics, proton pump inhibitors, serotonin antagonists, somatostatin analogs Haloperidol 0.5–2 mg PO/SC bid Ondansetron 4–8 mg PO bid/tid Dronabinol 2.5–5 mg PO bid/tid
Nociceptive pain Neuropathic pain	Opportunistic infection Malignancy Nonspecific HIV-related ART CMV Herpes Others	Antibiotics Chemotherapy/radiation NSAIDS: naproxen 250–375 mg PO q6–8h Corticosteroids: prednisone 20–80 mg PO od Add ART Change ART Antivirals: ganciclovir, acyclovir Acyclovir 400–800 mg PO tid–5 times per day NSAIDs, opioids, cannabis, TCAs, corticosteroids, anticonvulsants Nortriptyline 10 mg PO qhs (max dose 75 mg/day) Gabapentin 300–1200 mg PO tid
Weight loss	HIV Opportunistic infection Malignancy Chronic illness	ART Antibiotics Chemotherapy/radiation Dietary support/elemental and polymeric diet Growth hormone 0.1 mg/kg/SC od Testosterone patches Megestrol acetate 400–800 mg PO od Prednisone 20–80 mg PO od Dexamethasone 4–16 mg PO od Dronabinol 2.5–5 mg PO bid/tid

Boldface text indicates best evidence available.

HIV/AIDS patients, the most common being distal sensory polyneuropathy (DSP). DSP involves the distal lower extremities, especially the plantar aspects of both feet.

Peripheral neuropathies can be similar to DSP and may be caused by several antiretroviral medications, including didanosine, zalcitabine, and stavudine.

Clinical Pearls

- Most pain syndroms in patients with HIV are neuropathic rather than nociceptive

Another notable qualification specific to the HIV population is the increased incidence of opportunistic infections. HIV/AIDS patients are at particular risk for opportunistic infections of the central nervous system, such as cryptococcal meningitis, progressive multifocal leukoencephalopathy, and toxoplasmosis. These can cause an array of symptoms, including spastic paraplegia or paraparesis, loss of bowel and bladder function, painful muscle spasms, and dementia. The decision process of determining how to treat specific symptoms must be consistent with the goals of care and must follow the wishes of the patient and family.

Symptomatic complaints in the HIV/AIDS population may be due to HIV, antiretroviral treatments, or chronic illness.

Psychosocial and Spiritual Issues

The psychosocial context of HIV/AIDS is complex and is critical for palliative care providers to understand. HIV can be associated with a stigma, which may lead to concerns about confidentiality and inadequate care. In addition, AIDS tends to be more prevalent in vulnerable populations, including in those who are of low socioeconomic status or use intravenous drugs. Substance abuse has been reported to be around 50% in the US HIV-positive population, and clinicians should be aware of the high rate of concurrent psychiatric diagnoses and substance use disorders in the North American HIV community.[6]

Suicidal ideation is more common in these patients than in the general population. It was reported more frequently in patients who were not heterosexual, who described more symptoms of depression, and who rated HIV-related symptoms and medication side effects as more severe.[7]

Another study showed that patients who strive for spiritual growth in the context of their illness experience less negative affect, highlighting the importance of spiritual care as well as attention to symptoms.[8]

Patients with HIV/AIDS are less likely to have discussed advance directives and do-not-resuscitate (DNR) orders with their physicians than other patient populations with advanced illnesses. This tendency is increased for those who are non-white, use intravenous drugs, or are less educated.[9]

However, HIV-infected adults and adolescents have expressed a preference to initiate conversations about end-of-life care earlier in the disease process, rather than at a time of acute deterioration.[10] Earlier discussions have led to increased communication, decreased conflict and stress, and increased consistency with patient preferences.[10]

Clinical Pearls

- Patients with HIV/AIDS require a flexible approach to advance care planning, with frequent review of the goals of care.

Patients with HIV/AIDS may have different concerns regarding end-of-life decision-making than patients with cancer or other illnesses, and physicians should consider disease-specific issues. These may include the concerns of same-sex partners regarding health power of attorney and survivorship.

In addition, the fluctuating, uncertain course of AIDS requires a flexible, patient approach to advance care planning, with frequent review of the goals of care.[11]

The Future Outlook for Palliative Care in HIV/AIDS

HIV/AIDS has evolved from a fatal illness into a complex, chronic disease, driving changes in health policy, health services, and resource allocation. Since the introduction of ART, financial support for these treatments has been given priority over other services provided. As healthcare systems adjust to this changing milieu, palliative care will need to remain flexible to provide integrated and comprehensive care for a population with diverse needs.

Palliative care remains important for patients with HIV/AIDS across the disease continuum, not only to improve adherence to active treatment but also to further patients' quality of life, address symptom or psychosocial issues, and coordinate end-of-life planning.

References

1. Global Health Observatory, World Health Organization (2012). *Data on the Size of the HIV/AIDS Epidemic.* http://www.who.int/gho/en/.
2. Konopnicki D, De Wit S, Clumeck N (2013). HPV and HIV coinfection: a complex interaction resulting in epidemiological, clinical and therapeutic implications. *Future Virology* 3: 903.
3. Ferrando SJ (2009). Psychopharmacological treatment of patients with HIV/AIDS. *Psychiat Ann* 43(5):223.
4. Selwyn PA (2005). Palliative care for patient with human immunodeficiency virus/acquired immune deficiency syndrome. *J Palliat Med* 8(6):1248–68.
5. Rabkin JG, McElhiney MC, Rabkin R, McGrath PJ (2010). Modafinil treatment for fatigue in HIV/AIDS: a randomized placebo-controlled study. *J Clin Psychiatry* 71(6):707–15.
6. Durvasula R, Miller TR (2014). Substance abuse treatment in persons with HIV/AIDS: challenges in managing triple diagnosis. *Behav Med* 40(2):43.
7. Carrico AW, Johnson MO, Morin SF, Remien RH, Charlebois ED, Steward WT, et al. (2007). Correlates of suicidal ideation among HIV-positive persons. *AIDS* 21(9):1199–203.
8. Perez JE, Chartier M, Koopman C, Vosvick M, Gore-Felton C, Spiegel D (2009). Spiritual striving, acceptance coping, and depressive symptoms among adults living with HIV/AIDS. *J Health Psychol* 14(1):88–97.
9. Wenger NS, Kanouse DE, Collins RL, Liu H, Schuster MA, Gifford AL, et al. (2001). End-of-life discussions and preferences among persons with HIV. *JAMA* 285(22):2880–7.
10. Lyon ME, Garvie PA, McCarter R, Briggs L, He J, D'Angelo LJ (2009). Who will speak for me? Improving end-of-life decision-making for adolescents with HIV and their families. *Pediatrics* 123(2):e199–206.
11. Selwyn PA, Forstein M (2003). Overcoming the false dichotomy of curative vs. palliative care for late-stage HIV/AIDS: "let me live the way I want to live, until I can't." *JAMA* 290(6):806–14.

Palliative Care in End-Stage Neurological Disease

Tobias Walbert

Introduction

Neurological disorders are among the leading causes of morbidity and death worldwide. While stroke is third leading cause of death, after heart disease and cancer, in the United States, other neurological diseases have a more chronic course that leads to protracted disability, morbidity, and, ultimately, death.

Unfortunately, for many of these disorders, such as Parkinson's disease, amyotrophic lateral sclerosis (ALS), and multiple sclerosis (MS), there is currently no cure available. Adequate symptom management and, later, palliative care have the potential to maintain good quality of life for patients for as long as possible and ease the burden on caregivers and patients alike.

This chapter outlines the principles of clinical symptom management for some of the most important neurological diseases.

Amyotrophic Lateral Sclerosis

Amyotrophic laterial sclerosis (ALS) is a progressive neurodegenerative disorder that results in muscle weakness, disability, respiratory insufficiency, and eventually death. The median survival duration for patients is approximately 3 years, yet 10% will survive for > 10 years.

Given its highly predictable course, palliative care and symptom management should begin in the early stages of the disease. Multidisciplinary ALS clinics involving specialized neurologists, physical therapists, occupational therapists, speech therapists, and social workers have resulted in improved quality of life and lengthened survival.

Practice guidelines for treating ALS and the management of symptoms have been published by the American Academy of Neurology and the European Federation of Neurological Societies (EFNS).[1–3]

Muscle Weakness

A major symptom in ALS, progressive muscle weakness, should be managed by regular exercise. Physical therapy to the point of exhaustion is considered counterproductive, however. The main focus should be on maintaining mobility and the highest possible degree of independence.

As weakness progresses, passive physiotherapy gains importance in preventing contractures and stiffness. Assistive devices such as canes, ankle–foot orthoses, crutches, and walking frames should be used to maintain patients' mobility.

Dysarthria

Speech impairments affect up to three-quarters of ALS patients and frequently cause major distress for them and their caregivers. For this reason, a speech and language therapist is an important member of the care team and should be involved early after disease onset to continuously evaluate the patient for dysphagia and dysarthria.

Patients should be introduced early to alternative communication devices such as alphabet boards and computer-based systems that can be operated by hand or eye control.

Sialorrhea

Another common symptom in ALS is drooling, which is caused by a combination of facial muscle weakness and a reduced ability to swallow. Sialorrhea has been linked to aspiration pneumonia.

Treatment with anticholinergic agents is generally tried first. The treatment with botulinum toxin has been shown to be effective in a controlled trial in ALS and parkinsonism.[4] Irradiation of the salivatory glands might be tried if pharmacological interventions fail.[3]

Pharmacological treatment may include the following:
- Atropine drops, 0.5% or 1%, three or four times a day sublingually (advantage: short duration of action, less dry mouth)
- Glycopyrrolate 1–2 mg PO twice to three times daily, or 0.1–0.2 mg SC/IM q4–8h (can be nebulized as well)
- Botulinum toxin type B, 2500 units into bilateral parotid and submandibular glands

- Transdermal hyoscine patch (scopolamine) 1.5 mg, every 3 days
- Amitriptyline 10–150 mg PO daily at bedtime or alternatively 10 mg PO three times daily. The starting dose is 10–25 mg and is increased slowly as needed.

Pseudobulbar Affect (Emotional Lability)

Excessive laughing or crying affects 20%–50% of patients with ALS. Emotional lability is caused by bilateral corticobulbar tract degeneration and is not considered to be an emotional disorder per se.

Antidepressant medications have been used in the past, but their effectiveness has not been established. The combination of dextromorphan and quinidine has been shown to decrease rates of emotional outbursts and improve quality of life.[5]

The following treatments are used to ameliorate pseudobulbar affect:
- Dextromorphan/quinidine (30 mg/30 mg) PO twice daily
- Amitriptyline 10–150 mg PO daily at bedtime. The starting dose is 10–25 mg PO and is increased slowly as needed.
- Fluvoxamine 100–200 mg PO daily.

Muscle Spasticity

Increased muscle tone may be useful to help patients maintain antigravity power as weakness due to ALS progresses. However, spasticity may cause painful spasms. The muscle relaxants baclofen and tizanidine are roughly equivalent in efficacy in reducing muscle spasms and have similar rates of adverse events.

Baclofen can be associated with motor weakness. The side effect of tizanidine of dry mouth might actually help manage sialorrhea (see earlier discussion).

There is less evidence to support the use of dantrolene to manage spasticity than that for baclofen or tizanidine.[1]
- Baclofen starting at 5–10 mg twice daily to three times daily and increased slowly to doses up to 120 mg/day as needed. Baclofen pumps are usually not considered.
- Tizanidine 2–4 mg PO twice daily up to a total dose of 24 mg daily.

Muscle Cramps

Muscle spasms or cramps due to ALS can be associated with severe pain and discomfort. The American Academy of Neurology evaluated the use of pharmacological agents for muscle cramps in a practice guideline.[6]

Quinine sulfate is considered the most effective treatment option but should not be used routinely because of the potential for toxicity (cardiac arrhythmias, thrombocytopenia, severe hypersensitivity reactions, and potentially serious drug interactions). The EFNS guideline also recommends the use of levetiracetam based on a small[7] open label trial.[3]

Vitamin E, gabapentin, and magnesium have been used frequently but have failed to demonstrate efficacy in small clinical trials, whereas the following pharmacological agents have been shown to be beneficial:
- Quinine sulfate 325 mg twice a day
- Calcium channel blocker (such as diltiazem) 30 mg PO daily at night
- Naftidrofuryl, 300 mg PO twice daily; this drug is not available in the United States.

Pain

Neuropathic pain is not a characteristic feature of ALS. However, many patients suffer from pain secondary to muscle spasms, cramps, and contractures, as well as musculoskeletal pain caused by reduced mobility.

Frequent changes in position are essential to prevent the skin from breaking down. Physical therapy might help to avoid joint stiffness. Other management options include the use of nonopioid analgesics, opioid analgesics, or anti-inflammatory drugs.

Psychosocial Symptoms

Most patients with ALS describe depressive symptoms, and approximately 10% are estimated to develop major depression. Both patients and caregivers should be offered counseling, and pharmacological treatment should be considered.

There are no data to suggest that one antidepressant class is more efficacious than another in ALS. However, tricyclic antidepressants (TCAs) such as amitryptiline have side effects that can help alleviate other symptoms of ALS, including drooling, pseudobulbar affect, and insomnia.

Several antidepressant options are available:

- Amitriptyline 10–25 mg by mouth at bedtime, with slow titration to 100 or 150 mg as needed and tolerated
- Sertraline 50–200 mg by mouth daily
- Paroxetine 20 mg daily to 40 mg by mouth daily.

Insomnia

Sleep difficulties are mostly secondary to other problems associated with ALS. Causes of insomnia include anxiety, depression, dysphagia, dyspnea, and the inability to change posture, which can result in discomfort and pain. Thus, identification and treatment of the underlying causes is crucial to treating the insomnia.

Sedatives may be helpful; fear of respiratory depression is generally not justified.

Dysphagia

Difficulty swallowing is one of the most common symptoms of ALS, and patients should be screened for symptoms in the office setting at least once every 3 months.[2] Adjusting the consistency of the diet and teaching specific swallowing techniques are helpful in preventing aspiration in the early stages of the disease.

Choking due to food intake or weight loss of 10% or more of body weight should trigger a conversation about the placement of a percutaneous endoscopic gastrostomy (PEG) tube. For optimal safety and efficacy, PEG should be offered when the patient's vital capacity is above 50% of predicted.[1,2,4] Studies have shown that PEG tube placement prolongs survival, but there are insufficient data on its impact on quality of life.

Dyspnea

At the onset of respiratory symptoms indicating hypoventilation, or when a patient's forced vital capacity (FVC) drops below 50%, the patient should be counseled about noninvasive mechanical ventilation as well as the terminal phase of the disease. Deciding whether and when to initiate noninvasive ventilation is critical because of the risk of sudden death or ventilator dependence.

Besides assessment of vital capacity, nocturnal oximetry and polysomnography are helpful in detecting nocturnal hypoventilation. Patient survival is extended most when ventilation is initiated before vital capacity drops below 50%.

If patients decline noninvasive ventilation or do not tolerate it, options such as invasive ventilation or hospice referral should be discussed at this point.

Terminal Phase

As ALS progresses, the goal of patient care should focus on effective and compassionate care rather than maximizing function. Patients who are not ventilated mechanically usually transition from sleep into coma due to increasing hypercapnia.

The following treatment is available if the patient develops dyspnea or becomes restless:

- Morphine 2.5–5 mg PO, SC, or IV every 4 hours as needed for dyspnea
- Lorazepam sublingual (start with 1–2.5 mg) or midazolam PO or SC (start with 1–2 mg) for anxiety
- Chlorpromazine 12.5 mg every 4–12 hours PO, IV, or PR for terminal restlessness or confusion.

Palliative Care in the Stroke Patient

Stroke is the third leading cause of death in the United States, making the need for hospice care for many victims essential.[8] The severity of the stroke, and thus the need for rehabilitative or palliative care, depends on its location within the brain and the severity of the damage to the brain tissue.[9]

A stroke takes time to manifest its full effect, and some early symptoms might be transitory. The physician might consider a referral to hospice if the patient remains comatose or has a severely reduced level of consciousness (obtundation) with abnormal muscle contraction (myoclonus) for 3 days or longer.

Patients who survive 4 weeks and regain significant function during that time are more likely to need active rehabilitation than palliative care. Most recently, the American Heart Association/American Stroke Association published guidelines on how to integrate palliative care and address end-of-life issues in stroke. Some of the specific challenges in stroke patients are discussed in the following text.[9]

Dysphagia

Approximately one in three patients presents with swallowing problems immediately after the onset of a stroke. Limited oral intake is linked to malnutrition, poor outcome, and increased mortality.[9] In turn, poor nutritional status may lead to skin breakdown, muscle weakness, and decreased ability to participate in rehabilitation programs. Patients who do not tolerate solid food and liquids orally should receive nasogastric (NG), nasoduodenal, or PEG tube feedings to maintain hydration and nutrition while recovering from their strokes.[10] NG tube feeding is preferred in the first 2 to 3 weeks after stroke onset, as approximately 50% of all dysphagic patients will recover their ability to swallow within this time. However, 15% of patients are expected to have persistent dysphagia at 1 month, and NG or PEG tube placement should be discussed with the patient and the family. Dysphagic stroke patients who receive feeding via a nasogastric tube rather than a PEG tube have better functional outcomes but do not live significantly longer.[11]

The question of whether a patient with a poor prognosis and extensive brain damage should receive artificial nutrition is a very important one and should be discussed openly with the patient's family or power of attorney.

Reduced Communication

A stroke patient's ability to communicate might be hindered by aphasias, dysarthrias, or neuropsychological deficits such as agnosia, apraxia, neglect, and reduced visuospatial orientation. Stroke patients with aphasia were found to receive less pain medications than patients without aphasia.[12] Speech pathologists might be able to improve communication and implement coping strategies.

Incontinence and Bowel Management

Approximately half of stroke patients have symptoms of incontinence during the initial hospital stay, but only 20% are affected by urinary incontinence and 10% by fecal incontinence 6 months after their intial stroke. The use of in-dwelling catheters is associated with higher rates of infection and should be restricted as much as possible. Fecal incontinence can lead to decubitus ulcers and skin damage. Limited mobility and reduced oral intake increase the risk for constipation.

Pain

Pain in stroke patients may be directly related to the intracranial damage or to the results of plegia, such as contractures, pressure sores, or arthralgias caused by immobility. While pain is not commonly seen in the acute stroke setting, almost 50% of stroke survivors report new pain within 6 months after having had a stroke.[9]

Especially difficult to treat is the shoulder–hand syndrome (also called hemiplegic shoulder pain). In this complex regional pain syndrome, the paretic upper arm frequently appears painful, edematous, with altered heat and tactile sensations, and has a slightly dystrophic skin. Early mobilization has been shown to prevent shoulder–hand syndrome, which otherwise affects up to 80% with hemiplegia.

Ice, heat, and soft tissue massage, as well as oral analgesics (NSAIDs) have been used to achieve temporary pain control. Other treatment options include psychotherapy, regional anesthesia, neuromodulation, and sympathectomy. Short courses of oral steroids or intra-articular steroid injections might be also effective in treatment of the syndrome.

Approximately 10% of patients suffer from central post-stroke pain, which is a neuropathic pain syndrome characterized by unilateral pain and dysesthesia associated with impaired sensation. The pain is thought to be due to a lesion in the spinothalamic tract or the thalamus itself. This pain is typically resistant to opioids.

Several antidepressants and anticonvulsant drugs commonly used in neuropathic pain have been studied, but only amitriptyline and lamotrigen have been effective. Levetiracetam, gabapentin, pregabalin, carbamazepine, and venlafaxine have not resulted in significant pain relief when studies.

Palliative Care in Demyelinating Disease (Multiple Sclerosis)

Multiple sclerosis (MS) is the most frequent inflammatory demyelinating disorder of the central nervous system. While its exact cause is unknown, the clinical picture reflects the pathological mechanism of inflammation, demyelination, and axon degeneration.

Although new immunomodulatory therapy is able to slow disease progression, symptom management and palliative care remain important in the later stages of the disease.

The severity of MS can be divided into benign and malignant courses. *Benign MS* refers to disease in which the patient remains fully functional in all neurological systems 15 years after the disease onset. In *malignant MS*, patients display rapid disease progression, leading to significant neurological disability or death in a relatively short time. However, death due to MS is rare and is most likely to occur as a result of secondary complications such as aspiration pneumonia or pulmonary embolus.

Particularly after the onset of the chronic progressive phase of the disease, symptom management with the goal of improving or maintaining function and quality of life is paramount.[13]

Muscle Spasticity

Between 40% and 85% of patients with MS experience spasticity, which is associated with pain, spasms, gait disorders, and bladder dysfunction.

The mainstay of therapy is regular physical therapy to maintain strength and movement and to decrease spasticity. Physical therapy should be used in combination with drug therapy.

Available medications are only partially effective and can cause adverse effects such as sedation, weakness, and cognitive problems. Therefore, antispastic medication should be started at low doses and slowly titrated against the clinical effect.

- Baclofen: 5–25 mg 3–4 times daily PO (an intrathecal pump can be considered in severe cases)
- Tizanidine: 2–39 mg daily PO (titrated over 2–4 weeks; takes approximately 1 week to reach its full effect)
- Gabapentin: 600–900 mg three times daily PO
- Dantrolene: 25–200 mg twice daily PO

Fatigue

Fatigue has been reported for most patients with MS and is associated with high levels of disability. Underlying depression (causing fatigue) should be ruled out first.

Because fatigue can be greatly worsened by heat, cooling of the body or the extremities may alleviate the symptom. Multiple stimulants have been tested in mostly small studies, and research-derived evidence remains scarce.[14]

Medical options that can be tried include the following:

- Amantadine 100 mg twice daily PO (second dose taken in the afternoon to avoid insomnia)

- Modafinil 200–400 mg daily PO
- Methylphenidate 10–60 mg/day taken bid or tid
- Pemoline 20–60 mg daily PO.

Bladder Dysfunction

Bladder dysfunction develops in almost all MS patients, and bladder hyperreflexia affects approximately 60% of patients. The latter condition results in a sense of urgency, urge incontinence, and frequent micturition.

Assessment of the urinary system is important to improve these systems and to prevent urinary tract infections and skin breakdown secondary to urinary incontinence.

Behavioral intervention in the early stages of MS includes planning adequate fluid intake, with more intake in the morning than in the afternoon, and use of the bathroom every 2–4 hours.

Pharmacological management is described in Table 33.1.

Pain

Pain is a frequent symptom in MS, affecting 50%–75% of patients. Pain can present as directly MS-related neuropathic pain or as secondary to MS symptoms, such as spasticity or paresis. Neuropathic pain often affects the lower extremities. Trigeminal neuralgia is seen in 1% of patients with MS and is clinically indistinguishable from the idiopathic form.

The initial treatment for both forms is carbamazepine (Table 33.2). Tricyclic antidepressants can be used to treat neuropathic pain, but they must be started at low doses because their side effects might increase other symptoms in MS patients, such as fatigue.

Other medical options involve the use of anticonvulsants.

Table 33.1 Pharmacological Management of Bladder Dysfunction in Patients with MS

Indication	Medication	Dosage	Side Effects
Detrusor hyperreflexia (overactive bladder)	Tolterodine (anticholinergic)	1–2 mg IR bid PO or 2–4 mg ER daily PO	Dryness, drowsiness (fewer side effects than with oxybutnin)
	Oxybutinin (anticholinergic)	2.5 mg qd–tid PO (titration up to 20 mg/day)	Dryness, drowsiness
Urinary frequency	Imipramine (alpha-agonist and anticholinergic activity)	10–25mg bid–tid PO	Sedation, dizziness
Nocturia	Desmopressin (antidiuretic hormone)	0.2–0.4 mcg nasal spray qhs	Hyponatremia

Table 33.2 Pharmacological Pain Management for Patients with MS

Indication	Medication	Dosage	Side Effects
Trigeminal neuralgia	Carbamazepine	100–200 mg bid, increased to 600–800 mg daily as tolerated	Drowsiness, dizziness, nausea and vomiting
Neuropathic pain	Nortriptyline, desipramine (tricyclic antidepressants)	10–25 mg qhs, increased by 10–25 mg every 3–7 days as tolerated	Sedation, cognitive impairment
	Bupropion	100 mg bid, increased after 3 days to maximum of 150 mg/dose and 450 mg/day	Dry mouth, dizziness

Psychobehavioral Symptoms and Depression

Progressive MS requires patients to constantly adjust to new symptoms and limitations. The lifetime rate of depression in MS patient reaches 40%–50% by age 59 and is thought to be related to cerebral pathology and treatment with steroids.[11]

Treatment recommendations are based mainly on research in other chronic illnesses due to the lack of high-quality conclusive studies in MS.[15]

Antidepressants should be selected on the basis of their side-effect profiles. Selective serotonin reuptake inhibitors (SSRIs) cause less fatigue, but tricyclic antidepressants might be more helpful in managing neuropathic pain, sleep disturbances, or overactive bladder.

Denial and cognitive decline are frequently seen in the late stages of MS. Pathological laughing and crying are observed in 10% of patients, who might respond to amitryptiline. Cognitive deficits are detected in approximately half of patients, and 10% of patients with late-stage disease have moderate to severe dementia.

Management consists of cognitive training and teaching of compensatory strategies. Personality and cognitive changes can cause major distress for families and caregivers and require education and psychosocial intervention.

Palliative Care in Parkinson's Disease

Parkinson's disease (PD) is a chronic, progressive neurodegenerative disease defined by the classic triad of tremor, rigor, and akinesis. Patients are more likely to have idiopathic PD than an atypical or secondary parkinsonian syndrome when they present with unilateral onset, have resting tremors, and respond well to L-dopa.

In addition to the classic features, patients with PD may develop symptoms related to the disease itself or to the medications used to treat it.

Medical therapy involves a multispecialist team and good pharmacological knowledge to ensure maximal symptom control[16] (Table 33.3).

Psychosis and Hallucination

Psychosis is frequently seen in PD and is closely associated with visual hallucinations and delusions. Hallucinations occur especially in the advanced stages of the disease and affect up to 40% of patients.

Because these symptoms are often drug induced, the first step should include the critical reassessment of potentially offending antiparkinsonian drugs. Hallucinations often can be ameliorated by a dose reduction with limited loss of the drug-related benefit.

Antiparkinsonian drugs should be reduced or stopped in reverse order of their potency and effectiveness if hallucinations are causing significant disability. A proposed order would be anticholinergic drugs followed by amantadine, catechol-O-methyl transferase (COMT) inhibitors, and finally dopamine agonists.

Antipsychotic therapy with clozapine and quetiapine has limited effect on parkinsonism and is preferred over other atypical neuroleptics, such as risperidone and olanzapine. Typical neuroleptics, such as haloperidol, should be avoided. Clozapine is effective but is underused because of its side effect of agranulocytosis.

Table 33.3 Typical Non-Motor Symptoms and Signs of Parkinson's Disease

Symptom	Sign
Cognitive dysfunction	Dementia, confusion
Mood disorders	Depression, anxiety, apathy, or abulia
Autonomic dysfunction	Urinary urgency or frequency, constipation, orthostasis, erectile dysfunction
Pain and sensory disturbances	Secondary to dystonia, dyskinesia
Psychosis	Hallucinations, delirium
Sleep disturbances	Sleep interruption, PLMS, RBD
Fatigue	
Dermatological findings	Seborrhea

The patient's absolute neutrophil count must be closely monitored. Olanzapine is not effective and might even worsen patients' motor function.

Cognitive Dysfunction and Dementia

Cognitive dysfunction is common in PD, and severe dementia is a major cause of disability and mortality in patients with PD. As with other dementias, the treatment is symptomatic only and does not appear to modify the course of the disease or influence the prognosis.

The cholinesterase inhibitors donepezil and rivastigmine have modest benefit, but the latter especially can cause worsening of tremors.[17]

Depression

Approximately 40% of PD patients experience depression. Depressive symptoms are linked to increased motor disability and decreased quality of life. The tricyclic antidepressants amitriptyline and nortriptyline have been found to be effective in patients with PD; however, adverse events are thought to be lower with SSRIs.

Citalopram, sertraline, and controlled-release paroxetine do not appear to be effective in PD patients, according to results from small studies.

Adverse events are thought to be lower with SSRIs than with tricyclic antidepressants, but SSRIs should be avoided if a patient is also being treated with selegiline, a monoamine oxidase B inhibitor. This combination has been reported to exacerbate motor symptoms and to cause serotonin syndrome with severely disturbed mental, motor, and autonomic function.

Sleep Disorders

Most patients with PD suffer from sleep disorders, most commonly sleep fragmentation. Frequent awakening throughout the night and early-morning awakening are often caused by nocturia, difficulty turning over in bed, cramps, vivid dreams or nightmares, and neck or back pain.

A specific sleep disorder associated with PD is periodic limb movement disorder (PLMS). PLMS is estimated to occur in 30%–80% of patients with PD. This sleep disorder involves slow, rhythmic leg movements consisting of dorsal flexion of the feet and great toes and, occasionally, the knees and hips. PLMS responds to dopaminergic agents.

Another sleep disorder associated with PD is rapid eye movement (REM) sleep behavior disorder (RBD). Patients with RBD present with vigorous movements during REM sleep. Because of a lack of movement inhibition during REM sleep, they act out their dreams and present with vocalizations as well as kicking and punching motions of the limbs, sometimes injuring themselves or their bed partners.

Over one-third of patients who originally present with idiopathic RBD may eventually develop PD. Additional L-dopa or clonazepam are the agents of choice for treating RBD. Clonazepam (0.5 mg PO qhs, to be increased to 1–2 mg) is effective for nearly 90% of patients.

Clinical Pearls

- Most chronic neurological disorders such as ALS, end-stage Parkinson's disease, and secondary progressive MS have a predictable course of progression. Start the conversation about palliative measures early and remain involved.
- The management of neurological disorders is a team effort. Reach out early and involve other providers as needed.
- The central nervous system is complex and full of interactions. Many symptoms, especially fatigue, can be caused by medication side effects. Therefore, set treatment priorities together with the patient and check the medication list—sometimes less is more.
- Use medications' side effects to the patient's advantage. Many medications influencing the central nervous system have several effects that might be useful in treating more than one symptom. For example, amitryptiline might have a positive impact on the patient's mood and at the same time may decrease drooling.
- Almost all patients with chronic neurological disorders have psychobehavioral symptoms or show signs of depression. Screen for these disorders frequently and treat proactively.

References

1. Miller RG, Jackson CE, Kasarskis EJ, England JD, Forshew D, Johnston W, Kalra S, Katz JS, Mitsumoto H, Rosenfeld J, Shoesmith C, Strong MJ, Woolley SC (2009). Practice parameter update: the care of the patient with amyotrophic lateral sclerosis: multidisciplinary care, symptom management, and cognitive/behavioral impairment (an evidence-based review): report of the Quality Standards Subcommittee of the American Academy of Neurology. *Neurology* 73(15):1227–33.
2. Miller RG, Jackson CE, Kasarskis EJ, England JD, Forshew D, Johnston W, Kalra S, Katz JS, Mitsumoto H, Rosenfeld J, Shoesmith C, Strong MJ, Woolley SC (2009). Practice parameter update: the care of the patient with amyotrophic lateral sclerosis: drug, nutritional, and respiratory therapies (an evidence-based review): report of the Quality Standards Subcommittee of the American Academy of Neurology. *Neurology* 73(15):1218–26.
3. Andersen PM, Abrahams S, Borasio GD, de Carvalho M, Chio A, Van Damme P, Hardiman O, Kollewe K, Morrison KE, Petri S, Pradat PF, Silani V, Tomik B, Wasner M, Weber M (2012). EFNS guidelines on the clinical management of amyotrophic lateral sclerosis (MALS)—revised report of an EFNS task force. *Eur J Neurol* 19(3):360–75.
4. Molloy L (2007). Treatment of sialorrhoea in patients with Parkinson's disease: best current evidence. *Curr Opin Neurol* 20(4):493–8.
5. Brooks BR, Thisted RA, Appel SH, Bradley WG, Olney RK, Berg JE, Pope LE, Smith RA (2004). Treatment of pseudobulbar affect in ALS with dextromethorphan/quinidine: a randomized trial. *Neurology* 63(8):1364–70.
6. Katzberg HD, Khan AH, So YT (2010). Assessment: symptomatic treatment for muscle cramps (an evidence-based review): report of the Therapeutics and Technology Assessment Subcommittee of the American Academy of Neurology. *Neurology* 74(8):691–6.
7. Bedlack RS, Pastula DM, Hawes J, Heydt D (2009). Open-label pilot trial of levetiracetam for cramps and spasticity in patients with motor neuron disease. *Amyotroph Lateral Sc* 10(4):210–5.
8. Stevens T, Payne SA, Burton C, Addington-Hall J, Jones A (2007). Palliative care in stroke: a critical review of the literature. *Palliat Med* 21(4):323–31.
9. Holloway RG, Arnold RM, Creutzfeldt CJ, Lewis EF, Lutz BJ, McCann RM, Rabinstein AA, Saposnik G, Sheth KN, Zahuranec DB, Zipfel GJ, Zorowitz RD, American Heart Association Stroke Council, Council on Cardiovascular and Stroke Nursing, Council on Clinical Cardiology (2014). Palliative and end-of-life care in stroke: a statement for healthcare professionals from the American Heart Association/American Stroke Association. *Stroke* 45(6):1887–916.
10. Jauch EC, Saver JL, Adams HP, Jr., Bruno A, Connors JJ, Demaerschalk BM, Khatri P, McMullan PW, Jr., Qureshi AI, Rosenfeld K, Scott PA, Summers DR, Wang DZ, Wintermark M, Yonas H

(2013). Guidelines for the early management of patients with acute ischemic stroke: a guideline for healthcare professionals from the American Heart Association/American Stroke Association. *Stroke* 44(3):870–947.

11. Dennis M, Lewis S, Cranswick G, Forbes J (2006). FOOD: a multicentre randomised trial evaluating feeding policies in patients admitted to hospital with a recent stroke. *Health Technol Assess* 10(2):iii–iv, ix–x, 1–120.

12. Kehayia E, Korner-Bitensky N, Singer F, Becker R, Lamarche M, Georges P, Retik S (1997). Differences in pain medication use in stroke patients with aphasia and without aphasia. *Stroke* 28(10):1867–70.

13. Toosy A, Ciccarelli O, Thompson A (2014). Symptomatic treatment and management of multiple sclerosis. *Handbook Clin Neurol* 122:513–62.

14. Khan F, Amatya B, Galea M (2014). Management of fatigue in persons with multiple sclerosis. *Front Neurol* 5:177.

15. Minden SL, Feinstein A, Kalb RC, Miller D, Mohr DC, Patten SB, Bever C, Jr., Schiffer RB, Gronseth GS, Narayanaswami P (2014). Evidence-based guideline: assessment and management of psychiatric disorders in individuals with MS: report of the Guideline Development Subcommittee of the American Academy of Neurology. *Neurology* 82(2):174–81.

16. Miyasaki JM, Shannon K, Voon V, Ravina B, Kleiner-Fisman G, Anderson K, Shulman LM, Gronseth G, Weiner WJ (2006). Practice parameter: evaluation and treatment of depression, psychosis, and dementia in Parkinson disease (an evidence-based review): report of the Quality Standards Subcommittee of the American Academy of Neurology. *Neurology* 66(7):996–1002.

17. Zesiewicz TA, Sullivan KL, Arnulf I, Chaudhuri KR, Morgan JC, Gronseth GS, Miyasaki J, Iverson DJ, Weiner WJ (2010). Practice parameter: treatment of nonmotor symptoms of Parkinson disease: report of the Quality Standards Subcommittee of the American Academy of Neurology. *Neurology* 74(11):924–31.

Palliative Care in End-Stage Chronic Obstructive Pulmonary Disease

Simeon Kwan and Sriram Yennurajalingam

Introduction

Patients with end-stage chronic obstructive pulmonary disease (COPD) experience high symptom burden arising from severe dyspnea, fatigue, anxiety, depression, disability, and social isolation, resulting in poor quality of life. The caregiving burden for the family of a patient with end-stage COPD is significant. In this chapter, we discuss the key issues in assessing and managing end-stage COPD.

COPD, which affects 6% of the general population, is one of the leading causes of morbidity and mortality worldwide.[1] It is one of the five principal causes of mortality in the world according to the World Health Organization.[2] The incidence of COPD is increasing; it is estimated that COPD will become the fourth-leading cause of mortality by 2030.[1]

Prognostic Factors

Clinical Evaluation

According to the National Hospice and Palliative Care Organization, patients who meet any of the following criteria may be suspected of having end-stage COPD:

1. Disabling dyspnea at rest
2. Poor or no response to bronchodilators
3. A bed-to-chair existence
4. Repeated emergency room visits or hospitalizations for respiratory infection or failure
5. Hypoxemia at rest (partial pressure of oxygen < 55 mmHg)
6. Oxygen saturation < 88% while receiving supplemental oxygen
7. Hypercapnia (partial pressure of carbon dioxide > 50 mmHg)
8. Cor pulmonale
9. Right heart failure secondary to pulmonary disease
10. Unintentional progressive weight loss (> 10% over 6 months, serum albumin level < 2.5 g/dl)
11. Resting tachycardia (heart rate > 100 beats/minute).

The BODE index is used to determine the severity of disease in COPD patients[3] (see Table 34.1 for details of the BODE index).

Mortality

In general, it is difficult to predict mortality in patients with long-standing COPD, but the higher the BODE index, the higher the likelihood of death (see Table 34.2). Ultimately, patient satisfaction and quality of life are the key factors to guide decision-making. Additionally, patients with Global Initiative for Chronic Obstructive Lung Disease stages III or IV COPD have a much higher death rate (42.9 deaths per 1000 person years) than healthy individuals (5.4 deaths per 1000 person years; hazard ratio = 5.7).[4]

Table 34.1 Variables and Point Values Used for the Computation of the Body-Mass Index, Degree of Airflow Obstruction, Degree of Dyspnea, and Exercise Capacity (BODE) Index

Variable	Points on BODE Index			
	0	1	2	3
FEV_1 (% of predicted)	≥ 65	50–64	36–49	≤ 35
Distance walked in 6 min (m)	> 350	250–349	150–249	≤ 149
MMRC dyspnea scale	0–1	2	3	4
BMI	> 21	≤ 21		

Abbreviations: FEV_1, = forced expiratory volume in 1 second; MMRC = modified Medical Research Council.
Adapted from Celli BR, et al. (2004). The body-mass index, airflow obstruction, dyspnea, and exercise capacity index in chronic obstructive pulmonary disease. *New Engl J Med* 350(10):1005–12.

Table 34.2 Interpretation of the Body-Mass Index, Degree of Airflow Obstruction, Degree of Dyspnea, and Exercise Capacity (BODE) Index Scores

BODE Index Score	1-Year Mortality (%)	2-Year Mortality (%)	3-Year Mortality (%)
0–2	2	6	19
3–4	2	8	32
5–6	2	14	40
7–10	5	31	80

Morbidity

Patients with end-stage COPD may have to endure symptoms long term. Due to the difficulty of predicting mortality in end-stage COPD, morbidity and symptom management is of prime importance.

Acute Exacerbations

Usual management of acute exacerbations includes antibiotics, steroids, and BiPAP use. Almost 25% of COPD patients die within 1 year of hospitalization for an acute exacerbation. The median survival for COPD patients who have had an acute exacerbation after intensive care unit admission is 2 years, with a 50% likelihood of further hospitalization within 6 months.[4]

Circulatory Effects

COPD patients have a high risk of developing circulatory compromise that affects other organ systems. The risks of atherosclerosis and mortality are increased in COPD patients who smoke.[4]

Nutrition

In advanced COPD patients, the increased work required to breathe increases energy expenditure and may lead to cachexia. General health status can be further compromised by a lack of exercise due to low exercise tolerance and dyspnea. COPD patients who have a normal weight or are underweight have a significantly higher risk of death than patients who are overweight or obese.[4]

Palliative Care

Assessment

A pulmonologist, intensivist, primary care physician, or palliative care physician should direct palliative care in COPD patients according to the guidelines of the American Thoracic Society or the Canadian Thoracic Society. Patients should have access to an interdisciplinary palliative care team.[5] Comprehensive assessment involves accurately predicting the trajectory of functional decline to provide patients with early access to specialized palliative care services; performing detailed symptom assessment using validated symptom assessment tools such as the Edmonton Symptom Assessment Scale on a routine and consistent basis; screening patients for anxiety, depression, and spiritual or social distress; assessing caregiver burden in family members; evaluating patients for dyspnea (see Chapter 14), and managing it as appropriate in a palliative care setting with the goal of improving quality of life; and performing individualized diagnostic evaluations focused on determining the underlying cause of COPD and providing care accordingly.

End-of-life Decision-Making

Initiating end-of-life care planning should occur soon after the patient has been diagnosed with end-stage COPD. Early planning is essential due to the unpredictable speed at which end-stage COPD patients may deteriorate. Discussions about a patient's preferences for end-of-life care should include the patient, the patient's primary healthcare provider, and the patient's caregivers. Patients should be given information about the potential benefits and burdens of therapy. Other important decisions may involve the patient's preferences regarding resuscitation, intubation, mechanical ventilation, surrogate decision-makers, and advance directives, which should be discussed while the patient's health is stable.[4,6,7]

Psychosocial, Spiritual, and Family Distress

Although 37% of patients with advanced COPD are depressed, only 30% of these patients receive treatment for depression. Patients with end-stage COPD may benefit from antidepressive therapy if they have significant depressive symptoms.[4,6,8] Because COPD also affects quality of life, the patient's ability to perform activities of daily living independently or without dyspnea should be addressed.

Barriers to Providing Palliative Care

Several issues complicate or prevent the delivery of appropriate palliative care to COPD patients.

Inadequate communication between healthcare providers, patients, and families regarding end-of-life care, especially early in the course of the disease, can impede the delivery of appropriate palliative care. For example, when asking oxygen-dependent COPD patients about their avoidance of discussing end-of-life care, Curtis et al. found that more than 50% of patients provided responses such as "I'd rather concentrate on staying alive than talk about death" and "I'm not sure which physician will be taking care of me if I get very sick." Recent studies have underscored the need for clinicians to be able to communicate openly with their COPD patients regarding end-of-life decisions and comprehensive symptom management.

Predicting the disease course in COPD patients can be challenging because of the disease's variable trajectory, and as a result, patients with end-stage COPD often do not receive adequate palliative care services.[2] Various tools such as the BODE index, Hansen-Flaschen criteria, and Acute Physiology and Chronic Health Evaluation IV scores can be used to predict increased mortality in COPD patients who require intensive care unit admissions. Inadequate assessment and management of severe symptoms related to end-stage COPD can also complicate the delivery of palliative care.[4,6]

Communication

Discussions about end-of-life care can be difficult but are important aspects of the care provided to terminally ill patients and their families. Approximately 56% of terminally ill COPD patients want to know their life expectancy. In addition, many patients with end-stage COPD report wanting to discuss the following topics with their physician:

1. Diagnosis and disease progression
2. Effect of treatments on symptoms, quality of life, and life expectancy
3. Prognosis for survival and quality of life
4. Aspects of the dying process, specifically issues regarding breathlessness or suffocation)
5. Advanced planning for foreseeable medical needs and end-of-life care.[4,6,7]

Despite these desires, many physicians are unwilling to discuss these issues to avoid destroying their patients' hope.[7]

Management

Individualized treatment should be provided for patients with end-stage COPD. The underlying cause of COPD should be determined and care provided accordingly. COPD patients should be evaluated for dyspnea and cared for as appropriate in a palliative care setting with the goal of improving quality of life. Although only smoking cessation and long-term oxygen therapy (LTOT) have been shown to improve survival in COPD patients, other interventions may be beneficial in improving the quality of life of patients with end-stage COPD.[4,8]

Pharmaceutical Interventions

Pharmaceutical interventions for COPD are presented in Table 34.3. Inhaled corticosteroids have been shown to decrease mortality from all causes in COPD patients. The combination of long-acting agonists and steroids may provide a survival benefit, but this has not been tested in patients with end-stage COPD. Because they are an independent risk factor for death, oral corticosteroids should be limited to the short-term treatment of acute exacerbations in COPD patients.[4]

LTOT has been shown to prolong survival in severely hypoxemic patients (partial pressure of oxygen in arterial blood [PaO_2] < 55 mmHg).[9] Moderately hypoxemic patients with pulmonary hypertension, cor pulmonale, and/or secondary polycythemia may also benefit from LTOT. In COPD patients with mild hypoxemia (PaO_2 > 59 mmHg), the prescription of oxygen may improve quality of life and relieve dyspnea but should be determined on an individual basis.[4]

The sensation of dyspnea can be an incapacitating and distressing symptom in end-stage COPD.[4] The use of opioid medications in the relief of dyspnea is discussed further in Chapter 14.

Nonpharmaceutical Interventions

Patients with end-stage COPD may remain self-sufficient but have limitations in activities of daily living and quality of life. The use of nonpharmaceutical therapies has been shown to be effective in controlling the symptoms present in this group of patients.[10]

Noninvasive Positive Pressure Ventilation (NIPPV), in conjunction with LTOT and daytime exercise training, improves dyspnea and quality of life in COPD patients. Nocturnal NIPPV may be used to increase exercise tolerance during the day by resting the muscles at night. However, larger studies are needed to identify the patients who would most benefit from this approach.[8,10]

Regular exercise decreases the likelihood of hospitalization and mortality in COPD patients; in particular, whole-body strengthening exercises are helpful in successfully weaning patients off chronic ventilation.[10]

Neuromuscular electrical low-voltage stimulation has been shown to increase muscular oxidative capacity in COPD patients and can be used to treat debilitated patients.[10]

Poor caloric intake and high-energy requirements often lead to malnutrition in COPD patients. COPD patients with a BMI < 20 have lower survival and higher hospitalization rates than COPD patients with a BMI > 20. All

Table 34.3 Pharmaceutical Interventions for Chronic Obstructive Pulmonary Disease

Drug Class	Initial Dose	Indication	Caveats	Interactions	Common Side Effects
Short-acting β-agonists (albuterol)	MDI: 90 mcg/puff, 2 puffs every 4–6 hours PRN	Bronchospasm		Furosemide, haloperidol, methadone, duloxetine, moxifloxacin	Dizziness, dry mouth, nervousness
Long-acting β-agonists (salmeterol)	INH: 50 mcg every 12 hours	Bronchospasm, maintenance	Do not use for acute treatment	Carvedilol, flucanazole	Headache, sinus congestion, nervousness
Short-acting anticholinergics (ipratropium)	NEB: 0.5 mg every 6–8 hours	Bronchospasm	NEB: May mix with short-acting β-agonists	Tiotropium Bromide	Cough, dry mouth, headache, nausea, nervousness
Long-acting anticholinergics (tiotropium)	INH: 1 18-mcg capsule every 24 hours	COPD, maintenance	Do not use for acute treatment; must use dosing device	Metoclopramide	Blurred vision, dry mouth, GI intolerance

Methylxanthine (theophylline)	300–400 mg/day for 3 days, then 400–600 mg/day	COPD, maintenance	Must monitor blood levels; care with reduced clearance	Tramadol, metoprolol	Temporary changes in behavior, increased urination
Inhaled glucocorticosteroids (fluticasone)	44–220 mcg/spray, 2 puffs BID	COPD, maintenance	Titrate to lowest effective dose; taper to discontinuation		
Systemic glucocorticosteroids (prednisone)	60 mg/day for 3–10 days	Acute COPD exacerbation	Short-term use only	Furosemide, Fluoroquinolones	Difficulty sleeping, increased appetite, nervousness, hyperglycemia
Antibiotics	Patient- and agent-dependent	Infection	Use only for infection in acute exacerbation	Varies	Varies
Oxygen	Titrate to 90% saturation	Hypoxemia	Must demonstrate need		

Abbreviations: MDI = measured-dose inhaler; PRN = according to circumstances; INH = inhaler; NEB = nebulizer; GI = gastrointestinal; BID = twice per day.

COPD patients should undergo a thorough nutritional assessment and be cared for accordingly.[10]

Bullectomy in patients with a bulla that is compressing functional lung tissue, and lung volume reduction surgery in patients with upper lobe disease, may improve quality of life and exercise capacity.[10] However, due to the frailty of patients with limited life expectancy, the risks and benefits of surgery must be weighed carefully.[10]

Summary

Palliative care in COPD patients should focus on relieving dyspnea and optimizing quality of life. LTOT, inhaled corticosteroids, and inhaler anticholinergics have shown benefit in COPD patients. Attempts should be made to improve endurance and nutritional status.

Clinical Pearls

- Early and extensive communication regarding end-stage COPD and its implication on quality of life between the patient/family and the healthcare provider is critical.
- Discussions about end-of-life care preferences should be initiated after a patient recovers from acute exacerbation.
- Assess the perceived effect that COPD has on the patient's quality of life.

References

1. Global Initiative for Chronic Obstructive Lung Disease. *The Global Strategy for Diagnosis, Management and Prevention of COPD* (updated 2014). www.goldcopd.org.
2. Ek K, Andershed B, Sahlberg-blom E, Ternestedt BM (2014). "The unpredictable death": the last year of life for patients with advanced COPD: relatives' stories. *Palliat Support Care* (5):1213–22.
3. Celli BR, et al. (2004). The body-mass index, airflow obstruction, dyspnea, and exercise capacity index in chronic obstructive pulmonary disease. *N Engl J Med* 350(10):1005–12.
4. Ambrosino N, Simonds A (2007). The clinical management in extremely severe COPD. *Resp Med* 101:1613–24.
5. O'Donnell DE, Aaron S, Bourbeau J, et al. (2007). Canadian Thoracic Society recommendations for management of chronic obstructive pulmonary disease: 2007 update. *Can Respir J* 14(Suppl B):5B–32B.
6. Curtis JR (2006). Palliative care for patients with chronic obstructive pulmonary disease. *Resp Med: COPD Update* 2:86–90.
7. Disler RT, Currow DC, Phillips JL, Smith T, Johnson MJ, Davidson PM (2012). Interventions to support a palliative care approach in patients with chronic obstructive pulmonary disease: an integrative review. *Int J Nurs Stud* 49(11):1443–58.
8. Berman AR (2011). Management of patients with end-stage chronic obstructive pulmonary disease. *Prim Care* 38(2):277–97, viii–ix.
9. Bettoncelli G, Blasi F, Brusasco V, et al. (2014). The clinical and integrated management of COPD. *Sarcoidosis Vasc Diffuse Lung Dis* 31:3609.
10. Clini EM, Ambrosino N (2008). Nonpharmacological treatment and relief of symptoms in COPD. *Eur Respir J* 32:218–28.

Palliative Care in the Intensive Care Unit

Rony Dev

Overview

The aim of palliative care is to prevent unnecessary suffering experienced by patients facing an incurable illness. Patients admitted to the intensive care unit (ICU) often experience a high symptom burden secondary to their underlying disease and face the risk of dying. Painful invasive procedures and medical treatments not consistent with a patient's goals of care can add additional suffering for ICU patients.

In the United States, one in five deaths occurs in ICUs, which accounts for greater than 500,000 deaths annually.[1] Roughly, 5%–30% of patients die while hospitalized in an ICU, which would indicate a need to integrate palliative medicine with critical care.

The goal of relieving suffering in patients with complex illnesses can coexist with the curative treatment offered in an ICU. Often, it is difficult to distinguish between critical illness and terminal illness. Offering palliative care only at the time of withholding or withdrawing treatment may diminish the benefits of physical and psychosocial support that could be provided for ICU patients and their families. When critically ill patients are not responsive to curative treatment, the goal of comforting patients could and should always be continued.

In addition to assisting with symptom management in an ICU, palliative care providers can also assess and comfort family members whose loved ones are critically ill. By taking the time to listen to the concerns of family members and answer their questions, clinicians can assess levels of distress in family members and can offer interventions. After a patient has died, interventions to lessen the burden of bereavement should be initiated.

Communication and End-of-Life Discussions

Open and regular communication is essential for adequate palliation. For critically ill patients and their families, information regarding findings, medications, and expected changes may need to be repeated several times by healthcare professionals. In general, the use of graphs, question prompt lists, and recordings of consults can increase recall and satisfaction with information.

In the ICU setting, written materials including information leaflets have been shown to improve communication between healthcare providers and patients. However, patient and family satisfaction depends on their understanding, which may be limited.[2]

Family conferences can facilitate communication with patients and their caregivers. Results of prospective cohort trials in the ICU setting have shown that end-of-life family conferences are associated with improvement in family satisfaction, reduction in length of stay, and increased access to palliative care without an increase in mortality.[3]

Family members rate communication skills equal to or more important than a physician's clinical skills. Studies of communication have revealed the importance of the following: assurance of nonabandonment by healthcare providers, honoring patients' requests to be kept comfortable, and the healthcare team's support of decisions made by families regarding treatment preferences.[4] In addition, listening, acknowledging emotions, and explaining surrogated decision-making have been rated by families as critical to their satisfaction when their loved one is hospitalized.[5]

The VALUE mnemonic (Table 35.1) has been developed as a checklist to verify that adequate support in an end-of-life conference is provided for families of ICU patients. Survey responses from family members of 126 ICU patients in France who were randomized to receive either usual care or a communication-based intervention based on the VALUE strategy resulted in significantly decreased anxiety and depression.[3] In addition, family members who were surveyed 3 months after the patients had died showed decreased post-traumatic stress disorder.[3]

A summary of recommendations for optimal negotiation of the goals of care is provided in Box 35.1.

Table 35.1 VALUE Mnemonic

V	Value family statements
A	Acknowledge family emotions
L	Listen to the family
U	Understand the patient as a person
E	Elicit family questions

Adapted from Lautrette A, Darmon M, Megarbane B, et al. (2007). A communication strategy and brochure for relatives of patients dying in the ICU. *N Engl J Med* 356(5):469–78.

Box 35.1 Protocol to Negotiate Goals of Care

Recommendations include the following:
- Create the proper setting.
- Clarify what the patient and family already know.
- Explore the hopes and expectations of the patient and family.
- Suggest realistic goals.
- Use empathic responses.
- Make a plan and follow through with it.

Adapted from the Education on Palliative and End-of-life Care Project.

Interdisciplinary Team Collaboration

In addition to effective communication with patients and their families, communication provided by and within the interdisciplinary team of clinicians, nurses, respiratory therapists, pharmacists, social workers, and spiritual care support staff needs to be clear and consistent. Mixed messages by ICU clinicians were associated with increased anxiety and depression in family members.[6]

Observational research in the ICU setting has shown that increased interdisciplinary collaboration results in decreased ICU mortality, shorter length of stay in an ICU, lower rates of ICU readmission, and minimized stress in the workplace, for nurses in particular.[7]

Do Not Resuscitate (DNR) Orders

A DNR order is often implemented for patients with an advanced illness. It reflects a patient's preference for end-of-life care. A DNR order in place for critically ill patients is not to be confused with a patient's preference about other life-sustaining treatments, such as the administration of antibiotics, transfusion of blood products, and artificial nutrition or hydration. The establishing of goals of care consistent with patient preferences is critical for providing palliation at the end of life.

DNR orders often are not elicited by healthcare professionals. Reasons for clinicians not writing a DNR order include the belief that patients are not in imminent danger of dying, the belief that the primary care physician should be responsible for obtaining the DNR, and the lack of opportunity, or reimbursement for the time, to discuss end-of-life issues.[8] In addition, fear of litigation, discomfort, and lack of training for discussing end-of-life issues can result in avoidance of writing a DNR order.

Withdrawing Mechanical Ventilation

The withdrawing of mechanical ventilation can cause symptom distress in patients and stress on their family. Prior to withdrawal, appropriate communication with family members is critical to ensure that discontinuation of ventilation is in the best interest of the patient's overall well-being and is consistent with his or her goals of care.

The patient and family should be given reassurance that discontinuation of mechanical ventilation will be supervised by a qualified clinician and that any subsequent discomfort after withdrawal will be aggressively treated.

One protocol that has been studied[9] enables an ICU team to withdraw life-supporting mechanical ventilation in a way that minimizes unnecessary suffering (Figure 35.1). Incorporation of the protocol resulted in increased opioid and benzodiazepines use without an impact on the time to death.[9]

Figure 35.1. Protocol for withdrawing mechanical ventilation.

IMV = intermittent mandatory ventilation; PEEP = positive end expiratory pressure.

Adapted from Treece PD, Engelberg RA, Crowley L, et al. (2004). Evaluation of a standardized order form for the withdrawal of life support in the intensive care unit. *Crit Care Med* 32(5):1141–8.

Symptom Distress in ICU Patients

Patients hospitalized in an ICU may experience an increased symptom burden that can go undetected if not appropriately assessed. Both physical and psychological symptoms can be identified by careful and thorough symptom assessment.

In one study of 50 communicating patients hospitalized in an ICU, patients expressed a high level of distress, including symptoms of pain, thirst, insomnia, anxiety, depression, hunger, and dyspnea.[10]

In a recent retrospective review of 88 palliative medicine consults (6% of 1383 ICU admissions), interventions recommend included opioid adjustment (99%), initiation of steroids (70%), withdrawal of mechanical ventilation or bilevel positive airway pressure (BIPAP), discontinuation of total parenteral nutrition, addition of anti-emetics and antipsycotics, and discontinuation of benzodiazepines or other sedating medications. After the consultation, patients reported improved levels of pain, dyspnea, anxiety, and delirium.[11]

Symptom Assessment Scales for the ICU Patient

In order to provide effective analgesia with minimal side effects, daily bedside symptom assessments should be incorporated into routine practice. In the ICU, patients' pain is often not assessed adequately, and when it is assessed, assessment tools are infrequently used.[12]

When patients are able to communicate, their subjective rating of discomfort should be used to titrate medications to control symptoms. Studies show that when nurses assess pain, 35%–55% underrate the intensity of a patient's pain level. When assessing symptoms in patients able to communicate, a numeric pain scale between 0 and 10, a visual analog scale, or patient questionnaires may be used.

Symptom assessment can be complicated by the fact that many ICU patients are not able to communicate, since they are either intubated or too sedated. Examples of symptom assessment scales for noncommunicative patients include patient comfort, FLACC (face, legs, activity, cry, consolability), the Critical Care Pain Observation Tool (CPOT), and the Behavior Pain Scale (BPS) (facial expression, movement of upper limbs, and compliance with mechanical ventilation) (Table 35.2).[13]

In noncommunicative patients, both the BPS and CPOT have been validated and shown to be reliable; however, no scale has been incorporated as the standard pain assessment tool in the ICU setting. In one study of 230 ICU patients, incorporation of the BPS resulted in a decreased rate of severe pain, as well as a decrease in the duration of mechanical ventilation of patients.[14]

Table 35.2 Behavioral Pain Scale

Item	Description	Score
Facial expression	Relaxed	1
	Partially tightened (brow lowering)	2
	Fully tightened (eyelid closing)	3
	Grimacing	4
Upper limbs	No movement	1
	Partially bent	2
	Fully bent with finger flexion	3
	Permanently retracted	4
Compliance	Tolerating movement with ventilation	1
	Coughing but tolerating (most of the time)	2
	Fighting ventilator	3
	Unable to control ventilation	4

Scores from each of the three domains are summed, with a total score of 3 to 12.

Pain Secondary to Invasive Procedures

In addition to the symptom burden secondary to an underlying disease, critically ill patients may undergo invasive procedures that may be painful. ICU patients often experience a high level of discomfort during endotracheal tube placement and suctioning, arterial and central line placement, and arterial blood sampling.

A strategy of premedicating patients prior to painful procedures should be used to diminish patient discomfort.

Sedation Assessment

The provision of adequate pain control can be complicated by excessive sedation in critically ill patients. A balance between pain control and excessive sedation must be attained such that sedation should be tolerated only when its benefits outweigh the risks.

To attain a balance beneficial to patients, clinicians need to make frequent assessment of symptoms, carefully adjust opioids and sedatives while monitoring for side effects, and communicate with all members of the healthcare team, with careful attention to the bedside symptom assessment made by ICU nurses.

Examples of sedation scales that have been used in the ICU include the Ramsay Sedation Scale (Table 35.3), Richmond Agitation–Sedation Scale (Table 35.4), Motor Activity Assessment Scale, Vancouver Interactive and Calmness Scale, Adaptation to Intensive Environment, Minnesota Sedation Assessment Tool, and the Confusion Assessment Method (CAM).[13]

Benzodiazepines and propofol are commonly used sedatives in the ICU setting. Benzodiazepine use, however, has been shown to be a risk factor

Table 35.3 Ramsay Sedation Scale

Score	Definition
1	Anxious and agitated or restless or both
2	Cooperative, oriented, and tranquil
3	Responds to commands only
4	Brisk response to a light glabellar tap or loud auditory stimulus
5	Sluggish response to a light glabellar tap or loud auditory stimulus
6	No response to a light glabellar tap or loud auditory stimulus

Performed using a series of steps: observation of behavior (score 1 or 2), followed (if necessary) by assessment of response to voice (score 3), followed (if necessary) by assessment of response to loud auditory stimulus or light glabellar tap (score 4 to 6).

Table 35.4 Richmond Agitation–Sedation Scale

Score	Term	Description
+4	Combative	Overtly combative or violent, immediate danger to staff
+3	Very agitated	Pulls on or removes tube(s) or catheter(s) or exhibits aggressive behavior toward staff
+2	Agitated	Frequent nonpurposeful movement, patient–ventilator dyssynchrony
+1	Restless	Anxious or apprehensive but movements not aggressive or vigorous
0	Alert and calm	
–1	Drowsy	Not fully alert, but has sustained (> 10 seconds) awakening, with eye contact, to voice
–2	Light sedation	Briefly (< 10 seconds) awakens, with eye contact, to voice
–3	Moderate sedation	Any movement (but no eye contact) to voice
–4	Deep sedation	No response to voice, but any movement to physical stimulation
–5	Unarousable	No response to voice or physical stimulation

Performed using a series of steps: observation of behaviors (score +4 to 0), followed (if necessary) by assessment of response to voice (score –1 to –3), followed (if necessary) by assessment of response to physical stimulation such as shaking shoulder and then rubbing sternum if there is no response to shaking shoulder (score –4 to –5).
Reprinted with permission from Sessler et al. (2002). The F Agitation–Sedation Scale. *Am J Respir Crit Care Med* 166(10):1338–44.

for delirium for ICU patients, and recent studies support a reduction in reliance on benzodiazepines as a sedative.[15] The use of validated sedation scales and interruption of continuous sedation[16] with close monitoring of adverse events have shown improved clinical outcomes in ongoing clinical trials.

The sedative dexmedetomidine, an alpha-2-receptor agonist, promises to be an effective sedative for ICU patients without being associated with an increased risk for delirium,[15] but further research is needed.

Delirium

Delirium, defined as a disturbance of consciousness and cognition that fluctuates over time and develops acutely (hours to days), is often unrecognized by ICU healthcare providers. Prevalence of delirium in the ICU varies from 20% to 80% (see Table 35.5 for risk factors).[17] Delirium is associated with poor outcomes, including removal of Foley catheters, self-extubation, prolonged hospital stay, and even increased mortality.

Preliminary data confirming the increased risk of long-term cognitive impairment in delirious patients who survived ICU hospitalization have been brought to the attention of clinicians; however, more research is needed.

Analgesic and sedative medications are used to treat pain and anxiety in patients placed on mechanical ventilation; however, these medications have the potential to increase the likelihood of delirium.

Studies examining benzodiazepines have consistently shown an associated increased likelihood of delirium in ICU patients; however, data regarding opioids as a risk factor for delirium are less consistent. One study discovered higher opioid doses among ICU patients without delirium than with delirium.[18] Patients treated with meperidine were found to have an increased risk.

Providing adequate analgesia for ICU patients with close monitoring for signs and symptoms of delirium is warranted. Validated tools to screen for delirium in the ICU include the Intensive Care Delirium Screening Checklist (ICDSC) (Table 35.6)[19] and the Confusion Assessment Method for the ICU (CAM-ICU).[20]

A paucity of research exists on the prevention and treatment of delirium in ICU patients. Nonpharmacological strategies in non-ICU patients include frequent reorientation, restoration of normal sleep–wake cycles, early

Table 35.5 Risk Factors for Delirium in ICU Patients

Host Factors	Factors of Critical Illness	Iatrogenic Factors
Age (older)	Acidosis	Immobilization
Alcoholism	Anemia	Medications (e.g., benzodiazepines)
APOE4 polymorphism	Fever, infection, sepsis	Sleep disturbances
Cognitive impairment	Hypotension	
Depression	Metabolic disturbances	
Hypertension	Respiratory disease	
Smoking	High severity of illness	
Vision/hearing impairment		

Risk factors associated with delirium in both intensive care unit (ICU) and non-ICU studies.
APOE4 = apolipoprotein E4.[18]

Table 35.6 The Intensive Care Delirium Screening Checklist

Checklist Item	Description
Altered level of consciousness*	
A	No response
B	Response to intense and repeated stimulation
C	Response to mild or moderate stimulation
D	Normal wakefulness
E	Exaggerated response to normal stimulation
Inattentiveness	Difficulty following instructions or easily distracted
Disorientation	To time, place, or person
Hallucination-delusion-psychosis	Clinical manifestation or suggestive behavior
Psychomotor agitation or retardation	Agitation requiring the use of drugs or restraints, or slowing
Inappropriate speech or mood	Related to events or situation, or incoherent speech
Sleep–wake cycle disturbance	Sleeping <4 hours/day, waking at night, sleeping all day
Symptom fluctuation	Symptoms listed above occurring intermittently
Total score	0 to 8

* If A or B, then no other items are assessed that day.[20]

mobilization, removal of catheters, and minimizing unnecessary visual and auditory stimuli. These are often recommended for ICU patients but have not been well studied.

Specific to the ICU setting, correction of electrolyte abnormalities, treatment of underlying infections, correction of hypoxia and hypercapnia, treatment of hypoglycemia, and cautious use of opioids and sedatives are all critical to reducing the incidence of delirium.

Haloperidol is the initial recommended drug to treat delirium, resulting in a reduction of hallucinations, episodes of agitation, and unstructured thought patterns.[21] From clinical experience, the therapeutic dose of haloperidol ranges between 4 and 20 mg/daily.

Atypical antipsychotics may also be effective for the treatment of delirium; however, no placebo-controlled trials of either haloperidol or atypical antipsychotics have been conducted to help guide clinicians in the management of delirium in the ICU.

Benzodiazepines are often used to treat delirium tremens but are not recommended for treatment of delirium secondary to being a potential precipitating factor. Dexmedetomidine, a sedative, is also being evaluated for the treatment of delirium in the ICU, but definitive evidence is lacking. [22]

Conclusion

Critical care physicians and palliative care providers share a common goal of decreasing the suffering experienced by critically ill patients in the ICU, as well as that of their family members. With careful assessment of a patient's symptom distress and aggressive medical management with both a curative intent and the goal of patient comfort, the ICU team can provide the best possible care for patients and their families.

By integrating palliative care into the intensive care setting, improving symptom management, and providing clear and timely communication with patients and their families, healthcare providers can improve the overall care provided for ICU patients (see Box 35.2).

Box 35.2 Checklist for Palliative Care in the ICU

- Goals of care for the patient and/or family are addressed.
- Treatment is consistent with the patient's goals of care.
- Sedation assessment is done.
- Delirium screening is done.
- Symptom assessment is done.
- Pain and symptoms are adequately treated.
- Communication with the patient and/or family is carried out by the ICU team.
- Emotional and spiritual support is offered to the patient and/or family.

Clinical Pearls

- Clear and timely communication with ICU patients and their families is essential for palliation.
- Excessive sedation can result in increased morbidity and mortality in ICU patients.
- Mixed messages by the healthcare team can result in increased family distress.
- Delirium is often missed in ICU patients.

References

1. Angus DC, Barnato AE, Linde-Zwirble WT, et al. (2004). Use of intensive care at the end-of-life in the United States: an epidemiologic study. *Crit Care Med* 32(3):638–43.
2. Azoulay E, Pochard F, Chevret S, et al. (2002). Impact of a family information leaflet on effectiveness of information provided to family members of intensive care unit patients: a multi-center, prospective, randomized, controlled trial. *Am J Respir Crit Care Med* 165(4):438–2.
3. Lautrette A, Darmon M, Megarbane B, et al. (2007). A communication strategy and brochure for relatives of patients dying in the ICU. *N Engl J Med* 356(5):469–78.
4. Stapleton RD, Engelberg RA, Wenrich MD, et al. (2006). Clinician statements and family satisfaction with family conferences in the intensive care unit. *Crit Care Med* 34(6):1679–85.
5. Curtis JR, Engelber RA, Wenrich MD, et al. (2005). Missed opportunities during family conferences about end-of-life care in the intensive care unit. *Am J Respir Crit Care Med* 171(8):844–9.

6. Pochard F, Azoulay E, Chevret S, et al. (2001). Symptoms of anxiety and depression in family members of intensive care unit patients: ethical hypothesis regarding decision-making capacity. *Crit Care Med* 29(10):1893–7.

7. Curtis JR, Shannon SE (2006). Transcending the silos: toward an interdisciplinary approach to end-of-life care in the ICU. *Intensive Care Med* 32(1):15–7.

8. Eliasson AH, Parker JM, Shorr AF, et al. (1999). Impediments to writing do-not-resuscitate orders. *Arch Intern Med* 159(18):2213–7.

9. Treece PD, Engelberg RA, Crowley L, et al. (2004). Evaluation of a standardized order form for the withdrawal of life support in the intensive care unit. *Crit Care Med* 32(5):1141–8.

10. Nelson JE, Meier DE, Oei EJ, et al. (2001). Self-reported experience of critically ill cancer patients receiving intensive care. *Crit Care Med* 29(2):277–82.

11. Delgado-Guay MO, Parsons HA, Li Z, et al. (2008). Symptom distress, interventions, and outcomes of intensive care unit cancer patients referred to a palliative care consult team. *Cancer* 115(2):437–45.

12. Gelinas C, Fortier M, Viens C, et al. (2004). Pain assessment and management in critically ill intubated patients: a retrospective study. *Am J Crit Care* 13:126–35.

13. Sessler CN, Grap MJ, Ramsay MA (2008). Evaluating and monitoring analgesia and sedation in the intensive care unit. *Crit Care* 12(Suppl3):S2.

14. Chanques G, Jaber S, Barbotte E, et al. (2006). Impact of systematic evaluation of pain and agitation in an intensive care unit. *Crit Care Med* 34(6):1691–9.

15. Pandharipande PP, Pun BT, Herr DL, et al. (2007). Effect of sedation with dexmedetomidine vs. lorazepam on acute brain dysfunction in mechanically ventilated patients: the MENDS randomized controlled trial. *JAMA* 298(22):2644–53.

16. Kress JP, Pohlman AS, O'Connor MF, et al. (2000). Daily interruption of continuous sedative infusions in critically ill patients undergoing mechanical ventilation. *N Engl J Med* 342(20):1471–7.

17. Girard TD, Pandharipande PP, Ely EW (2008). Delirium in the intensive care unit. *Crit Care* 12(Suppl 3):S3.

18. Ouimet S, Kavanagh BP, Gottfried SB, et al. (2007). Incidence, risk factors and consequences of ICU delirium. *Intensive Care Med* 33(1):66–73.

19. Bergeron N, Dubois MJ, Dumont M, et al. (2001). Intensive Care Delirium Screening Checklist: evaluation of a new screening tool. *Intensive Care Med* 27(5):859–64.

20. Ely EW, Inouye SK, Bernard GR, et al. (2001). Delirium in mechanically ventilated patients: validity and reliability of the confusion assessment method for the intensive care unit. (CAM-ICU). *JAMA* 286(21):2703–10.

21. Jacobi J, Fraser GL, Coursin DB, et al. (2002). Clinical practice guidelines for the sustained use of sedatives and analgesics in the critically ill adult. *Crit Care Med* 30(1):119–41.

22. Reade MC, Finfer S (2014). Sedation and delirium in the intensive care unit. *N Engl J Med* 370(5):444–54.

Chapter 36

Research in Terminally Ill Patients

**Sriram Yennurajalingam
and Eduardo Bruera**

Introduction

Palliative care is an approach that aims to improve the quality of life of patients facing the problems associated with life-threatening illness. Generally, palliative care provides prevention and relief of suffering by means of early identification and assessment and control of symptoms (physical and psychological).

However, palliative care also relies on proper decision-making; good communication; addressing of family, caregiver, and spiritual issues; and a support system to help the family cope during the patient's illness and in their own bereavement.[1] These areas require a solid body of knowledge, which in turn depends on good research.

This chapter summarizes practical issues and gives a brief overview of the conducting of palliative care clinical trials.

Challenges in Conducting Palliative Care Research

Research in the palliative care clinical setting is greatly needed to address gaps in knowledge. Such research would help clinicians develop appropriate measures for assessing the symptoms and unmet needs of patients with life-limiting illness and those of their families; would determine active and effective treatments; and would determine the efficient use of resources for patients with terminal illness.

Unfortunately, research in palliative care is limited and challenging, owing to the severity of patients' illnesses, the presence of coexisting symptoms, polypharmacy, and other logistical factors inherent to treating palliative care patients (see Box 36.1).

Conducting clinical research on patients receiving palliative care presents many challenges, including the following:

1. Patients at various stages of the disease trajectory have comorbidities that tend to confound the outcomes for a given research question tested, especially during the last months, weeks, or days of life.
2. It may be ethically challenging to investigate the effectiveness of treatment when suffering worsens.
3. Even when a patient or family member agrees to participation in a clinical trial, attrition occurs because of disease progression, transfer of the patient to a different facility, loss of patient or family interest, or the patient's death.

These factors affect not only sample homogeneity but also the sample size and the ability of the investigator to complete the clinical trial in a timely manner. Other challenges in clinical trial research include the small number of palliative care researchers and limited funding.

Box 36.1 Challenges in Conducting Palliative Care Research

- *Severity of illness*: unstable patient population (owing to unstable disease and general medical condition); limited patient and family participation (due to lack of interest or time, logistics, or perception of increased burden as a result of participation; concerns about or aversions to randomization); may result in attrition or slow accrual
- *Heterogeneous* (confounding variables): patients having various comorbidities; polypharmacy, including disease-specific treatments; complications
- *Limited resources*: research faculty and personnel, funding, collaboration
- *Ethical concerns*: use of placebo in a vulnerable population
- *Complexity in attribution* of treatment-related adverse events because of disease progression
- *Limited consensus* on prioritization, definitions, objectives, and end points in the research community (e.g., fatigue trials).

Palliative Care Research

Prior to embarking on new research, it is important to develop research queries. Once queries are generated, they should be prioritized.

Experience, expertise, and the practice of evidence-based medicine in palliative care are used to define and refine the questions to be asked. The process of framing a research direction can be summarized by the acronym *PICO* (problem, intervention, comparison, and outcome).[2]

The *problem* is defined as a patient population or condition that is being investigated. The *intervention* commonly includes treatment, diagnostic tests, prognostic factors, and exposure to risks. It is common for the intervention to be kept as simple as possible and for external extraneous variables to be minimized.

A *comparison* is defined as an alternate intervention with which to compare the intervention of interest. To give a patient a placebo when there is a proven treatment variable would be unethical. In palliative care, it is always pertinent and important to compare an intervention or treatment with the standard of care rather than with a placebo, owing to ethical considerations.

An *outcome* is a measurable study end point. For example, a logical study end point for the treatment of fatigue near the very end of life would be the use of a validated tool, such as the Functional Assessment of Chronic Illness Therapy fatigue subscale.

Palliative care studies include ethnographic studies and observational studies. *Ethnographic studies* describe people through writing (e.g., case reports). *Observational studies* include descriptive, analytical, cross-sectional, and cohort studies; surveys; controlled clinical trials; and experimental studies.

Palliative care studies can also be classified into qualitative and quantitative studies. *Qualitative studies* include analysis of language, behavior, or recordings. Such studies may also include data-collecting interviews, the use of focus groups, analyses of primarily involved grounded theory, and content analysis, as well as schematic analysis.

Quantitative studies look for whether a given event regarding disease is a random event or chance event. These require statistical analysis of numerical data.

Furthermore, palliative care studies can be prospective or retrospective. A *prospective study* is designed to address a particular research question via defined eligibility criteria, statistical analysis, and evaluation of outcome in a controlled setting. A *retrospective study* is a review of previously collected patient data—for example, toxicity and patient survival.

Clinical trials are categorized by phase. A *phase I* trial focuses on safety, optimal dose, and dosing schedule or method. A *phase II* trial focuses on initial efficacy response of a therapy, effect on a particular tumor type (in cancer care), or state of disease.

Phase III trials are usually randomized, controlled studies or studies that compare experimental treatment drugs or therapy to current standards. *Phase IV* is a further evaluation of an approved strategy—for example, evaluating the long-term toxicity of a given treatment over a period of years.

Phase I clinical trials present unique challenges. They may create an ethical dilemma of therapeutic intent versus understanding the safety of a given drug. There is also extensive use of pharmacokinetics and molecular markers or biomarkers in phase I trials, leading to a significant amount of patient burden. The use of phase I trial design in palliative care, especially in terminally ill patients with good performance status, needs to be individualized, especially with regard to ethical issues and quality of life.

Most clinical trials in palliative care are phase II, in the early stages of studying a given drug's efficacy. The major complication of a phase II trial is the use of a placebo. Placebos are important in palliative care and symptom control; in fact, the placebo effect usually ranges from 30% to 50%.[3]

At the same time, given the focus on quality of life and the need for immediate relief of symptoms, patients and their caregivers and healthcare providers are reluctant to use a placebo, as they want the patient to receive a potentially effective treatment instead of no treatment.

The other major challenges with phase II trials, as well as phase III trials, are blinding, attrition, and dropout rates. These impact both the understanding and effectiveness of a given treatment as well as the timely completion of a trial.

Protocol Development

A well-written protocol is essential for the successful outcome of any research trial. A protocol that is complete and clearly defined will be successful and easy to execute. A protocol should be viewed as an instruction manual or road map that clearly defines how the study will answer a research question and how the trial is being conducted. The following elements of a protocol are important for proper execution.

The *objectives* should be consistent with the phase of the protocol.

The *background* should give information on the disease being studied. It should contain the rationale for the study, the hypothesis (the formal prediction), and an assumption of something that is observed in clinical practice and needs to be clearly defined. The background should be followed by intervention information or, in the case of a treatment trial, drug information.

The research *design* should include a well-characterized patient population to be evaluated. This should be included in the subject information, along with the setting where the treatment or trial is being conducted (for example, the hospital—outpatient or inpatient—or hospice).

The *eligibility criteria* should include the inclusion and exclusion criteria for the trial and should be followed by a well-defined treatment plan. The *treatment plan* includes the outcome measures and assessment tools used to evaluate these outcomes. The outcome measures should also include the toxicity of a given treatment.

The time points of assessment and the outcome measures should be as minimal as possible so as to reduce patient and caregiver burden. Always consider conducting some of the assessment via telephone or online, if appropriate or feasible, given the frail nature of the patient population, to avoid missing data.

This should be followed by *statistical considerations*, which should provide detailed information on how the primary and secondary outcomes would be tested and analyzed. There should also be information on interim analysis. The sample size should be set with consideration of the attrition rate, which is approximately 30% in palliative care populations.

References should be provided throughout the protocol so as to base evidence on statements made. The *appendices* should include any questionnaires and side effects of the measures used.

The most important part of the protocol is the *informed consent* document. It should clearly state the purpose of the trial; the appendices that the patient may obtain; dated information about how long a given questionnaire should take to answer; and the time, effort, and financial requirements of participating in the trial. The informed consent document should also mention clearly any potential side effects or injury.

A *protocol* should be written with all the collaborators, including the principal investigator, the mentor, if pertinent, a biostatistician, and the interdisciplinary team (which may include the bedside nurse, the social worker, and the basic scientist, if pertinent).

Before initiation of the study, it is important to have the protocol reviewed by peers, the hospital, or a scientific committee. Many institutions have an institutional review board that considers the science and patient safety before approving a trial.

It is also essential to have a study management plan that basically establishes standards that will ensure compliance with federal regulations, good clinical practice, and assurance and accountability requirements. This ensures proper conduct of the study, provides the general rules of the study and the key roles of the study personnel, and provides for patient confidentiality and a monitoring and auditing plan.

The most important aspect prior to activation of the study is the meeting with the biostatistician. This meeting should also involve the principal investigator, co-investigators, collaborators, the data collection and management team, and the regulatory management team. A clear timeline of activation, implantation, and analysis of a given protocol should be documented.

An important consideration is proper training of all personnel. This includes orientation of the collaborators and proper training of the research nurse and investigators about adverse events and deviations that need to be filed in a timely manner. The data manager should enter the data in a timely fashion.

Another important consideration is financial—specifically, that reimbursement of the patient is clearly documented in the form of a contract.

Developing appropriate skills, applying ethical principles to the conduct of research, and, above all, processing good research questions with a productive protocol and study management will help improve the standards of palliative care treatment.

Recruiting and Retention in Clinical Trials: Measures to Facilitate Accrual and Completion

One of the most challenging aspects of conducting a successful clinical trial is accrual. Various measures have been described in the literature.[3–8] Patient-related factors that facilitate enrollment include the following:

- Fear of a breach of privacy or autonomy or suspicion regarding the research itself may impede authorization.
- The research team's ability to explain the possible outcomes as potentially beneficial for future patients may trigger an altruistic tendency in the patients (a desire to create a legacy) and may prompt patients to enter the trial. Investigators should explain that the discernable benefits of participation in a clinical trial are the possibility of new treatment for a refractory symptom, the possibility of the research team adding an extra dimension of care for patients, and a meaningful task for the patient.

Measures for Successful Recruitment

1. Establish a study identity.[4,5]
2. Emphasize the benefits of participation.[6]
3. Minimize the burden for participants.
4. Involve the caregivers during the informed-consent process, along with the patient.
5. Provide incentive (but not through coercion).
6. Retain a control group.
7. Retain project staff and participants.
8. Offer support.
9. Be flexible.
10. Maintain tracking systems.

Ethics in Palliative Care Research

Key factors in the ethical conduct of research in palliative care, in which participants are particularly vulnerable because of their desperate need for treatment options, must be considered:

1. The objectives of clinical trials in the terminally ill should take into consideration the possibility of minimal potential harm (including research-related distress and burden on the patient and caregiver) and a possible improvement in quality of life.
2. Informed consent for clinical trials must include understanding of the purpose of the research, any foreseeable risks, any possible benefits, any appropriate alternative procedures or treatments, confidentiality of records, participation being voluntary, ability to withdraw at any time, and that continuing care is not dependent on participation in the trial. The informed consent may sometimes need the participation of caregivers. Precaution should be taken to ensure the decision-making capacity of the participant. Surrogate consent needs to be obtained in certain situations (e.g., child, delirium studies).
3. Ethical conduct of research studies is reviewed by an institutional review board or research ethics committee.

References

1. World Health Organization (2009). *WHO Definition of Palliative Care*. Retrieved November 18, 2009, from http://www.who.int/cancer/palliative/definition/en/
2. NHS-Executive-Anglia-and-Oxford (1999). Asking the question: finding the evidence in evidence based health care. In: *An Open Learning Resource for the Health Care Practitioners*, Vol. 2. Luten: Chiltren Press, pp. 3–16.
3. de la Cruz M, Hui D, Parsons HA, Bruera E (2010). Placebo and nocebo effects in randomized double-blind clinical trials of agents for the therapy for fatigue in patients with advanced cancer. *Cancer* 116(3):766–74.
4. Davis LL, Broome ME, Cox RP (2002). Maximizing retention in community-based clinical trials. *J Nurs Scholarsh* 34:47–53.
5. Coday M, Boutin-Foster C, Goldman Sher T, Tennant J, Greaney ML, Saunders SD, et al. (2005). Strategies for retaining study participants in behavioral intervention trials: retention experiences of the NIH Behavior Change Consortium. *Ann Behav Med* 29(2 Suppl.):55–65.
6. Wright JR, Whelan TJ, Schiff S, Dubois S, Crooks D, Haines PT, et al. (2004). Why cancer patients enter randomized clinical trials: exploring the factors that influence their decision. *J Clin Oncol* 22:4312–8.
7. White C, Hardy J (2010). What do palliative care patients and their relatives think about research in palliative care? A systematic review. *Support Care Cancer* 18(8):905–11.
8. Bruera E (2006). Practical tips for successful research in palliative care. In: Bruera E, Higginson IJ, Ripamonti C, Von Gunten C (eds.), *Textbook of Palliative Medicine*. London: Hodder Arnold, pp. 202–7.

Prevention and Management of Burnout and Compassion Fatigue in Healthcare Providers

Mary L. S. Vachon

Reviews of the literature[1-3] have shown that staff in hospice and palliative care experience less stress and burnout than those in other areas of healthcare, although there is some evidence that this may be changing.[4-7] The finding of less stress may stem from the recognition early in the field that there needs to be support within the system.[1] Recently, however, palliative care staff are more apt to report challenges with overwork,[5,6] and palliative care registrars reported problems with the perception of low prestige of their specialty, as well as issues with nursing staff.[5]

This chapter defines the terms associated with stress, and reviews the rates of burnout and compassion fatigue in palliative care. It examines the sources of stress associated with burnout and compassion fatigue, signs and symptoms, protective factors that may mitigate stress, and strategies to prevent and treat burnout and compassion fatigue.

Burnout and Job Engagement

- *Burnout* is a form of mental distress manifested in "normal" persons who did not suffer from prior psychopathology, who experience decreased work performance resulting from negative attitudes and behaviors.[8]
- *Burnout* is a psychological syndrome in response to chronic interpersonal stressors on the job. The three key dimensions are *emotional exhaustion (EE), cynicism and detachment from the job (depersonalization) (DP)*, and a *sense of ineffectiveness and a lack of personal accomplishment (PA)*.[9]
- *Job engagement* is the opposite of burnout. Engagement is a persistent, positive-affective-motivational state of fulfillment in employees that is characterized by vigor, dedication, and absorption.[10]
- *Engagement* is associated with a sustainable workload, feelings of choice and control, appropriate recognition and reward, a supportive work community, fairness and justice, and meaningful and valued work.

Other Frameworks for Understanding Person–Job Interaction

Although burnout is by far the most researched approach to understanding stress in hospice and palliative care, other concepts are also of interest. These include the following:

- *Stress*, which is "experienced when the demands from the work environment exceed the employee's ability to cope with (or control) them."[11]

  - *Compassion fatigue* is almost identical to post-traumatic stress disorder, except that it applies to those emotionally affected by the trauma of another (usually a client or family member).[12] Compassion fatigue is also known as secondary or vicarious traumatization.[12,13]

  - Current thinking regarding the construct of compassion fatigue is that there is a domain of compassion fatigue which occurs when there is a combination of burnout and experiences that lead to the development of secondary traumatic stress.[14]

  - *Compassion satisfaction (CS)*[15] is satisfaction derived from the work of helping others. It may be the portrayal of efficacy. Caregivers with CS derive pleasure from helping others, like their colleagues, feel good about their ability to help and make a contribution. There may be a balance between compassion fatigue and compassion satisfaction. Caregivers may experience compassion fatigue, yet they like their work because they feel positive benefits from it. They believe that what they are doing is helping others and may even be redemptive.

  - *Moral distress* in the workplace occurs when there is an experience of incoherence between one's beliefs and one's actions, and possibly also outcomes (i.e., between what one sincerely believes to be right, what one actually does, and what eventually transpires).[16] "Moral distress may also arise . . . for one or more of the following reasons: an error in judgment, some personal failing (for example, a weakness or crimp in one's character such as a pattern of 'systemic avoidance'), or other circumstances truly beyond one's control."[17]

Rates of Burnout and Compassion Fatigue

Shanafelt and Dyrbye[18] reviewed studies of burnout among oncology-focused medical specialties and found a point prevalence of 25%–35% among medical oncologists, 38% among radiation oncologists, and 28%–36% among surgical oncologists. A review of 10 studies[19] (total $n = 2,357$) identified a range of 8%–51% of oncology staff suffering severe burnout on at least one of the burnout components, with overall EE and DP prevalence rates of 36% and 34%, respectively, only slightly higher than the norms on the Maslach Burnout Inventory of 33%.

Comparing oncology and palliative care staff, Ramirez et al.[20] found that palliative care physicians were significantly less likely than their oncology colleagues to report EE (15%), DP (8%), or low PA (25%). In a Japanese survey,[21] palliative care physicians were also less likely to report EE (15% vs. 23%) or DP (8% vs. 10%), but both groups were significantly above the norm in reporting low feelings of personal accomplishment (PA) (53% vs. 65%). A more recent study of palliative care staff in Minnesota[22] ($n = 567$) found higher levels of burnout than compassion fatigue, but the palliative care staff had less symptoms of burnout or compassion fatigue than the norms for the ProQOL-RIII scale, which measures compassion fatigue, compassion satisfaction, and burnout.

In a somewhat larger Canadian study of palliative care staff, including physicians ($n = 630$),[23] participants had higher scores for compassion satisfaction, slightly higher scores for compassion fatigue, and comparable levels of burnout compared with the norms. Another smaller Canadian study ($n = 63$),[7] however, showed greater stress in caregivers who spent more of their time working with palliative patients.

Who Is at Risk of Burnout?

Burnout has been associated with the following variables:

- Younger age[7,8,24]
- Being under age 55[20]
- Being single[21]
- Personality characteristics associated with burnout include neuroticism, lower levels of hardiness and self-esteem;[8,10,] the profession of medicine with its delay of satisfactions;[27,28] the compulsive triad in physicians of doubt, guilt feelings, and an exaggerated sense of responsibility[27,28]
- Work–home interference[6]
- Highly motivated health professionals with intense investment in their profession are at a greater risk for the development of burnout[29]
- Research is much stronger for the association between burnout and a wide range of job characteristics, including chronically difficult job demands, an imbalance between high demands and low resources, and the presence of conflict (whether between people, between role demands, or between important values), than for personal variables.[10]

What Protects Against Burnout and Compassion Fatigue?

- Having spiritual beliefs[7,14]
    - Supportive spouses or partners[25,26]
    - Both hardiness and a sense of coherence were each associated with resilience in palliative care nurses.[27]
- Caregivers who engage in self-care and have some form of spiritual practice are more empathic,[28] are less prone to burnout[7,29] and compassion fatigue,[7,14,32] and have greater compassion satisfaction.[7,14,30]
- Having a supportive work environment, awareness of personal triggers, development of effective communication skills, professional supervision processes, effective ways of managing one's own loss and grief experiences, and participating in interventions aimed at repairing the effects of compassion fatigue.[31]

Signs and Symptoms of Burnout

See Box 37.1 for the signs and symptoms of burnout.

Box 37.1 Signs and Symptoms of Burnout

Physical
Fatigue
Physical and emotional exhaustion
Headaches
Gastrointestinal disturbances
Weight loss
Sleeplessness
Hypertension
Myocardial infarction

Psychological
Anxiety
Depression
Boredom
Frustration
Low morale
Irritability
May contribute to alcoholism and drug addiction

Occupational
Depersonalization in relationships with colleagues, patients, or both
Emotional exhaustion, cynicism, perceived ineffectiveness
Job turnover
Impaired job performance
Deterioration in the physician–patient relationship and a decrease in the quality and quantity of care
Increase in medical errors

Social
Marital difficulties.

A Model for Understanding Occupational Stress

Research on burnout has focused on the degree of match or mismatch between the person and six domains of the job environment. The greater the gap or mismatch between the person and the environment, the greater the likelihood of burnout. The greater the match or fit, the greater the likelihood of engagement with work. Six areas of work life encompass the major organizational antecedents of burnout. These include workload, control, reward, community, fairness, and values.[9]

Burnout arises from chronic mismatches between people and their work settings in some or all of these areas. The area of values may play a central mediating role for the other areas,[8] although, for individuals at risk of burnout, fairness in the work environment may be the tipping point determining whether people develop job engagement or burnout.[8]

Emotion–work variables (e.g., requirements to display or suppress emotions on the job, requirements to be emotionally empathic) have been found to account for additional variance in burnout scores over and above job stressors.[9] Box 37.2 shows the hospice/palliative care research within this model.

Box 37.2 Factors Related to Burnout and Job Engagement in Hospice/Palliative Care

Workload

- Excessive workload exhausts the individual to the extent that recovery may become impossible. Emotional work is especially draining when the job requires people to display emotions inconsistent with their feelings.[9]
- Workload relates to the exhaustion component of burnout.[9]
- Palliative care physicians had less stress from workload than colleagues in clinical and radiation oncology,[20] but a more recent study showed that those who spent more of their workday dealing with the dying had higher stress and more depersonalization.[7]
- Workload was related to stress and burnout in oncology and palliative staff in a Canadian study.[6]
- Appropriate workload was correlated with job satisfaction in Canadian palliative care nurses.[32]

Control

- Control is related to inefficacy or reduced personal accomplishment. Mismatches often indicate that individuals have insufficient control over the resources necessary to do their work or insufficient authority to pursue the work in what they believe is the most effective manner.[8]
- From the 1970s stress has resulted from a lack of knowledge of interpersonal skills and a lack of communication skills and/or management skills.[1,3,20,21]

Box 37.2 (Continued)

- When caregivers have less control they are less satisfied with their work.[33]
- When staff have more autonomy they have greater job satisfaction.[32]

Reward

- Lack of reward may be financial when one does not receive salary or benefits commensurate with one's achievements, or lack of social rewards when one's hard work is ignored and is not appreciated by others. The lack of intrinsic rewards (e.g., doing something of importance and doing it well) can also be a critical part of this mismatch.[10]
- If palliative care nurses felt there was a balance between their rewards and efforts, they had high job satisfaction. If there was an imbalance between rewards and efforts, they had distress.[32]

Community

- This mismatch arises when people lose a sense of personal connection with others in the workplace.[10]
- Problems with colleagues have been reported in many studies.[1,2,5,24,29,33]
- "Our personal identity is formed and shaped as a result of our interaction with other people as well as the expression of our basic genetic makeup. We, therefore, seek out and develop formal and informal social groups and networks in both our private and our working life which supplement the relationships we already have within our family unit."[34]
- Social support from people with whom one shares praise, comfort, happiness, and humor affirms membership in a group with a shared sense of values.[9]
- The quintessential feature of a small, well-balanced team is leadership that is shared or rotates, depending on the issue involved.[34]
- In a healthy team there is room for disagreement.
- Factors crucial to communication in a new German palliative care team were close communication, team philosophy, good interpersonal relationships, high team commitment, autonomy, and the ability to deal with death and dying. Close communication was by far the most frequently mentioned criteria for cooperation. Team performance, good coordination of workflow, and mutual trust underpin the evaluation of efficient teamwork. Inefficient teamwork is associated with the absence of clear goals, tasks, and role delegation, as well as a lack of team commitment.[35]

Fairness

- This mismatch arises when there is not perceived fairness in the workplace. Fairness communicates respect and confirms people's

Box 37.2 (Continued)

self-worth. Mutual respect between people is central to a shared sense of community.[8]

- For individuals at risk of burnout, fairness in the work environment may be the tipping point determining whether people develop job engagement or burnout.[8]
- Palliative care nurses reported workplace politics involving behaviors or actions by organizations and/or individuals that were perceived by participants as being destructive, blocking, or incongruent to equitable health care.[33]

Values

- Palliative care staff found their work rewarding.[1,2,4,6,24,29]
- Teamwork depends to a certain extent on people being able to subscribe to a *shared* set of values that reinforce the team's way of working and reduce the likelihood of clashes with personal values.[34]
- Individuals need to reconcile their individual moral values with those required by, or most readily identified with, their professional role, and their membership in a larger moral unit—the team. There can be challenges if individuals do not agree with a strong philosophy or ethos of the team.[34]
- A team may decide to change or modify its philosophy in light of external factors; an individual may feel that his or her personal philosophy no longer fits with the team's.[34]

Emotion–Work Variables: Issues of Death and Dying

- Emotion–work variables (e.g., requirements to display or suppress emotions on the job, requirements to be emotionally empathic) account for additional variance in burnout scores, over and above job stressors.[9]
- The care of the dying can be stressful.[6,7,14,22,23,29]
- In Japanese oncologists and palliative care physicians, insufficient confidence in the psychological care of patients was associated with physician burnout rather than involvement in end-of-life care.[21] Japanese oncologists and palliative care physicians who were less confident in dealing with psychologic care and demonstrated higher levels of EE were more likely to choose continuous deep sedation for patients with refractory physical and psychologic distress.
- Palliative care takes caregivers into emotional realms that are neither easy nor comfortable. The caregiver may be permanently changed through this encounter.[36] Caregivers need to be prepared to do this work and need self-awareness to effectively function in the field.[29]
- Palliative care/hospice staff providing assistance with provision of relief from physical, emotional, and/or spiritual pain or distress, or psychosocial support to patients and/or families, or emotional support to other team members, had higher levels of compassion fatigue and burnout and no significant difference in levels of

Box 37.2 (Continued)

compassion satisfaction compared to those who did not provide the service.[23]

- Constantly confronting the death of others causes caregivers to repeatedly re-evaluate their own mortality and re-examine the meaning of life and death.
- Multiple losses and constant exposure to death and loss may leave staff with grief overload and considerable distress. However, participating in the death of some patients may also result in intense positive experiences that promote professional development.[1,2,4,24,29]
- Melanie Vachon and her colleagues found that the connections nurses make with their patients in confronting death can involve both suffering and meaning.[37]
- Reactions to grief (e.g., altered treatment decisions, mental distraction, emotional and physical withdrawal from patients) suggest that the failure of oncologists to deal appropriately with grief from patient loss may negatively affect not only oncologists personally but also patients and their families.[38]

Coping and Avoiding Burnout

Recognizing that one cannot give from an empty cup and that avoiding burnout and compassion fatigue is both an individual and organizational responsibility, studies have found the following to be effective in coping and avoiding burnout and compassion fatigue:

- Physical well-being, professional relationships, taking a transcendental perspective, talking with others, hobbies, clinical variety, personal relationships, personal boundaries, "time away" from work, passion for one's work, realistic expectations, the use of humor and laughter, and remembering patients.[39]
- Protective practices to counter isolation (in professional, personal, and spiritual realms), developing mindful self-awareness, consciously expanding perspective to embrace complexity, active optimism, holistic self-care, maintaining clear boundaries, exquisite empathy (highly present, sensitive, heartfelt empathic engagement), professional satisfaction, and creating meaning.[42]
- Resilience, spirituality, and emotionality were negatively and significantly correlated with compassion fatigue, with the subscale of religiosity being positively correlated.[30]
- A sense of competence, control, or pleasure in one's work; team philosophy, building, and support; control over aspects of practice; lifestyle management; and a personal philosophy of illness, death, and one's role in life.[24]
- Recovery from burnout is possible, with prospective studies in medical students and residents suggesting that approximately 12%–27% recover over the following 12 months. However, recovery requires deliberate and sustained effort to identify and address the factors contributing to burnout.[18]
- A review of burnout interventions identified 25 relevant studies.[41] Most (80%) programs led to reduced burnout. Person-directed interventions reduced burnout in the short term (6 months or less), while a combination of person- and organization-directed interventions had longer lasting effects (> 12 months).
- Caregivers need to be "connected" in order to continue to practice end-of-life care.[29]
- Box 37.3 shows a list of lifestyle practices to promote wellness and prevent burnout.

Box 37.3 Lifestyle Management

Recognize and monitor symptoms
Good nutrition
Meditation
Spiritual life
Grieving losses, personally and as a team
Decrease overtime work
Exercise: aerobic, yoga, qi gong, tai chi
Time in nature: walking, gardening
Music: singing, listening to music, playing an instrument
Energy work: reiki, healing touch, therapeutic touch
Maintain sense of humor
Balance work and home lives to allow sufficient "time off"
Go on a retreat
Have a good social support system, personally and professionally
Seek consultation if symptoms are severe
Discuss work-related stresses with others who share the same problems
Visit counterparts in other institutions; look for new solutions to problems
Remember the Serenity Prayer at work. (God grant me the serenity to accept the things I cannot change, the wisdom to change the things I can, and the wisdom to know the difference.) Sometimes work-related problems can be solved; other times, leaving the work environment and taking the wisdom gained is a good solution.

Adapted from Kearney MK, Weininger RB, Vachon MLS, Mount BM, Harrison RL (2009). Self-care of physicians caring for patients at the end of life: "being connected ... a key to my survival." *JAMA* 301:1155–64.

Educational Interventions

Stress and burnout were more prevalent in physicians who did not feel they had adequate communication skills and had difficulty with psychosocial communication. Reviews of the impact of communication skills training on burnout have reached varied conclusions, with the most recent finding inadequate evidence to support a positive impact.[42]

Accelerated Recovery Program for Compassion Fatigue

The Accelerated Recovery Program (ARP) for Compassion Fatigue was established in 1997 as "a five-session individual treatment model for treating professional care-providers who had become overwhelmed by the demands of their work."[43] The idea was that secondary exposure to serious illness, trauma, or injury resulted in a wound in caregivers that required further intervention. "The stages of the treatment process focus on issues such as the therapeutic alliance between clinician and patient, clinicians' quantitative assessment of their own distress, anxiety management skills, the importance of narrative regarding personal and work-related experiences, and issues related to the exposure and resolution of secondary traumatic stress (STS). A key component of this training is cognitive restructuring for self-care and the integration of new concepts and skills. In addition, the ARP provides an aftercare resiliency plan emphasizing resiliency skills, self-management and self-care skills, connection with others, skills acquisition, and conflict resolution."[43]

In the ARP, self-reflective and self-care skills are taught to establish a non-anxious presence and self-validated caregiving. "Non-anxious presence is the ability to sit comfortably with the emotional strain on exposure to patient distress and remain a compassionate witness."[43] This model may involve a paradigm shift for physicians from being a hero to being a healer. "It is within this 'healer' paradigm that maintaining a non-anxious presence can make sense for physicians. Here they can learn that being non-anxious can be healing *in and of itself* to a patient possibly facing the most terrifying time in his or her life. Through this practice physicians may also learn a more spiritual lesson: that healing and being successful as a healer does [sic] not necessarily mean the cure of disease."[43] Self-reflection and self-care lead to an increased ability to attend to one's own needs or those of others, while feeling replenished. This leads to improved self-validated caregiving, and non-anxious presence while caring for others and self.

Meaning-Centered and Mindfulness-Based Intervention

Very important, systematic research is being done in Quebec by Lise Fillion and her colleagues, including Melanie Vachon (no relation to the author). Fillion and her colleagues are working with meaning-centered interventions, combined with mindfulness meditation, in palliative care as well as intensive care units. The work is based in part on the Being with Dying (BWD) program earlier developed by Roshi Joan Halifax and her colleagues.[44] In a synopsis of their work,[45] Fillion, Truchon, L'Heureus, et al. note their goal in their research and cite their multiple previous references:

> In the current context of labor shortages and limited access to palliative care, a major challenge arises in making organizational choices that take into account the evolution in the working community, new occupational requirements, as well as the improved management of workplaces and well-being of personnel. The researchers' primary objective is to improve the conditions in which palliative care is provided by validating a conceptual framework that results in a better understanding of the work satisfaction and well-being of nurses in this field. The results of this study will offer decision-makers a choice of models of services to be favoured and a better understanding of the aspects to be considered before implementing training services or programs for caregivers and managers.[45]

The recommendation of complementing MCI with mindfulness is in line with the Being with Dying intervention (BWD).[44,46] The BWD program is an eight-day residential program based on scientific data that

> . . . encompasses ethical, spiritual, psychological, existential and social aspects of care of the dying. It includes mindful and compassionate approaches to end-of-life care, compassion-based ethics and communication strategies in EOLC, clinician self-care and contemplative interventions appropriate for clinicians/caregivers and dying people. The program builds on reflective practices that can regulate attention and emotion, cultivate compassion, aid in the development of a meta-cognitive perspective, promote calm and resilience, reduce stress, and foster emotional balance, embodiment and compassion. The training also emphasizes basic neuroscience research in relation to the clinical, contemplative and conceptual content of the training.[44]

The premise of BWD, which is based on the development of mindfulness and receptive attention through contemplative practice, is that cultivating the stability of mind and emotions enables clinicians to respond to others and themselves with compassion. The program provides skills, attitudes, behaviors, and tools to change how caregivers work with the dying and bereaved. Roshi Joan Halifax and her colleagues developed the GRACE process used in the program to prime compassion in clinicians for compassion-based clinician-patient interactions. The acronym GRACE stands for the following elements:

- Gather your attention.
- Recall your intention.
- Attune by checking in with yourself, then the patient.
- Consider what will really serve your patient by being truly present with your patient and letting insights arise.
- Engage, enact ethically, and then end the interaction.

The program was developed to help prevent burnout and secondary trauma in caregivers including doctors, nurses, human rights activists, and others working in stressful situations. The practice offers "a simple and efficient way to open to the experience of the suffering of others, to stay centered, and to develop the capacity to respond with compassion." Roshi Joan Halifax defines compassion as "the capacity to be attentive to the experience of others, to wish the best for others, and to sense what will truly serve others. Ironically, in a time when we hear the phrase 'compassion fatigue' with increasing frequency, compassion as we are defining it does not lead to fatigue. In fact, it can actually become a wellspring of resilience as we allow our natural impulse to care for another to become a source of nourishment rather than depletion."[46] She notes that compassion makes it possible for us to help others in a more skillful and effective way. Recent research studies show that compassion helps us as well by reducing physiological stress and promoting physical and emotional well-being.[46]

Clinical Pearls

- Research over five decades shows that palliative care practitioners generally experience less stress and burnout and, more recently, less compassion fatigue than other healthcare practitioners, but this may be changing.
- Caregivers often feel job engagement and compassion satisfaction in their work with clients. They like what they do and feel good about it.
- Spirituality can protect caregivers from burnout and compassion fatigue.
- Appropriate lifestyle balance, finding meaning in one's life and one's work, and self-awareness can make one a happier person and more effective caregiver.
- Interventions must be at both the personal and organizational levels.
- Important interventions based on scientific understanding of the brain and the mind–body connection is now being done to enable caregivers to be more compassionate, but to practice true compassion, one must start with self-compassion.

References

1. Vachon MLS (1995). Staff stress in hospice/palliative care: a review. *Palliat Med* 9:91–122.
2. Vachon MLS (2011). Four decades of selected research in hospice/palliative care: have the stressors changed? In: I. Renzenbrink (ed.), *Caregiver Stress and Staff Support in Illness, Dying, and Bereavement*. Oxford: Oxford University Press, pp. 1–24.
3. Pereira SM, Fonseca AM, Carvalho AN (2011). Burnout in palliative care: a systematic review. *Nursing Ethics* 18, 317–26.
4. Vachon MLS. Huggard PK, Huggard JA (2015). Reflections on occupational stress in palliative care nursing: is it changing? In: Ferrell B, Coyle N, Paice J (eds.), *Oxford Textbook of Palliative Nursing*, 4th edition, pp. 969–986. New York: Oxford University Press.
5. Berman R, Campbell M, Makin, W, Todd C. (2007). Occupational stress in palliative medicine, medical oncology and clinical oncology specialist registrars. *Clin Med* 7: 235–42.
6. Dougherty E, Pierce B, Ma C, Panzarella T, Rodin G, Zimmermann C (2009). Factors associated with work stress and professional satisfaction in oncology staff. *Am J Hosp Pall Med* 26:105–11.
7. Koo K, Zeng L, Zhang L, DasGupta T, Vachon MLS, Holden L, Jon F, Chow E, Di Prospero L (2013). Comparison and literature review of occupational stress in a palliative radiotherapy clinic's interprofessional team, the radiation therapists, and the nurses at an academic cancer centre. *J Med Imaging and Rad Sci* 44: 14–22.

8. Maslach C, Leiter M (2008). Early predictors of job burnout and engagement. *J Appl Psychol* 93:498–512.

9. Maslach C, Schaufeli WB, Leiter MP (2001). Job burnout. *Ann Rev Psychol* 52:397–422.

10. Maslach C. (2003) Job burnout: new directions in research and intervention. *Curr Dir Psychol Sci* 12:189–92.

11. European Agency for Safety and Health at Work (2000). *Safety at Work*. Retrieved November 13, 2008, from http://agency.osha.eu.int/publications/factsheets/8/en/facts8_en.pdf.

12. Figley CR (ed.) (1995). *Compassion Fatigue: Coping with Secondary Traumatic Stress Disorder in Those Who Treat the Traumatized*. New York: Brunner/Mazel.

13. Figley CR (ed.) (2002). *Treating Compassion Fatigue*. New York: Brunner-Routledge.

14. Huggard PK, Stamm BH, Pearlman LA (2013). Physician stress: compassion satisfaction, compassion fatigue and vicarious traumatization. In: Figley CR, Huggard PK, Rees C (eds.), *First Do No Self-Harm*. New York: Oxford University Press, pp. 127–45.

15. Stamm BH. (2002) Measuring compassion satisfaction as well as fatigue: developmental history of the compassion satisfaction and fatigue test. In: Figley CF (ed.), *Treating Compassion Fatigue*. New York: Brunner-Routledge, pp. 107–19.

16. Jameton A (1984). *Nursing Practice: The Ethical Issues*. Englewood Cliffs, NJ: Prentice Hall.

17. Webster GC, Baylis FE (2000). Moral residue. In: Rubin SB, Zoloth L (eds.), *Margin of Error: The Ethics of Mistakes in the Practice of Medicine*. Hagerstown: University Publishing Group, pp. 217–230, 218.

18. Shanafelt T, Dyrbye L (2012). Oncologist burnout: causes, consequences and responses. *J Clin Oncol* 30(11): 1235–41.

19 . Trufelli DC, Bensi CG, Garcia JB, et al. (2008). Burnout in cancer professionals: a systematic review and meta-analysis *European J Cancer Care* 17(6):524–31.

20. Ramirez AJ, Graham J, Richards MA, Cull A, Gregory WM (1996). Mental health of hospital consultants: the effect of stress and satisfaction at work. *Lancet* 16:724–8.

21. Asai M, Morita T, Akechi T, et al. (2007). Burnout and psychiatric morbidity among physicians engaged in end-of-life care for cancer patients: a cross-sectional nationwide survey in Japan. *Psycho-Oncology*. 16:421–8.

22. Whitebird RR, Asche SE, Thompson, GL, Rossom R, Heinrich R (2013). Stress, burnout, compassion fatigue, and mental health in hospice workers in Minnesota. *J Palliat Med* 16:12:1534–9.

23. Slocum-Gori S, Hemsworth D, Chan WWY, Carson A, Kazanjian A (2013). Understanding compassion satisfaction, compassion fatigue and burnout: a survey of the hospice, palliative care workforce. *Palliat Med* 27:2:172–8.

24. Vachon MLS (1987). *Occupational Stress in the Care of the Critically Ill, the Dying and the Bereaved*. New York: Hemisphere.

25. Spickard A Jr, Gabbe SG, Christensen JF (2002). Mid-career burnout in generalist and specialist physicians. *JAMA* 288:1447–50.

26. Shanafelt T, Chung H, White H, Lyckholm LJ (2006). Shaping your career to maximize personal satisfaction in the practice of oncology. *J Clin Onc* 24:4020–6.

27. Ablett JR, Jones RSP (2007). Resilience and well-being in palliative care staff: a qualitative study of hospice nurses' experience of work. *Psycho-Oncology* 16:733–40.

28. Shanafelt TD, West C, Zhao X, Novotny P, Kolars J, Habermann T, Sloan J (2005). Relationship between increased personal well-being and enhanced empathy among internal medicine residents. *J Gen Int Med* 20:559–64.

29. Kearney MK, Weininger RB, Vachon MLS, Mount BM, Harrison RL (2009). Self-care of physicians caring for patients at the end of life: "being connected … a key to my survival." *JAMA.* 301:1155–64.

30. Huggard P (XXXX). Compassion fatigue and dying and death: what strategies will prevent the development of compassion fatigue and what is the evidence for their effectiveness? In: Hinerman N, Fisher R (eds.), *Making sense of death and dying*. Oxfordshire: Inter-Disciplinary Net.

31. Najjar N, Davis LW, Beck-Coon K, Doebbeling CC (2009). Compassion fatigue: a review of the research to date and relevance to cancer-care providers. *J Health Psychol* 14:267–77.

32. Fillion L, Tremblay I, Truchon M, et al. (2007). Job satisfaction and emotional distress among nurses providing palliative care: empirical evidence for an integrative occupational stress-model. *Int J Stress Manag* 14:1–25.

33. Glass N, Rose J (2008). Enhancing emotional well-being through self-care the experiences of community health nurses in Australia. *Holist Nurs Pract* 22:6:336–47.

34. Speck P, ed. (2006). *Teamwork in Palliative Care: Fulfilling or Frustrating?* Oxford: Oxford University Press, p. 7–23.

35. Jünger S, Pestinger M, Elsner F, Krumm N, Radbruch L (2007). Criteria for successful multiprofessional cooperation in palliative care teams. *Palliat Med* 21:1–8.
36. Boston P, Towers A, Barnard D (2001). Embracing vulnerability: risk and empathy in palliative care. *J Palliat Care* 17:248–53.
37. Vachon M, Fillion L, Achille M (2012). Death confrontation, spiritual-existential experience and caring attitudes in palliative care nurses: an interpretative phenomenological analysis. *Qual Res Psychol* 9:151–72.
38. Granek L, Tozer R, Mazzotta P, et al. (2012). Nature and impact of grief over patient loss on oncologists' personal and professional lives. *Arch Intern Med* 172(12):964–6.
39. Swetz KM, Harrington SE, Matsuyama RK, Shanafelt TD, Lyckholm LJ (2009). Strategies for avoiding burnout in hospice and palliative medicine: peer advice for physicians on achieving longevity and fulfillment. *J Pall Med* 12:9: 773–7.
40. Harrison R, Westwood M (2009). Preventing vicarious traumatization of mental health therapists: identitiying protective practices. *Psychother Theory Res Pract Train* 46(2):203–19.
41. Awa WL, Plaumann M, Walter U (2010). Burnout prevention: a review of intervention programs. *Pt Ed Counsel* 78(2):184–90.
42. Moore PM, Rivera Mercado S, Grez Artigues M, Lawrie TA (2013). Communication skills training for healthcare professionals working with people who have cancer (Review). *The Cochrane Library*, vol 3. http://www.thecochranelibrary.com. JohnWiley & Sons.
43. Baranowsky A, Schmidt D. (2013). Overcopers: medical doctor vulnerability to compassion fatigue. In: Figley CR, Huggard PK, Rees C (eds.), *First Do No Self-Harm*. New York: Oxford University Press, pp. 203–15, 211, 212.
44. Halifax J (2013). Being with Dying—Curriculum for the Professional Training Program in Compassionate End-of-Life Care. In: Singer T, Bolz M (eds.), *Compassion: Bridging Practice and Science*. Munich: Max Planck Society, pp. 467–478, 467.
45. Fillion L, Truchon M, L'Heureux M, Dallaire C, Langlois L, Bellemare M, Dupuis R (2013). To improve services and care at the end of life: understanding the impact of workplace satisfaction and well- being of nurses. Rapport R-794, Montréal, IRSST. http://www.irsst.qc.ca/-projet-vers-l-amelioration-des-services-et-des-soins-de-fin-de-vie-mieux-comprendre-l-impact-du-milieu-de-travail-sur-la-satisfaction-et-le-bien-etre-des-0099-6050.html.
46. Halifax J (2014). G.R.A.C.E.: training in cultivating compassion in interactions with others. Upaya Zen Center, Upaya blog, February 12.

Index